主审 童 建
主编 曹 毅 李建祥 张 洁

毒理学教程

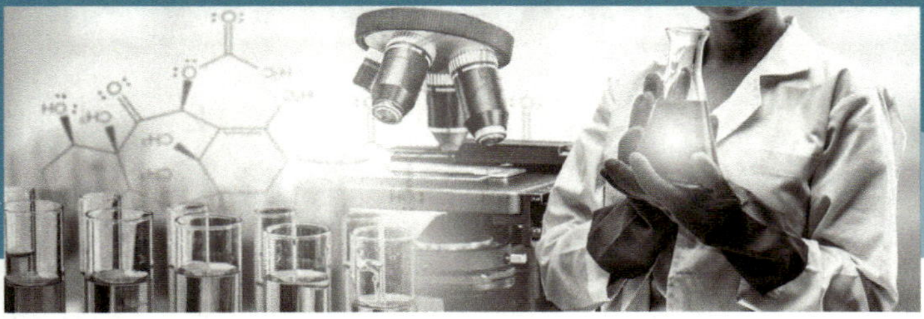

Textbook of Toxicology

苏州大学出版社
Soochow University Press

图书在版编目(CIP)数据

毒理学教程 = Textbook of Toxicology : 英文 / 曹毅，李建祥，张洁主编. -- 苏州 : 苏州大学出版社，2024. 12. -- ISBN 978-7-5672-5024-6

Ⅰ. R99

中国国家版本馆 CIP 数据核字第 2024MH0117 号

书　　名: 毒理学教程
DULIXUE　JIAOCHENG

主　　编: 曹　毅　李建祥　张　洁
责任编辑: 闫莹莹
装帧设计: 吴　钰

出版发行: 苏州大学出版社(Soochow University Press)
社　　址: 苏州市十梓街 1 号　**邮编**: 215006
印　　装: 苏州市古得堡数码印刷有限公司
网　　址: www. sudapress. com
邮　　箱: sdcbs@ suda. edu. cn
邮购热线: 0512-67480030
销售热线: 0512-67481020

开　　本: 787 mm×1092 mm　1/16　**印张**: 22. 75　**字数**: 526 千
版　　次: 2024 年 12 月第 1 版
印　　次: 2024 年 12 月第 1 次印刷
书　　号: ISBN 978-7-5672-5024-6
定　　价: 88. 00 元

凡购本社图书发现印装错误，请与本社联系调换。服务热线:0512-67481020

Preface

Toxicology is a fundamental discipline in both public health and preventive medicine, as well as a critical foundation for students of medicine, pharmacy, and food safety. Modern toxicology primarily studies the adverse effects of exogenous factors (chemicals, physical factors, and biological agents) on biological systems and their underlying mechanisms, encompassing the science of safety evaluation and risk assessment.

Toxicology possesses the attributes of both a fundamental and an applied discipline, holding profound significance for training public health and medical professionals. It has extensive applications in the assessment and management of health-related products, such as chemicals, drugs, health foods, and cosmetics. Toxicology is becoming increasingly prominent for the development of disciplines related to public health and preventive medicine, as well as for promoting social and economic progress.

Since 2006, Soochow University has embarked on the course of Fundamentals of Toxicology, which is a bilingual one for undergraduate students majoring in Preventive Medicine. Starting from 2014, the course has transitioned to be taught in English only. Over years of implementing both bilingual and full English teaching, it has been recognized the importance and urgency of an up-to-date bilingual textbook. In 2008, Soochow University collaborated with renowned domestic universities such as Capital Medical University, Peking University, and Fudan University to compile the inaugural bilingual textbook, "Essentials of Toxicology", tailored to meet the demands of bilingual teaching for domestic students. This textbook was officially published as a national planning textbook under the "11th Five-Year Plan", and a revised edition was released in 2016. Both editions have significantly advanced of bilingual toxicology teaching at Soochow University and some other domestic universities.

As toxicology disciplines continue to evolve rapidly, the textbook must incorporate emerging concepts and technologies. Additionally, ongoing reforms in teaching methods, including problem-based learning (PBL), digital transformation, and research-oriented teaching, pose fresh challenges to the format and content of bilingual textbooks. Against this background, the teaching team at Soochow University has compiled this new toxicology coursebook as a full English teaching material.

The compilation of this textbook follows several key principles: firstly, it emphasizes systematicity, logic, and scientific nature of the textbook to meet the requirements of the toxicology teaching syllabus for undergraduate students, the public health physician qualification examination and the postgraduate entrance examination; secondly, it adheres to the basic principles of "three fundamentals" (basic theories, basic knowledge, and basic skills) and "five properties" (ideological, scientific, advanced, enlightening, and applicable), focusing on cultivating students' basic theoretical foundation and skills in toxicology; thirdly, it integrates Soochow University's characteristics in toxicology teaching, paying attention to introducing new developments in toxicology, adds chapters on radiation toxicology, chronotoxicology, and nanotoxicology; fourthly, it emphasizes applicability and readability of the textbook for the students.

This textbook consists of 19 chapters, including 11 chapters on general toxicology, 5 chapters on target organ toxicology, and 3 chapters on special toxicology. Primarily designed for full English instruction in Preventive Medicine, this textbook can also be utilized for pharmacy, health inspection, and health management courses. Furthermore, it can serve as a valuable reference for graduate students and other professionals in related fields.

In the process of compiling this textbook, we received invaluable guidance and assistance from Soochow University Press. Twelve teachers from the Department of Toxicology at Soochow University invested considerable time and effort in its creation. In particular, Dr. Song Xiaoyao, who served as the secretory for this textbook, has devoted tremendous efforts to coordinating and organizing the entire project. We offer our deepest respect and gratitude to all involved in this challenging task. We acknowledge that there may be errors or insufficiencies in this textbook, and sincerely welcome constructive feedback and suggestions from all teachers, students and colleagues, as it will greatly aid in our efforts to improve and refine future editions.

Cao Yi

December 2024

Contents

CHAPTER 1

Introduction to Toxicology

Definition of Toxicology

The term "Toxicology" originates from the ancient Greek words "toxikon" and "logos", with its original meaning of the "scientific description of poisons". The traditional definition of toxicology involves the study of the adverse effects of exogenous chemicals (xenobiotics) on living organisms. Modern toxicology, building upon the foundation of traditional toxicology, has expanded its scope, methodologies, and objectives beyond the traditional definition. The contemporary definition of toxicology is the study of the adverse effects and biological mechanisms of various chemical, physical, and biological agents on living systems, along with evaluation and risk assessment. Toxicology can be more precisely defined as the study of the detection, occurrence, characterization, effects, and management of harmful agents.

In today's world, there are over 80, 000 commercial and industrial chemicals in use, with approximately 500 - 1, 000 new chemicals entering the environment each year. Due to this increasing diversity and prevalence of potential chemical exposures for humans, toxicology has gained significant importance in quantitatively estimating the potential health effects and environmental impact of various exposure scenarios, such as pesticide residues on food, contaminants in drinking water, and airborne dust in the workplace.

Scope of Toxicology

Three Main Specialized Areas

The field of toxicology is typically divided into three main specialized areas: descriptive toxicology, mechanistic toxicology, and regulatory toxicology. Although all three categories have distinctive characteristics, each contributes to the others, and all are vitally important to chemical risk assessment.

Descriptive toxicology focuses on toxicity testing to systematically identify and characterize the adverse effects of chemical, physical, and biological agents. It provides essential information for safety evaluation and regulatory requirements. It may involve studying the effects of substances such as drugs, food additives, and environmental pollutants on humans, as well as assessing their potential impacts on various other organisms and entire ecosystems. By conducting systematic experiments, researchers determine the levels of exposure that cause adverse effects, identify the target organs or systems affected, and observe the onset, progression, and reversibility of toxicity. The data generated serves as the foundation for establishing safe exposure limits and for guiding further research into the mechanisms of toxicity.

Mechanistic toxicology delves into identifying and understanding the mechanisms by which chemicals exert toxic effects on living organisms. In risk assessment, mechanistic data play a crucial role in demonstrating whether observed adverse outcomes in laboratory animals are directly relevant to humans. Mechanistic data may also aid in the development of safer alternative chemicals and rational therapies for chemical poisoning and diseases. An understanding of the mechanisms of toxic action contributes to advancements in basic physiology, pharmacology, cell biology, and biochemistry.

Regulatory toxicology involves decision-making based on data from descriptive and mechanistic studies, determining whether a drug or chemical poses an acceptably low risk for its intended use and establishing standards for acceptable chemical levels in various environments.

Other Specialized Areas of Toxicology

In addition to the primary categories mentioned above, toxicology encompasses various specialized fields based on the types of chemicals involved or the application of toxicological knowledge. Forensic toxicology deals with medicolegal aspects of chemical effects on humans and animals, playing a vital role in postmortem investigations. Clinical toxicology focuses on diseases caused by toxic substances and the treatment of chemical poisonings. Environmental toxicology examines the impact of chemical pollutants on biological organisms and ecosystems. Drug toxicology is crucial in preclinical safety assessments of potential pharmaceuticals and the study of high-dose drug effects. Occupational toxicology addresses chemical exposures and diseases in the workplace, influencing the development of safety procedures and exposure limits. These specialized areas, while distinct, are interconnected and collectively contribute to the comprehensive understanding and management of chemical risks in our increasingly complex world.

Multidisciplinary Nature of Toxicology

Relationship to Other Sciences

Although generally accepted as a specific scientific field during the 20th century, toxicology is not a discipline in its own but comprises many different disciplines at present. Toxicology is a highly eclectic interdisciplinary science with contributions from and to a broad spectrum of other sciences. At one end of the spectrum are those sciences that contribute their methods and philosophical concepts to serve the needs of toxicologists, either in research or in the application of toxicology to human affairs. At the other end of the spectrum are those sciences to which toxicology contributes.

In the first group, chemistry, biochemistry, physiology, immunology, pathology, epidemiology, biomathematics, and ecology have historically influenced toxicology, providing methods and philosophical concepts. Molecular biology has, in the last few decades, contributed to dramatic advances in toxicology.

In the group of sciences to which toxicology contributes significantly are such aspects of medicine as public health, occupational health, internal medicine, forensic medicine, and pharmacy. Toxicology also contributes in an important way to veterinary medicine, and to such aspects of agriculture as the development and safe use of agricultural chemicals. The contributions of toxicology to environmental studies have been becoming increasingly important in recent years.

The field most closely related to toxicology is pharmacology. In many countries, toxicology as a discipline has developed from pharmacology. Pharmacology and toxicology both study the effect of chemicals on living organisms and have often used identical methods. However, fundamental differences have developed with advances in these sciences. Pharmacology focuses on chemicals with beneficial effects (drugs) at low doses, whereas toxicology studies the adverse health effects occurring with the same chemicals at high doses. Today, the main interest of research in toxicology has shifted to studies on the long-term effects of low-dose chemical exposures, such as cancer or other irreversible diseases. Moreover, most chemicals of interest to toxicologists are not used as drugs.

Toxicology is unique in its position as a recognized scientific discipline encompassing both basic and applied issues. Few fields can claim such a direct link between fundamental science and practical applications.

Toxicology Is Both a Science and an Art

Toxicology, like medicine, is both a science and an art. The science of toxicology involves the observational and data-gathering phase, while the art of toxicology consists of the utilization of the data to predict outcomes of exposure in human and animal populations. In most cases, these phases are linked because the facts generated by the science of toxicology are used to develop extrapolations and hypotheses to explain the adverse effects of chemical agents in situations where there is little or no information. For instance, the observation that TCDD (2, 3, 7, 8-tetrachlorodibenzo-p-dioxin) causes liver cancer in female rats is based on scientific observation, but predicting similar effects in humans is an artistic inference. It is crucial to distinguish facts from predictions in toxicology. Failing to differentiate between the science and the art may lead to confusing facts with predictions and incorrectly attributing equal validity to both. In toxicology, as in all science, theories are more certain than hypotheses, which in turn are more certain than speculations, opinions, conjectures, and guesses.

Historical Aspects of Toxicology

Antiquity and Middle Ages

The history of toxicology spans millennia, tracing its roots to the earliest human civilizations. Primitive humans recognized and utilized natural poisons from animals and plants for hunting, warfare, and even assassination. The term "toxicology" originates from the Greek words "toxikon", referring to a poisonous substance used on arrowheads, and "logia", meaning "the study of". The word "toxikon" itself is derived from "toxikos", meaning "pertaining to a bow".

Ancient civilizations demonstrated a sophisticated understanding of poisons. The Ebers Papyrus (circa 1, 500 BC) contains information on numerous recognized poisons. Hippocrates, the ancient Greek physician who lived around 400 BC, showcased a professional awareness of poisons and the fundamental principles of toxicology in his writings. He addressed topics such as poisoning treatment by influencing absorption and mentioned clinical toxicology principles related to bioavailability in therapy and overdosage.

During this era, the use of poisons for murder, suicide, and political assassinations was prevalent. For example, it is well known that Socrates (circa 469 – 399 BC) committed suicide by taking hemlock as a state-sanctioned execution method. King Mithridates Ⅵ of Pontus did numerous acute toxicity experiments on unfortunate criminals to search for antidotes to poisonous substances. He regularly protected himself with a mixture of 50 different antidotes.

Dioscorides (40–90 AD), a Greek physician serving in the court of the Roman emperor Nero, was the first to attempt a classification of poisons and completed with descriptions and illustrations. His categorization into plants, animals, and mineral poisons remained a standard for 16 centuries and is still recognized as a practical classification system today.

During the Middle Ages, particularly in Italy, the art of poisoning for political purposes developed into a dark and infamous practice. Notable families, such as the Borgias, gained infamy for their involvement in poisoning during the 15th and 16th centuries.

Age of Enlightenment

During the late Middle Ages, Paracelsus (1493–1541) emerged as a significant figure in the history of science and medicine. Between the time of Aristotle and the Age of Enlightenment, there was little substantial change in the biomedical sciences. However, Paracelsus initiated a view that became a lasting contribution to the field of toxicology (Figure 1–1). Paracelsus believed that experimentation is essential in studying the effects of chemicals

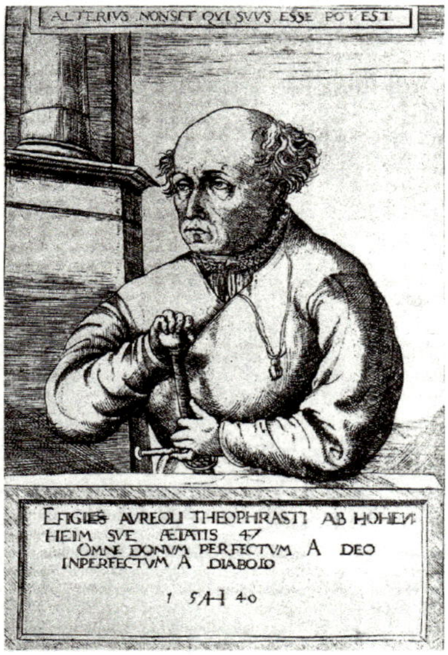
ALTERIVS NONSIT QVI SVVS ESSE POTEST
EFIGIES AVREOLI THEOPHRASTI AB HOHEN-
HEIM SVE AETATIS 47
OMNE DONVM PERFECTVM A DEO
INPERFECTVM A DIABOLO

Figure 1–1 P. A. Paracelsus (1493–1541)

This Swiss physician and scientist questioned and rejected the irrational medicine of his time. He especially realized the crucial importance of dose in relation to both the adverse and the beneficial effects of chemicals.

on living organisms. He emphasized the importance of distinguishing between the therapeutic and toxic properties of chemicals. He argued that the therapeutic and toxic properties of chemicals could be indistinguishable except by dose. Additionally, Paracelsus summarized his views in the following famous phrase: "All substances are poisons; there is none that is not a poison. The right dose differentiates a poison from a remedy." This statement is properly regarded as a landmark in the development of the science.

The industrial revolution led to a marked increase in occupational diseases, prompting the emergence of pioneering figures in the field of occupational toxicology. One such notable figure was Bernardino Ramazzini, who in 1700 published the comprehensive work *Discourse on the Diseases of Workers*. This seminal publication laid the foundational standards for the discipline of occupational medicine, marking a significant milestone in the establishment of occupational toxicology.

In 1795, Percival Pott made a crucial contribution by identifying the link between soot exposure and scrotal cancer in chimney sweepers. This was the first reported instance of a specific environmental factor, in this case, polyaromatic hydrocarbons, being associated with carcinogenicity.

Moving into the nineteenth century, a period characterized by industrial and political revolutions, the field of toxicology continued to evolve. The development of organic chemistry played a pivotal role during this era. In 1800, organic chemistry was still in its infancy, but by 1825, notable advancements had been made, including the synthesis of phosgene and mustard gas. Unfortunately, these chemicals were later employed as war gases during World War I, underlining the dual-edged nature of chemical innovation.

Another significant figure in the history of toxicology was Mathieu Joseph Bonaventure Orfila (1787–1853), a Spaniard who worked at the University of Paris in the early nineteenth century. He is regarded as the "father of modern toxicology" (Figure 1–2). Orfila played a crucial role in establishing toxicology as a separate scientific discipline. Through numerous

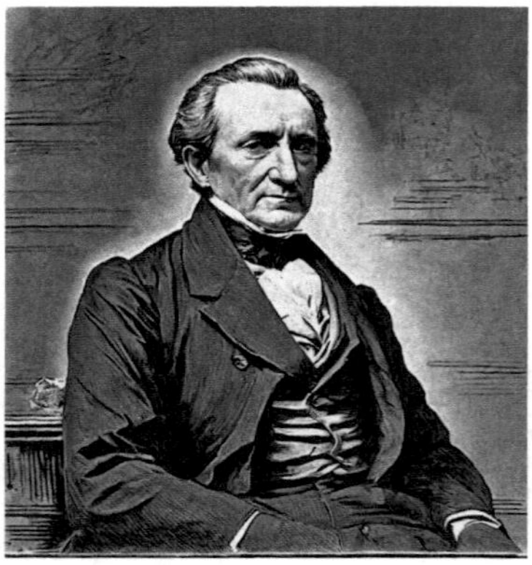

Figure 1–2 **M. J. B. Orfila (1787–1853)**

A Spanish chemist and physician, he can properly be called "the father of modern toxicology". His two-volume work, published as an English translation in 1817, was the first textbook of toxicology.

quantitative toxicological studies on experimental animals, he elucidated the relationship between the dose of a toxic agent and the resulting biological effects. Moreover, Orfila made substantial contributions to the field of forensic toxicology by applying analytical chemistry methods to detect poisons in autopsy materials and exhumed bodies. Additionally, Orfila critically evaluated the treatment procedures used at that time for treating poisoning, many of which were found to be ineffective. Many of his recommendations regarding the elimination of poisons from the body and the use of artificial respiration remain valid today.

Many German scientists contributed greatly to the growth of toxicology in the late nineteenth and early twentieth centuries. The notable figures among them were Oswald Schmiedeberg (1838 – 1921) and Louis Lewin (1850 – 1929). Schmiedeberg's research focused on the synthesis of hippuric acid in the liver and the detoxification mechanisms of the liver in several animal species. Lewin made contributions to the chronic toxicity of narcotics and other alkaloids.

Modern Age

The twentieth century witnessed a rapid evolution of toxicology, with exponential growth particularly evident in the post-World War Ⅱ era. This period saw a marked increase in the production of drugs, pesticides, munitions, synthetic fibers, and industrial chemicals, necessitating a more comprehensive understanding of their potential toxicological impacts.

Prohibition of alcoholic beverages in the United States opened the door for early studies of neurotoxicology. It was discovered that triorthocresyl phosphate (TOCP) and methanol are neurotoxicants. Concurrently, Mueller's discovery of DDT and other organohalides such as hexachlorobenzene and hexachlorocyclohexane in the late 1920s led to the widespread use of insecticidal agents, further expanding the scope of this field.

The tragic event of sulfanilamide in glycol solution led to the passage of the Copeland Act in 1938. This legislation mandated safety testing of drugs prior to marketing and led to the formation of the U. S. Food and Drug Administration (FDA). The sulfanilamide disaster played a critical role in the further development of toxicology, resulting in work by Eugene Maximillian Geiling at the University of Chicago that elucidated the mechanism of toxicity of both sulfanilamide and ethylene glycol. Simultaneously, Arnold Lehman's group at the FDA conducted studies on glycols and other chemicals, developing crucial toxicological methods and standards. Their work established foundational concepts such as the median lethal dose (LD_{50}), no observed adverse effect level (NOAEL), and acceptable daily intake (ADI).

In 1945, Sir Rudolph Peters studied the mechanism of action of arsenical war gases and so was able to devise an effective antidote known as British Anti-Lewisite. Another seminal event in toxicology that occurred during the World War Ⅱ era was the discovery of organophosphate cholinesterase inhibitors. The importance of the early research on the organophosphates has taken on special meaning in the years since 1960, when these non-bioaccumulating insecticides were gradually replaced DDT and other organochlorine insecticides.

The 1940s saw groundbreaking research in chemical carcinogenesis, notably Elizabeth and James Miller's seminal work on reactive intermediates and mixed-functional oxidases at the University of Wisconsin. This research laid the foundation for many contemporary studies in the field.

The 1960s were a tumultuous time for society, and toxicology was swept up in the tide. Starting with the tragic thalidomide incident and the publication of Rachel Carson's *Silent Spring* (1962), the field of toxicology developed at a feverish pitch. The end of the 1960s witnessed the "discovery" of TCDD as a contaminant in the herbicide Agent Orange. The discovery of a high-affinity cellular binding protein designated the "Ah" receptor and the work on genetics of the receptor have revolutionized toxicology.

The expansion of legislation, journals, and new societies involved in toxicology was exponential during the 1970s and 1980s and showed no signs of slowing down.

Modern toxicology, which is more than 100 years old, is both an experimental and an applied science. It is a predictive science that has evolved remarkably since the time of Orfila, particularly in the past 70 years. Recent additions to the discipline include studies of regulatory toxicology for safety evaluation and risk assessment.

As we progress through the 21st century, toxicology continues to be shaped by expanding knowledge in immunology, genetics, and molecular biology. These advancements promise to deepen our understanding of chemical-biological interactions and refine our ability to predict and mitigate toxic effects. The field remains dynamic, adapting to new challenges posed by emerging technologies and environmental concerns, while continuously improving its methodologies to ensure public health and environmental safety.

Methods and Types of Toxicology Studies

It is essential to rely on human data generated under similar exposure conditions to assess the potential human hazard of a specific chemical. Unfortunately, such data are rarely available. The human data that are most typically available are generated from human populations in some occupational or clinical settings in which the exposure was believed at least initially to be safe. The exceptions, of course, are those infrequent, unintended poisonings or environmental releases. Thus, toxicology study data can originate from five distinct categories: basic animal toxicology tests, less conventional alternative tests (mainly in vitro methods), epidemiological studies, clinical exposure studies, and accidental acute poisonings.

Each type of toxicology study has inherent advantages and disadvantages. No single test system is likely to be ideal for assessing the potential human hazard of a chemical. It is imperative to assess the strengths and weaknesses of each test system to conclude its effectiveness. Table 1-1 summarizes the advantages and disadvantages of toxicology studies by category.

Table 1-1 Some Advantages and Disadvantages of Toxicology Studies by Category

Type of Study	Advantages	Disadvantages
In vivo methods	Easily manipulated and controlled Evaluate effects on intact animals and assess organ system interactions Widest range of potential effects to study The chance to identify and elucidate mechanisms of adverse effects	Test species response is of uncertain human relevance Exposures levels may not be relevant to the human exposure level Structural and biochemical differences between test animals and humans that make extrapolation from one to the other difficult
In vitro methods	Less expensive and quick to perform Easier to control for host factors Conservation of animal resources and ethically more acceptable Possible to use human tissue	Cannot fully approximate the complexities that take place in whole organisms Inability to detect delayed and/or chronic toxic effects
Epidemiological studies	The direct observation of effects in humans Real-life exposure conditions relevant to chemical-induced health effects The full range of human susceptibility may be measurable The chance to study the interactive effects of other chemicals	Often costly and time-consuming Many confounding risk factors are present Exposures may have been poorly documented Determining crude endpoints of exposure such as mortality and morbidity Post facto—not necessarily designed to be protective of health
Clinical (human) exposure studies	The conditions of these studies are better defined and controlled Most relevant species (humans) to study Exposure conditions may be altered during the exposure interval in response to the presence or lack of an effect, making NOAELs* easier to obtain	May be costly to perform The most sensitive group (e. g. young, elderly, infirm) may often be inappropriate for study Primarily limited to examining safe exposure levels or minimally serious effects Usually limited to shorter exposure intervals
Accidental acute poisonings	Exposure conditions are realistic Require very few individuals to perform Inexpensive than other human studies	Accurate exposure information may be lacking The knowledge gained from these studies may be of limited relevance to other human exposure situations

* NOAELs: no observed adverse effect levels.

In Vivo Methods

"In vivo studies" are those performed using any intact higher organisms (most commonly, mammals) as a model system. Eight different species are usually used in toxicological whole animal studies. The most commonly used species in toxicological whole animal studies, in descending order of using frequency, are rats, mice, rabbits, guinea pigs, hamsters, dogs, ferrets, and monkeys. There are two main principles underlying all animal experiments in toxicology. The first is that the effects produced by a chemical in laboratory animals, when properly qualified, are applicable to humans. The second is that experimental animals are given chemicals in large amounts (high doses) necessary and valid to discover possible hazards in humans because the incidence of an effect in a population is greater as the dose increases.

In Vitro Methods

"In vitro (test) systems" are those that do not employ intact higher organisms as models for predicting potential human effects. There is a wide range of such test systems, which include isolated perfused organs, organ culture, tissue slices, cell cultures (primary cell cultures, established cell lines), tissue homogenates, subcellular fractions, purified enzymes, and lower organisms (prokaryotes). The term "in vitro system" is frequently used for all short-term tests for mutagenicity (e. g. Ames assay). "In vitro systems" have a number of limitations which prevent them from being acceptable models. At the same time there are substantial potential advantages in using "in vitro systems". The advantages of using cell or tissue culture in toxicological testing are accurate dosing, quantitation of results, and so on.

Epidemiological Studies

Epidemiology and toxicology are fundamentally different. Epidemiology is observational, constrated with the experimental nature of toxicology. Despite many problems inherent to epidemiological studies including various biases, confounding factors, and inadequate quantitation of exposures, these studies offer a major advantage over those conducted with animals: providing the actual health experiences of human beings subjected to real-life exposures.

Epidemiological studies in toxicology can be broadly categorized into cohort studies, case-control studies, and cross-sectional studies. Cohort studies follow groups of individuals over time, case-control studies compare groups with and without a specific health outcome, and cross-sectional studies examine the prevalence of outcomes and exposures at a single point in time. Each type has its own strengths and is suited to different research questions.

Epidemiological data from well-conducted human studies are the most convincing evidence of a causal association between chemical exposure and disease, and therefore can be very useful for identification of the potential human hazard. Such data are useful in confirming the safety indicated by animal studies after the establishment of NOAEL. The data are also useful in subsequent periodic reviews, and might facilitate a reevaluation of the safety standard.

Clinical (Human) Exposure Studies

In addition to epidemiological surveys of populations exposed to a toxic chemical under normal usage conditions, clinical experimental exposure studies in human volunteers serve as a crucial source of human toxicological data. Although an experiment is defined as observations under controlled exposure conditions, there is sometimes a gray area distinguishing an experiment with human subjects from observations on human subjects under natural conditions. These investigations are often ethically restricted to examining mild, temporary effects of short-term exposures in a limited number of subjects.

Certain types of information about the effects of chemicals can only be gleaned through direct observations on humans. Carefully controlled experiments frequently yield valuable insights at doses well below anticipated "safe" levels. Examples may include measuring subtle changes in reaction time, behavioral functions, and sensory responses.

Accidental Acute Poisonings

Accidental acute poisonings are a significant source of data in clinical toxicology. These studies are typically case reports or a small case series, and thus, measures of individual variations in response may be difficult to estimate. While invaluable for identifying novel toxic agents and understanding their clinical manifestations in humans, such opportunistic observations have inherent limitations for quantitative risk assessment. A primary challenge is the frequent uncertainty regarding the exact dose of the toxicant to which the individual was exposed. The amount ingested, inhaled, or absorbed is often unknown or must be roughly estimated from the patient's recall or circumstantial evidence, which complicates the establishment of a clear dose-response relationship. Furthermore, the clinical picture can be confounded by numerous factors, including the co-ingestion of other substances such as alcohol or other drugs, the presence of underlying diseases, and significant delays between exposure and medical intervention. These variables can modify the toxicokinetics and toxicodynamics of the substance in question, making it difficult to attribute specific effects solely to the poison of interest. Reporting bias also plays a role, as more severe or unusual cases are more likely to be documented and published, potentially skewing the perception of the substance's typical effects and overall lethality. Therefore, while case reports of accidental poisonings are crucial for hazard identification and guiding clinical management, the data derived from them must be interpreted with considerable caution due to the lack of controlled experimental conditions and the presence of multiple, often unquantifiable, confounding variables.

Challenges and Future Prospects

During the past several decades, toxicology has developed more rapidly than any other science in a comparable period of time. From a discipline largely descriptive of deleterious effects on intact animals, toxicology now embraces all aspects of modern biology from molecular biology to highly sophisticated instrumental analysis. The philosophical basis has shifted from routine risk analysis based primarily on mortality or pathological endpoints to an analysis of mechanisms of toxic action and the development of new paradigms of risk assessment that include mechanistic considerations. Toxicology's advances are often based on utilizing concepts and techniques developed from basic biomedical research. The field of toxicology has developed a well-characterized set of techniques to assess the behavioral and histopathological consequences of chemical exposure in various animal models. These techniques are suitable for determining crude endpoints of exposure such as death but not optimal for assessing the more subtle effects of very low level of multi-agent chemical exposure, nor do they offer mechanistic explanations at the molecular level. More recently, in vitro techniques using mammalian cell culture, including human cells, have been developed. These approaches offer high-throughput, inexpensive assays using defined cell types. We now know that gene activity is exquisitely sensitive to environmental perturbations and that genetic regulation is responsive long before the elaboration of long-term pathologies. It is therefore possible to develop a predictive toxicology based on analyses of the genome, proteome and metabolome.

At the beginning of the twenty-first century, the practice of toxicology is undergoing many changes, and still, toxicology faces many challenges. These challenges emanate from the swift evolution of technology, particularly in biotechnology and bioinformatics, necessitating a continual reassessment of procedures for chemical safety evaluation.

Toxicogenomics: A Revolutionary Paradigm

The dynamic landscape of toxicology has been profoundly shaped by the remarkable strides in molecular biology over the past two decades, giving rise to the groundbreaking subdiscipline of toxicogenomics. This field harnesses the prowess of functional genomics technologies, encompassing transcriptomics, proteomics, and metabolomics, to delve into the intricate study of adverse effects induced by xenobiotic substances, elucidating their correlation with the structure and activity of the genome.

In its broadest sense, toxicogenomics includes studies of the cellular products controlled by the genome. The new "global" methods of measuring families of cellular molecules, such as RNA, proteins, and intermediary metabolites have been termed "-omic" technologies, based on their ability to characterize all, or most, members of a family of molecules in a single analysis. With these new tools, we can now obtain complete assessments of the functional activity of biochemical pathways, and of the structural genetic (sequence) differences among individuals and species, that were previously unattainable. The advent of high-throughput and multi-endpoint analysis, exemplified by gene expression arrays and advanced methods for protein and cellular small molecule analysis, has propelled significant breakthroughs in understanding the molecular mechanisms underpinning xenobiotic-induced damage to cells and tissues.

In addition to studying gene expression changes, toxicogenomics also encompasses epigenetic modifications induced by toxicants. These epigenetic changes can have long-lasting effects on gene expression and may even be passed on to subsequent generations, adding another layer of complexity to toxicological assessments.

These technologies have immense transformative potential. They can help develop novel, sensitive biomarkers to monitor subtle changes in gene expression. Such advances also enable better understanding of how genetic variation affects toxicological outcomes and identification of highly responsive subgroups within the human population.

The biological response to environmental exposure is so complex and involves so many interactive factors and networks that the use of a "systems toxicology" analytical approach is required. Systems toxicology investigates the interaction between xenobiotics and biological systems through monitoring the changes of molecular expression (transcript, protein and metabolite profiling) and conventional toxicological parameters, and then iteratively integrating various response data with bioinformatics and computational techniques. Toxicology is gradually evolving into a systems toxicology that will eventually allow us to describe all the toxicological reactions and predict the modes of action that occur within a living system.

Hormesis: A Key Concept in Toxicology

There is an old saying that a little dirt is good for you. It has been suggested that early exposure of the immune system to foreign agents such as bacteria helps to protect young children from infectious diseases later in life. There is growing evidence that this belief may have more widespread relevance in that low levels of chemicals may not only be harmless but positively beneficial. There is some scientific basis for this concept of "hormesis" in that exposure to low levels of chemicals will stimulate the body and individual cells to increase protective measures. This means that extrapolating from a high dose of a chemical to a very low dose to determine a threshold and calculate risk may not be appropriate, especially if a linear model is used which implies there is no safe dose (for example, for a carcinogen). Acceptance of the existence and dominance of hormetic dose responses has the potential to markedly change the fields of toxicology, risk assessment, and risk communication. One of the most significant implications is that it challenges the linear no threshold (LNT) model, which assumes that carcinogens can act without thresholds. If this hormetic model were accepted and implemented, it would have a major impact on a large number of environmental and occupational health standards.

3R's Principle of Humane Animal Use in Research and Alternatives

Since the early 1980s, public perception of the value of animal testing has been strongly influenced by what is now called the animal rights movement. This movement advocates for the ethical treatment of animals and opposes the use of animals for scientific research, education, and entertainment. This concern about animal welfare and the effort of technological improvements have led to increasing use of alternative methods and models. Alternative methods in the wider sense of the word are procedures that result in a reduction of the number of animals, and permit a lessening of pain and anxiety. The historical beginnings of this concept date to 1959 when Russell and Burch first proposed what have come to be called the 3R's principle of humane animal use in research: replacement, reduction, and refinement. Replacement means utilizing methods which do not use intact higher (vertebrate) animals in place of those that do. Reduction refers to the use of fewer animals. Refinement entails the modification of existing procedures so that animals are subjected to less pain and distress. The 3R's principle is widely accepted as guiding principle for the ethical use of animals in research and are incorporated into many national and international regulations and guidelines.

Validation of new or revised alternative methods, in terms of comparability of response with routine "in vivo (test) systems", is usually necessary for their regulatory acceptance. Significant progress has been made in recent years regarding the scientific principles and processes for adequate validation of in vitro and other alternative methods proposed for regulatory applications. However, the use of alternative methods is not only driven by ethical considerations, but also by scientific and practical advantages. It can be predicted that the use of alternative techniques for the purpose of developing the understanding of mechanisms of toxicity will greatly expand in many areas with the progress of the science of toxicology.

Predictive Toxicology and QSAR

Predictive toxicology is an emerging interdisciplinary science with contributions from chemistry, biology, and medicine as well as statistics and computer science. In predictive toxicology, the major efforts are made to develop procedures (algorithms in computer science terms) that are able to predict adverse effects (the output) from chemical and biological information (the input). The key problem in predictive toxicology is to identify the parameters that are relevant for a particular adverse effect. Methods for parameter selection are therefore an important research topic in predictive toxicology. For the prediction algorithm, there are two strategies: expert systems and data-driven approaches. More recently, techniques originating from artificial intelligence research have been used in predictive toxicology.

The primary aim of predictive toxicology is the prediction of toxic activities of untested compounds. This enables one to evaluate potential side effects of candidate structures even without synthesizing them. The prioritization of compounds for experiment toxicity assays is another important application of predictive toxicology. One of examples of the creative use of predictive toxicology methods is to provide information for the design of less dangerous, but equally efficient compounds (computer-aided drug design). Predictive toxicology can also serve as a tool for the generation and verification of scientific hypotheses. One of the most widely used methods in predictive toxicology is quantitative structure-activity relationship (QSAR), which is a mathematical model that relates the chemical structure of a compound to its biological activity.

The examination of the toxicodynamics models and toxicity models for both prokaryotic and eukaryotic cells shows that a combination of TS (topostructure) and TC (topochemical) descriptors is capable of producing predictive models of reasonable quality. In the post-genomic era, relevant genomic sequence and proteomics information can be condensed into descriptors and used in QSAR model development. Instead of developing models based on chemodescriptors derived from molecular structure (chemoinformatics) or biodescriptors derived from genomics or proteomics (bioinformatics) alone, we need to develop an integrated approach (I-QSAR) with a combination of both classes of descriptors.

Health Effects of Chemical Mixtures and Technological Advances

In most cases, exposure of humans to chemicals occurs not to one single substance but to mixtures. Thus, the interactions between the constituents of the mixture must also be considered in evaluating the potential effects of exposure to any chemical mixtures. Given the different types of mixtures for which health risk assessments are performed, as well as the many factors that impact the overall toxicity of such mixtures, no single approach is suitable to conduct every health risk assessment. The risk assessment process must encompass all available toxicological data and scientific evidence on the plausible toxicities of chemical mixtures.

Comprehensive experimental research is essential to elucidate the complex toxicological mechanisms of chemical mixtures and advance our understanding of their molecular toxicology. Such studies should investigate not only the direct interactions between mixture components, but also how different components compete for or modulate the same biological targets. This includes competitive inhibition of metabolic enzymes, competitive binding to receptors and transporters, and synergistic or antagonistic effects on cellular pathways and gene expression. Understanding these molecular level interactions will enable the development of biologically-based predictive models for the toxicity of mixtures.

Recent regulatory frameworks have evolved beyond traditional chemical mixtures assessment to emphasize cumulative risk evaluation across multiple environmental media. This approach recognizes that humans are simultaneously exposed to chemicals through air, water, soil, food, and consumer products. Traditional medium-by-medium risk assessments fail to capture the true cumulative exposure burden, making cross-media evaluation essential for realistic health risk characterization.

The term "silico toxicology" refers to the use of advanced computer simulation tools such as reaction network modeling that will, to a great extent, replace mechanistic and animal experimental studies, which may be impractical or impossible to perform in animal laboratories for complex biological systems involving chemical mixtures and multiple stressors. These techniques, in combination, will equip the field of toxicology with the much-needed speed and predictability, and replace the classical time-consuming, less-predictive testing methods. Bioinformatics and data analysis will play a key role in the future of toxicology, a field which is largely driven by issues that relate to human exposure to chemical mixtures and their health consequences.

Artificial Intelligence in Toxicology

Artificial intelligence (AI) is a rapidly developing subdiscipline of computer science with the goal of designing and creating machines or computational models that can perform a variety of cognitive tasks at a level comparable to or even exceed human intelligence. The term "artificial intelligence" can have different meanings in different fields. In the field of toxicology, it refers to the applications of various machine learning methods in the prediction and evaluation of chemical toxicokinetics (e. g. absorption, distribution, metabolism, and excretion) and toxicity properties.

Machine learning is a subarea of artificial intelligence, and it refers to mathematical or computer algorithms designed to teach or train a computational model to solve a problem or perform complex tasks based on some input parameters. Machine learning is generally categorized into 3 types: supervised learning, unsupervised learning, and reinforcement. In recent years, machine learning and artificial intelligence approaches are increasingly applied in different subject areas of toxicology, including neurotoxicology, cardiovascular toxicology, nanotoxicology, toxicokinetics, dermatoxicology, carcinogenesis and so on.

Significant progress has been achieved in integrating machine learning and artificial intelligence approaches with traditional toxicology approaches, such as physiologically based pharmacokinetics (PBPK) models, quantitative structure-activity relationship (QSAR) models, adverse outcome pathway (AOP) analysis, high-throughput screening, toxicogenomics. These integrations are further enhanced by the availability of big data resources, and comprehensive toxicological databases. By leveraging machine learning and artificial intelligence approaches, now it is possible to develop PBPK models for hundreds of chemicals efficiently. They also allow the creation of in silico toxicity prediction models with accuracy comparable to which in vivo animal experiments. Additionally, researchers can now rapidly analyze diverse data types, including toxicogenomics and high-content imaging data, to generate new insights into toxicity mechanisms. These achievements were impossible with traditional manual approaches. To advance this field of toxicological sciences unceasingly, several challenges should be considered: ① not all machine learning models are equally useful for a particular type of toxicology data, and thus it is important to test different methods to determine the optimal approach; ② current toxicity prediction is mainly on bioactivity classification (yes/no), so additional studies are needed to predict the intensity of effect or dose-response relationship; ③ as more data become available, it is crucial to perform rigorous data quality check and develop infrastructure to store, share, analyze, evaluate, and manage big data; ④ it is important to convert machine learning models to user-friendly interfaces to facilitate their applications by both computational and bench scientists.

(Cao Yi)

CHAPTER 2

Essential Concepts of Toxicology

Toxic Agents, Toxicity and Adverse Effects

Toxic Agents and Their Classification

One could define a ***poison*** as any agent capable of producing a deleterious response in a biological system, seriously injuring function or producing death. This is not a useful working definition, however, for the simple reason that virtually every known chemical has the potential to produce injury or death if it is present in a sufficient amount (dose). At sufficiently high doses, any chemical may be described as toxic. The importance of dose is clearly seen with molecular oxygen or dietary metals. Oxygen at a concentration of 21% in the atmosphere is essential for life, but 100% oxygen at atmospheric pressure causes severe lung injury in rodents and often results in death. Some metals such as iron, copper, and zinc are essential nutrients. When they are present in insufficient amounts in the human diet, specific disease patterns develop, but in high doses they can cause fatal intoxications. Similarly, once a medication exceeds the safe dosage for use, it can cause toxic or side effects.

Therefore, all toxic effects are products of the amount of chemical to which the organism is exposed and the inherent toxicity of the chemical; they also depend on the sensitivity of the biological system. The ***toxicity*** of a chemical could be defined as the ability to cause a deleterious effect on a biological system or route of exposure. Among chemicals there is a wide range of doses or dosages (mg/kg) needed to produce toxic effects, serious injury, or death. Table 2-1 shows the dosages of chemicals that cause death in 50% of treated animals (LD_{50}).

Table 2-1 **Approximate Acute LD_{50} Values of Some Representative Chemicals**

Agent	LD_{50}/(mg/kg) *	Animal	Route
Ethyl alcohol	10, 000	Mouse	Oral
Sodium chloride	4, 000	Mouse	IP
Ferrous sulfate	1, 500	Rat	Oral
Morphine sulfate	900	Rat	Oral
Phenobarbital sodium	150	Rat	Oral
Picrotoxin	5	Rat	SC
Strychnine sulfate	2	Rat	IP
Nicotine	1	Rat	IV
d-Tubocurarine	0. 5	Rat	IV
Hemicholinium-3	0. 2	Rat	IV
Tetrodotoxin	0. 10	Rat	IV
Dioxin (TCDD)	0. 001	Guinea pig	IV
Botulinum toxin	0. 00001	Rat	IV

* LD_{50} is the dosage (mg/kg body weight) causing death in 50% of exposed animals.
IP, SC, and IV stand for intraperitoneal, subcutaneous, and intravenous injection, respectively.

Toxic agents are chemicals of all kinds, both synthetic and natural ones. The term ***toxin*** generally refers to toxic substances of animals, plants, fungi, or bacterial origin that are produced naturally. The term ***toxicant*** is used in speaking of toxic substances that are produced by or are a byproduct of anthropogenic (human-made) activities.

Toxic agents may be classified in terms of their target organs (e. g. liver, kidney, hematopoietic system), use (e. g. pesticide, solvent, food additive), source (animal or plant toxins), adverse effects (e. g. cancer, mutation), chemical stability or reactivity (explosive, flammable, oxidizer), general chemical structure (e. g. aromatic amine, halogenated hydrocarbon), or poisoning potential (extremely toxic, very toxic, slightly toxic, etc.). Classification of toxic agents based on their biochemical mechanisms of action (e. g. alkylating agent, cholinesterase inhibitor, methemoglobin producer) is usually more informative than classification by general terms such as irritants and corrosives. However, more descriptive categories such as air pollutants, occupation-related exposures, and acute and chronic poisons may be more useful to associate toxic chemicals that result in similar adverse events or are encountered under specific conditions. There is no single classification that is applicable to the entire spectrum of toxic chemicals. Instead, a combination of classification systems is generally needed to best characterize toxic substances. Classification systems that take into consideration both the chemical and the biological properties of an agent and the exposure characteristics are most likely to be useful for legislative or control purposes. For example, in relation to the way humans are exposed to them, the toxic substances fall into several classes: drugs, pesticides, food additives, hazardous wastes and pollutants, industrial chemicals, household products, and natural toxins. Collectively, these chemicals are frequently referred to as ***xenobiotics***, where "xeno-" means foreign and "-biotic" means anything affecting biology. They are all foreign to the body and biologically active with the potential to interact with organisms. The concept that contrasts with exogenous chemicals is endogenous chemicals. ***Endogenous chemicals*** refer to substances that already exist within an organism or are formed as products or intermediates during metabolic processes. Toxicology has strengthened research on endogenous toxins, such as oxygen-free radicals, nitrogen-free radicals, and the toxicity and mechanisms of action of homocysteine. Toxicology research focuses on the harmful effects of exogenous or endogenous chemicals on the body, rather than their beneficial effects such as nutritional or therapeutic effects.

Toxicity and Its Classification

Toxicity

Toxicity refers to the inherent ability of a chemical substance to cause harmful effects on an organism under specific conditions. Toxicity is an innate and intrinsic characteristic of a substance, determined by measuring the magnitude of its toxic effects on an organism under specific conditions, such as evaluating the acute toxicity of a toxin through standardized tests. The magnitude of toxicity of chemical sabstances depends on the chemical structure of the substances. Clearly, it is necessary to systematically study the interrelationship between the chemical structure and physicochemical properties of chemical substances and their toxicity.

According to the different levels of exposure and duration of toxic substances (such as high-dose acute exposure, low-dose chronic exposure, or long-term exposure to low doses), toxicity can be classified as acute toxicity, subchronic toxicity, and chronic toxicity, or as short-term toxicity and long-term toxicity. Based on the types of toxic effects induced, toxicity can also be classified as general toxicity and specific toxicity (including teratogenicity, carcinogenicity, and mutagenicity).

Selective Toxicity

Selective toxicity means that a chemical produces injury to one kind of living matter (such as a cell or organism) without harming another form of life even though the two may exist in intimate contact. Selective toxicity generally refers to the difference in toxicity of a chemical substance among different species. It is now recognized that selective toxicity can occur between species, as well as between individuals within the same species (with certain individuals being more susceptible, such as high-risk populations), or between different organs or systems within the same individual (with specific organs being the target organs).

Firstly, the chemical is equally toxic to both organisms but accumulates preferentially in the target; secondly the chemical alters a unique cellular or biochemical feature that is absent or irrelevant in the unaffected species. As a result, selective toxicity appears. One source of variation that can lead to selectivity is differences in the absorption, biotransformation, or excretion of the toxicant. The selective toxicity of an insecticide spray may be partly due to a larger surface area per unit weight that causes the insect to absorb a proportionally greater dose than does the mammal being sprayed. The effectiveness of radioactive iodine in the treatment of hyperthyroidism (as well as its thyroid carcinogenicity) is related to the selective ability of the thyroid gland to accumulate iodine. Another major reason why chemicals are toxic to one, but not to another type of tissue is that there are differences in metabolism or transport that dictate accumulation of the ultimate toxic compound in various tissues.

Target Organ

Most chemicals that produce systemic toxicity do not cause a similar degree of toxicity in all organs; instead, they usually elicit their major toxicity in only one or two organs. Selective damage to certain organs or tissues by a systemically distributed chemical is termed organ-specific or tissue-specific toxicity; the organs damaged are referred to as ***target organs*** of toxicity of the particular chemical. The target organ of toxicity is not often the site of the highest concentration of the chemical. The target organ most frequently affected in systemic toxicity is the central nervous system(CNS). Next are the circulatory system; the blood and hematopoietic system; visceral organs such as the liver, kidney, and lung; and the skin. Muscle and bone are the least. With substances that have a predominantly local effect, the frequency with which tissues react depends largely on the portal of entry.

Toxicity Classification

Toxicity classification refers to the categorization of substances based on their level of toxicity to humans or other living organisms. There are several different systems used to classify toxicity, but one of the most used is the Globally Harmonized System of Classification and Labelling of Chemicals(GHS). In addition to acute toxicity, the GHS also has categories for chronic toxicity, carcinogenicity, reproductive toxicity, and other hazards that may be associated with exposure to certain substances.

Adverse Effects and Types of Toxic Effects

Adverse Effects

The spectrum of undesired effects of chemicals is broad. Some effects are deleterious, and others are not. In therapeutics, for example, each drug produces a number of effects, but usually only one effect is associated with the primary objective of the therapy; all the other effects are referred to as undesirable or side effects of that drug for that therapeutic indication. However, some of these side effects may be desired for another therapeutic indication. Some side effects of drugs are never desirable and are always deleterious to the well-being of humans. These are referred to as the adverse or toxic effects of the drug.

Distinction between adverse and non-adverse effects from exposure to a chemical is sometimes difficult but always significant in toxicology. ***Adverse effects*** are defined as pathological lesions, or biochemical, metabolic or genetic changes that affect the performance of the organism, impair the ability to adapt to environmental alteration, or cause changes in the genetic information transmitted to offspring. However, ***non-adverse effects*** may be deduced as the absence of biological changes that impair the capacity of the organism to adapt and compensate for maintaining homeostasis, enhance the susceptibility of the organism to the deleterious effects of other environmental influences, or have a significant impact on the well-being, growth, development, and life span.

The ***spectrum of toxic effect***, also known as the spectrum of adverse effect, is composed of a series of different biological effects exhibited by exogenous chemicals on organisms as the dose increases. It can manifest as: ① Increased organism burden caused by exogenous chemicals; ② Unexplained physiological and biochemical changes; ③ Subclinical alterations; ④ Clinical poisoning; ⑤ Death. Organism burden refers to the quantity and distribution of chemicals and/or their metabolites in the body. Subclinical alterations, clinical poisoning, and death are considered adverse effects (toxic effects). The spectrum of toxic effect may also include carcinogenic, mutagenic, and teratogenic effects.

Adaptation and Tolerance

Adaptation and tolerance are concepts related to toxicity, which refer to the appropriate responses of organisms to environmental changes or external stimuli, but their meanings are different.

Adaptation is the process by which organisms undergo adaptive adjustments to environmental changes through mechanisms such as genetic variation and natural selection, in order to enhance their chances of survival and reproduction. Adaptations can be physiological, involving changes in morphology, structure, and function, or behavior, involving changes in behavioral patterns and habits. Adaptation allows organisms to better adjust to their environment and increase their chances of successful survival.

Tolerance is the ability of organisms to resist harmful factors or external stimuli. Tolerance can be physiological, involving enhanced metabolic capabilities to detoxify toxins, or behavior, involving the search for or selection of suitable environments to avoid harmful factors. Tolerance enables organisms to survive in environments with harmful factors and reduces the likelihood of damage.

Adaptation and tolerance are important strategies for the survival and reproduction of organisms in different environments. They help organisms adapt to and cope with environmental changes and pressures.

Types of Toxic Effects

The toxic responses that form the study of toxicology span a broad biologic and physiologic spectrum (broad range of potentially adverse effects). The nature and magnitude of toxic effects depend on many factors such as the physicochemical properties of the chemical and its toxicokinetics, and the adaptive and protective mechanisms of the host. The latter factors include physiological mechanisms such as adaptive enzyme induction, DNA repair, and others. Effects of interest may range from something relatively minor such as irritation or tearing, to a more serious response like acute and reversible liver or kidney damage, to an even more serious and permanent disability such as cirrhosis of the liver or liver cancer. Toxic effects may be divided according to timescale (immediate versus delayed), general locus of action (local, systemic, organ specific), basic mechanisms of toxicity (reversible versus irreversible), or certain specific states of response (hypersensitivity and idiosyncratic reactions).

Immediate Toxic Effects Versus Delayed Toxic Effects

Immediate toxic effects can be defined as those that occur or develop rapidly after a single administration of a substance, whereas ***delayed toxic effects*** are those that appear long after the initiation and/or cessation of exposure to the toxicant. Carcinogenic effects of chemicals usually have a long latency period, often 20 to 30 years. An example is vaginal/cervical cancer during adulthood resulting from in utero exposure to diethylstilbestrol (DES).

Reversible Toxic Effects Versus Irreversible Toxic Effects

Some toxic effects of chemicals are reversible, and others are irreversible. ***Reversible toxic effects*** are those that diminish once exposure to a toxicant is stopped. The degree of reversibility of toxicity depends on a number of factors, including the extent of exposure (time and amount of toxicant), the type of injury and the capacity of the affected tissue to regenerate or repair injury. For example, kidney damage caused by xenobiotics is often, after survival of the acute phase of the intoxication, without further consequence due to the high reserve capacity of the kidney.

Irreversible toxic effects are often caused by the covalent binding of toxic chemicals to biological macromolecules. Under extreme conditions, the modified macromolecule is not repaired; after excretion of the toxic agent, the effect persists. Further exposure to the toxic agent may lead to additive effects. Carcinogenic and teratogenic effects of chemicals, once they occur, are usually considered irreversible toxic effects. Injury to the central nervous system is largely irreversible since the differentiated cells of the nervous system cannot divide and dead cells cannot be replaced.

Local Toxic Effects Versus Systemic Toxicity

Local toxic effects refer to those that occur at the site of first contact between the biological system and the toxicant. Local effects may be produced by skin contact with a corrosive agent, by inhalation of irritant gases, or by ingestion of tissue-damaging materials. These types of toxic responses are usually restricted to the tissues with direct contact with the agent. However, life-threatening intoxications may occur if vital organs like the lung are damaged. For example, inhaled phosgene damages the alveoli of the lung and causes lung edema. The massive damage to the lung results in the substantial mortality observed after phosgene intoxication.

In contrast to local toxic effects, ***systemic toxic effects*** are characterized by the absorption of the chemical and its subsequent distribution from the port of entry to a distant site where toxic effects are produced. With the exception of highly reactive xenobiotics, which primarily exert local effects, the majority of chemicals act systemically. In some cases, the two kinds of effects can both be observed. In the event of a pronounced local toxic effect, systemic toxic effects may also be observed.

Allergic Reactions

A ***Chemical allergy*** is an immunologically mediated adverse reaction to a chemical resulting from previous sensitization to that chemical or to a structurally similar one. The term ***hypersensitivity*** is most often used to describe this allergic state, but ***allergic reaction*** and ***sensitization reaction*** also describe this situation when preexposure to the chemical is required to produce the toxic effect. Once sensitization has occurred, allergic reactions may result from exposure to very low doses of chemicals, and therefore population-based dose-response curves for allergic reactions have seldom been obtained. For a given allergic individual, however, allergic reactions can be dose-related. Sensitization reactions are sometimes very severe and may be fatal.

Most chemicals and their metabolic products are not sufficiently large to be recognized by the immune system as foreign substances and thus must first combine with an endogenous protein to form an antigen (or immunogen). A molecule that must combine with an endogenous protein to elicit an allergic reaction which is called a hapten. The hapten-chemical complex (antigen) is then capable of eliciting the formation of antibodies, and usually is required for the synthesis of significant amounts of antibodies at least 1 or 2 weeks. Subsequent exposure to the chemical results in an antigen-antibody interaction, which provokes the typical manifestations of allergy. These may affect various organ systems and range in severity from skin pruritus to fatal anaphylactic shock. The pattern of allergic response differs in various species. In humans, involvement of the skin (e. g. dermatitis, urticaria, and itching) and of the eyes (e. g. conjunctivitis) is most common.

Idiosyncratic Reactions

Chemical ***idiosyncratic reactions*** refers to an abnormal reactivity to a chemical. The response observed is usually qualitatively similar to that observed in most individuals but may take the form of extreme sensitivity to low doses or extreme insensitivity to high doses of the chemical. This response is genetically determined, and a good example would be sensitivity to nitrates due to deficiency in NADH-methemoglobin reductase.

Mode of Action and Adverse Outcome Pathways

Mode of Action

Mechanisms of action refer to the detailed molecular and biochemical changes that are required for a molecule to cause damage. This is a precise determination of "how" and the "extent" to which molecular events cause toxicity. At times when these fundamental mechanisms are unknown, toxicologists describe the mode of action for a toxicant as an instead. The ***mode of action (MOA)*** describes the functional or anatomical changes caused by a toxicant at a cellular level, such as key events and processes leading to molecular and functional effects that would in general explain the overall process of cancer development. In many cases these could be plausible hypothesized MOAs for both specific toxicity endpoints, but the detailed mechanistic nuances of the pathway might not yet be fully known. The term "mode of action" is more often used in regulatory toxicology and has been described as a biologically plausible sequence of key events leading to an observed effect supported by robust experimental observations and mechanistic data. Of particular interest in the determination of a MOA is the evaluation of biological plausibility and coherence with existing data, as well as temporal and dose-response relationships in evaluating the strength and specificity of the association. In investigating MOA, a number of considerations are made regarding three points: ① key events, ② associative events, ③ modulating factors. *Key events* are causal precursors that are necessary for the adverse outcome. An example of a key event might be the formation of a specific DNA adduct. *Associative events* are processes that are not required for the MOA but can serve as indicators or surrogate markers for the key events. An example of an associative event could be cellular proliferation in a nontarget tissue. Also important are *modulating factors* that can alter the dose-response relationship or likelihood of inducing a key event leading to an adverse outcome. The generation of reactive oxygen species, or oxidative stress, is considered one type of modulating factor. Others include altered cellular communication, activation of certain transcriptional pathways, immune responsiveness, life stage and genetic variation.

Adverse Outcome Pathways

Adverse outcome pathways (AOPs), are being recognized as a new construct for organizing biological information. AOPs provide a conceptual framework and practical tool to portray and associate sequential biological events at the molecular, cellular, and organ levels following exposure to a chemical that ultimately results in toxicity to an organism (Figure 2-1).

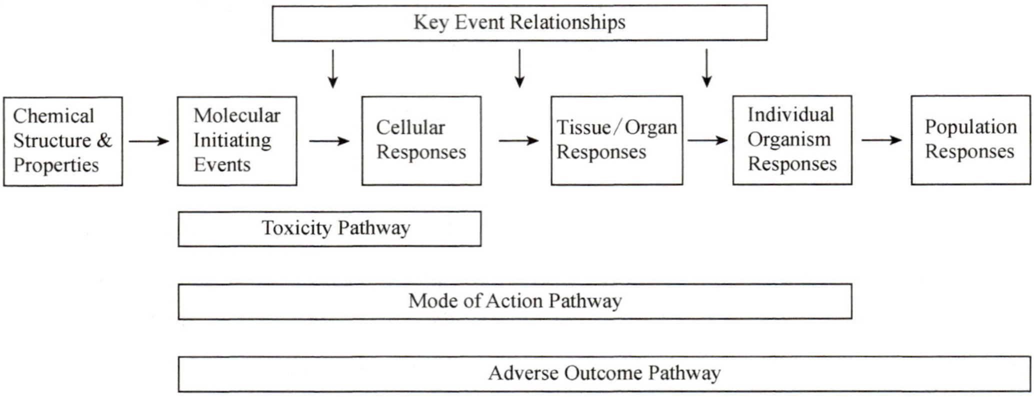

Figure 2-1 Key parts of AOPs

AOPs are composed of molecular initiating events (MIE), key events (KE), key event relationships (KER), and adverse outcomes (AO). In each AOP, a chemical's structural and properties are first evaluated using in silico approaches, which may include metabolism of the chemical to other forms or not. Then, the chemical is assessed for critical molecular initiating events, which include receptor/ligand interactions, macromolecule interactions, protein modifications and alkylation, nuclear receptor activation, and changes in membrane fluidity. As biological complexity increases, a series of responses will be identified at the cellular, organ, and organism levels. Each response will represent key linked events in the AOP that are essential for the progression of toxicity. Responses that include the MIE and the cellular response are typically classified as the toxicity pathway. The organism responses consist of target organ toxicities, malformations, cancer development, and/or lethality revealed from in vivo testing. Collectively, the MIE and KEs comprise the mode of action pathway. While

AOPs are similar to modes of action for a chemical, AOPs are anchored to the MIE, AO and specialized KEs of regulatory significance, which strengthen the certainty of the overall model. Most importantly, AOPs are not considered specific to a particular chemical. Likewise, AOPs are modular with KEs and KER potentially being used in multiple pathways. Researchers can build AOPs using the Adverse Outcome Pathway Knowledge Base (AOP-KB) from the Organization of Economic Cooperation and Development (OECD), an international organization that develops standardized testing guidelines.

Dose, Response and Dose-Response Curve

Dose and Response

Dose

Dose usually implies the ***exposure dose***, the total amount of chemical administered to an organism or incorporated into a test system. It usually appears in the form of quantity per unit body weight given on a single occasion (g/kg) or repeated daily (g/(kg · d)). However, dose may not be directly proportional to the toxic effects since toxicity depends on the amount of chemical absorbed. The concept of dose can be further defined in terms of internal (absorbed) dose, delivered target organ dose and biologically effective dose. ***Internal (absorbed) dose*** is the actual quantity of a toxicant that is absorbed into the organism and distributed systemically throughout the body. ***Delivered target organ dose*** refers to the amount of toxicant that gets to the target organ, causing a measurable effect. The amount of an internal dose necessary to elicit a response or health effect is referred to as the ***biologically effective dose***.

In order for the term "dose" to be meaningful, it is essential to provide information regarding the route, duration, and frequency of exposure. The major routes by which toxic agents gain access to the body are the oral, inhalation, dermal, and other parenteral routes (e.g. intravenous, intramuscular). The exposure of animals to chemicals is usually divided into four categories: acute, subacute, subchronic, and chronic. Acute exposure is defined as exposure to a chemical for less than 24 hours. Subacute exposure refers to repeated exposure to a chemical for less than 1 month, subchronic for 1 to 3 months, and chronic for more than 3 months, even up to years (Figure 2-2).

Single exposure to a chemical is observed in acute studies of short duration. Repeated exposures to chemicals can occur over a range of time periods spanning short, intermediary and long periods.

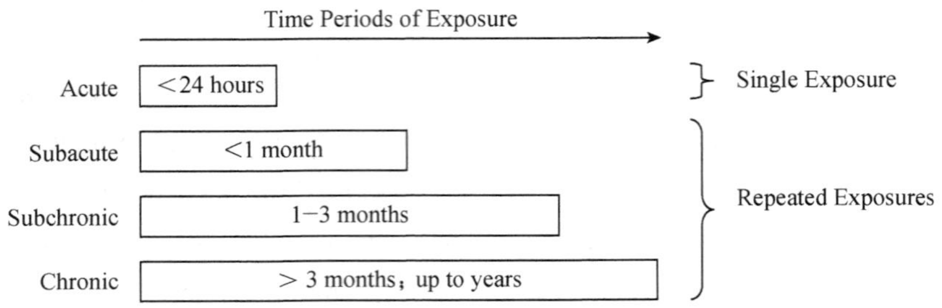

Figure 2–2 **Time periods of chemical exposure**

Two Different Types of Response—Graded Response and Quantal Response

From a practical point of view, there are two different types of response: graded response and quantal response. The ***graded response*** involves continual changes in effect with increasing dose. For example, effects on body weight, food consumption, enzyme inhibition or changes in physiological function such as heart rate. Graded response may be determined in an individual or in simple biochemical systems. An example of a graded toxic effect in an individual may be inflammation caused by skin contact with an irritant material. Low doses cause slight irritation; as the amount increases, irritation turns to inflammation and the severity of inflammation increases. Mortality and tumor formation are examples of ***quantal response*** in which the defined effect is either present or absent. The term"quantal response" is used to describe a specific type of biological response that can be quantified. This response is characterized by an "all-or-none" effect, whereby individuals within a given population either respond to a given stimulus or do not respond at all.

Dose-Response Relationships

The relationship between the "dose" and "response" to a chemical is the foundation of modern toxicology. ***Dose-response relationships*** are defined as the association between the amount of a toxicant administered and the extent to which changes are observed in a biological system. When describing chemical exposures, it is important to consider both the dose of the chemical administered or measured in the environment (external dose) as well as the amount of chemical absorbed and found at the site of biological activity (internal dose). There are a number of toxicokinetic factors that will be important in determining the internal dose of most chemicals, which often can vary between tissues. In addition to assessing internal doses, one's ability to quantify a biological response will depend upon defining an endpoint that can be quantified. Whatever response is selected for measurement, the dose-response relationship assumes a form that occurs so consistently as to be considered the most classic and fundamental concept in toxicology. Indeed, an understanding of this relationship is essential for the study of toxic chemicals.

Dose-response relationships are routinely divided into two types: ① the ***graded dose-response relationship***, which describes the response of an individual organism to increasing doses of a chemical, often refers to as a graded response because the measured effect is continuous over a range of doses; ② the ***quantal dose-response relationship***, which characterizes the distribution of individual responses to different doses in a population of organisms. This type of dose-response relationship is said to exist when changes in dose produce consistent, nonrandom changes in response.

Although the distinctions between graded and quantal dose-response relationships are useful, the two types of relationships are conceptually identical. The ordinate in both cases is simply labeled response, which may be the degree of response in an individual, or the fraction of a population responding at a particular level of effect, and the abscissa is the range of administered doses.

Major Assumptions in Establishing the Dose-Response Relationship

Prior to the utilization of dose-response relationships, it is essential to consider a number of fundamental assumptions. The first assumption is that the observed response is a direct consequence of the administered chemical, establishing a clear cause-and-effect relationship. The second assumption is that the magnitude of the response is in fact related to the dose. This assumes that there is a molecular target site (or sites) with which the chemical interacts to initiate the response, which is related to the concentration of the agent at the target site, which in turn is related to the dose administered. The third assumption is that a quantifiable method of measuring toxicity and a precise means of expressing the results of such measurement are both available. A given chemical may have a family of dose-response relationships, one for each toxic endpoint. For example, a chemical that produces cancer through genotoxic effects, liver damage through inhibition of a specific enzyme, and CNS effects through a different mechanism may have three distinct dose-response relationships, one for each endpoint.

Biological Variation: Hypersusceptible and Resistant Members

In practical terms, the biology experimenter finds that there are differences in susceptibility to chemicals among individual members of a supposedly homogeneous population of animals, a condition frequently refers to as "***biological variation***". Experiments have shown that typically this intraspecies variation follows a Gaussian distribution when a frequency histogram is made relating the frequency of quantal responses such as lethality and a given dose.

As can be observed in the upper panel of Fig. 2-3, only a limited number of animals exhibits a response to the lowest and highest doses. Larger numbers of animals responds to doses intermediate between those two extremes, and the maximum frequency of response occurrs in the middle portion of the dose range. Animals responding at the left end of the curve are referred to as hypersusceptible, and those at the right end of the curve are called resistant.

Dose-Response Curve

Frequency, Quantal Dose-Response Curve

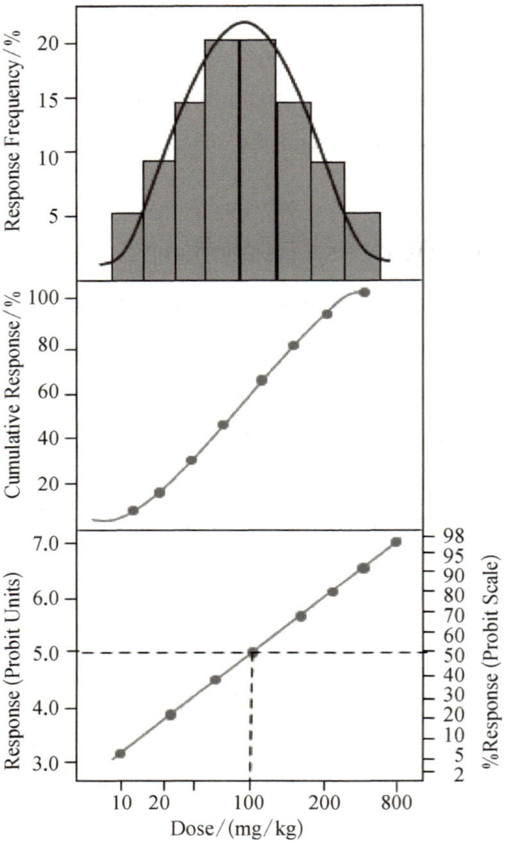

Figure 2-3 Diagram of quantal dose-response relationship

The bars in the frequency histogram in the top panel of Figure 2-3 represent the percentages of animals that died at each dose minus the percentages that died at the immediately lower dose. When a sufficiently large number of doses is used with a large number of animals per dose, a bell-shaped ***frequency-response curve*** known as a normal frequency distribution is observed.

The abscissa is the log dosage of the chemical. The ordinate of the top panel is mortality frequency producing a bell-shaped curve; in the middle panel a sigmoidal curve is produced when the ordinate is percent mortality; and in the bottom panel the response is linearized when the mortality is in probit units.

Cumulative, Quantal Dose-Response Curve

If the numbers of individuals responding at each consecutive dose are added together, a cumulative, quantal dose-response relationship is obtained as depicted in the middle panel of Figure 2-3. The typical dose-response curve is usually sigmoidal in shape. In toxicology, frequency-response curves, as shown in the top panel, are not commonly used to illustrate the dose-response relationship; instead, ***cumulative dose-response curves*** are generally used because an individual who responds at a low dose will, of course, also respond at higher doses. Thus, the frequency of responders at a given high dose includes all those that responded at that and all lower doses. A normally distributed sigmoidal curve such as this one approaches a response of 0 percent as the dose is decreased and approaches a response of 100 percent as the dose is increased, but theoretically it never passes through 0 and 100 percent.

Probit Transformation of the Dose-Response Curve

In toxicology, we often encounter normally distributed populations. Statistical analyses of such populations reveal that approximately 68. 3% of subjects exhibit responses within one standard deviation (SD) of the mean, while 95. 5% and 99. 7% fall within two and three SDs, respectively. Given that quantal dose-response phenomena typically follow a normal distribution, we can convert percentage responses to normal equivalent deviations (NEDs), which represent units of deviation come from the mean.

To facilitate calculations and avoid negative values, we add 5 to each NED, resulting in probit units (derived from "probability unit"). In this transformation, a 50% response corresponds to a probit of 5, while+1 SD and −1 SD deviations correspond to probits of 6 and 4, respectively.

When we plot the cumulative response on a probit scale against the logarithm of the dose, the sigmoidal dose-response curve transforms into a linear relationship, as illustrated in the lower panel of Figure 2-3. This probit transformation is crucial for determining the slope of the dose-response curve and deriving numerical values for various parameters.

To determine the LD_{50}, we draw a horizontal line from probit unit 5 (representing 50% mortality) to intersect the dose-effect line. From this intersection, we draw a vertical line to the abscissa, identifying the LD_{50}. Similarly, we can derive other percentile values, such as the LD_{95}(lethal dose for 95% of subjects) or LD_5(lethal dose for 5% of subjects), using the same method.

The linear transformation afforded by the probit analysis also enables additional mathematical procedures, including the calculation of confidence intervals. This approach enhances our ability to interpret and compare dose-response relationships across different toxicological studies.

Slope of the Dose-Response Curve

In toxicological assessments, while the LD_{50} is a crucial parameter, the slope of the dose-response curve often proves to be even more significant when comparing the relative toxicities of two compounds. The slope represents the relationship between the change in response and the change in dose, providing valuable insights into a compound's toxicological profile. Figure 2-4 illustrates the dose-response curves for two compounds with identical LD_{50} values but markedly different slopes. Compound A exhibits a relatively flat dose-response curve, whereas Compound B displays a steep one. These slope differences have important implications for toxicity interpretation. A steep dose-response curve, as seen in Compound B, indicates that the majority of the population responds over a narrow dose range. This characteristic suggests a more uniform response across the population and potentially more predictable toxic effects. Conversely, a flat dose-response curve, exemplified by Compound A, implies that a wide range of doses is required to affect the majority of the population. This pattern may indicate greater individual variability in response to the compound. When comparing these compounds, it becomes apparent that their relative toxicities vary depending on the specific endpoint of interest. At lower response levels, Compound B appears less toxic than Compound A, as evidenced by its higher LD_5 (the lethal dose for 5% of the population). However, this relationship inverts at higher response levels, with Compound B showing greater toxicity based on its lower LD_{95} (the lethal dose for 95% of the population). This example underscores the importance of considering the entire dose-response relationship, rather than relying solely on a single point estimate like the LD_{50}, when evaluating and comparing the toxicities of different compounds. Such comprehensive analysis is crucial for accurate risk assessment and the development of safe exposure guidelines in toxicology and related fields.

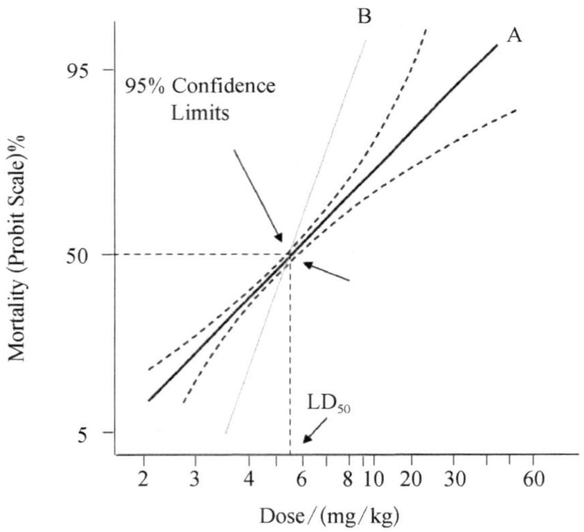

Figure 2-4 Comparison of dose-response relationship for two different compounds

Dotted lines represent the confidence limits for compound A.

Shapes of the Dose-Response Curves

Toxicology studies are designed to investigate responses across a wide range of doses. The shape of the dose-response curve has many important implications in toxicity assessment. Characterization of adverse responses at low doses often depends upon having sensitive measures that detect meaningful, biologic changes. It is often assumed that toxicants will elicit monotonic responses where increasing doses will cause a steady unidirectional change in response (e. g. increase or decrease). The typical dose-response curve can usually be described by a sigmoidal curve or linear extrapolation. Among monotonic dose-response curves, there are dose-dependent transitions that are important in the mechanism (s) of toxicity. Dose-response relationships also exist that are nonmonotonic, where multiple inflection points exist along the curve that change the shape. In some instances, the curve may be "J-shaped" or "U-shaped". As discussed below, essential nutrients can exhibit U-shaped and inverted U-shaped curves. Similarly, some chemicals are thought to confer benefit to the organism at low exposures (called "hormetic effects" or "hormesis") and harmful at higher doses. Still other dose-response curves resemble a "roller coaster" with multiple up and down inflection points. Long-standing regulatory approaches have focused on monotonic dose-response curves to extrapolate the effects anticipated at low doses. However, a review of regulatory framework has begun to examine nonmonotonic dose responses, particularly for endocrine active chemicals.

Essential Nutrients

For natural or endogenous chemicals that are required for normal physiological function and survival (e. g. vitamins and essential trace elements such as chromium, cobalt, zinc, manganese, and selenium), the graded dose-response relationship in an individual over the entire dose range can be U-shaped (Figure 2-5). That is, at very low doses, there is a high level of adverse effect, which decreases with an increasing dose. This region of the dose-response relationship for essential nutrients is commonly referred to as a deficiency. As the dose is increased to a point where the deficiency no longer exists, no adverse response is detected, and the organism is in a state of homeostasis. However, as the dose is increased to abnormally high levels, an adverse response, usually qualitatively different from that observed at deficient doses, appears and increases in magnitude with increasing dose.

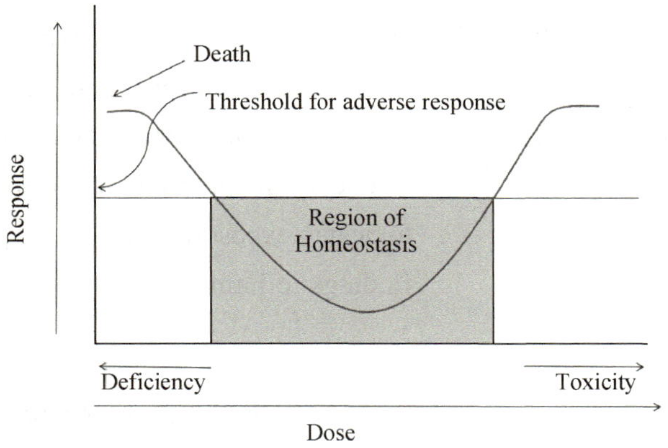

Figure 2-5 **Graded dose-response relationship for an essential substance**

It is generally recognized that, for most types of toxic responses, a threshold exists so that at doses below the threshold, no toxicity is evident. For essential substances, doses below the minimum daily requirement, as well as those above the threshold for safety, may be associated with toxic effects. The shaded region represents the region of homeostasis—the dose range that results in neither deficiency nor toxicity.

Hormesis

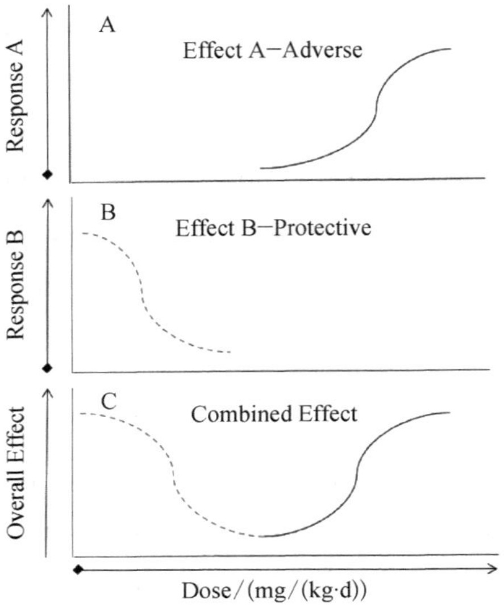

Figure 2-6 Hypothetical dose-response relationship depicting characteristics of hormesis

Hormetic effects of a substance are hypothesized to occur when relatively low doses result in the stimulation of a beneficial or protective response (B), such as induction of enzymatic pathways that protect against oxidative stress. Although low doses provide a potential beneficial effect, a threshold is exceeded as the dose increases and the net effects will be detrimental (A), resulting in a typical dose-related increase in toxicity. The complete dose-response curve (C) is conceptually similar to the graded dose-response relationship for essential nutrients.

Evidence suggests that some non-nutritional substances may also impart beneficial or stimulatory effects (e. g. of growth, reproduction, survival, or longevity) at low doses but that, at higher doses, produce adverse effects (Figure 2-6). This concept of "***hormesis***" also may result in a U-shaped dose-response curve. For example, chronic alcohol consumption is well recognized to increase the risk of esophageal cancer, liver cancer, and cirrhosis of the liver at relatively high doses, and this response is dose-related. However, there is also clinical and epidemiological evidence that low to moderate consumption of alcohol reduces the incidence of coronary heart disease and stroke. There are other agents that display hormesis for which the benefit of low doses is less intuitive. Several studies on animals and humans have suggested that low doses of ionizing radiation decrease cancer incidence and mortality while high doses lead to increased cancer risk. There are some evidences that hormesis may be applicable to a variety of types of chemical toxicants as a generalized phenomenon to a certain extent. Because of these phenomena, there is great interest in understanding biological responses at low doses of toxicant exposure and the applicability of these findings to human health.

Time Factor

Since toxic responses to a chemical are usually functions of both time and dose, in typical dose-response relationships, the maximum effect observed during the time of observation is plotted against the dose to give time-independent curves. The time-independent dose-response relationship may be used to study dose-response for both reversible and irreversible toxic effects. However, in risk assessments that consider the induction of irreversible effects such as cancer, the time plays a major role and has important influences on the magnitude or likelihood of toxic responses. Thus, for this type of mechanism of toxic action, ***dose-time-response relationships*** are better descriptors of toxic effects.

Biomarker

In dose-response relationship studies, the selection of exposure dose indicators and response indicators is crucial. Among them, the study and application of biological markers (biomarkers) are of significance in this regard. A ***Biomarker*** refers to a specific measurement or combination of measurements that can reflect the absorbed xenobiotics or their biological response by an organism, either within the organism or externally. Biomarkers can be divided into biomarkers of expasure, biomarkers of effects, and biomarkers of susceptibility.

Biomarkers of Exposure

Biomarkers of exposure refer to the measurement of the content of exogenous chemicals, their metabolites, or products resulting from their interaction with endogenous molecules. Biomarkers of exposure can serve as indicators of absorbed or target organ doses and provide information about exposure to exogenous chemicals. Examples include measurements of chemical prototypes, metabolites, adducts to hemoglobin, and DNA adducts.

Biomarkers of Effect

Biomarkers of effect refer to measurable physiological, biochemical, behavioral, or other changes in the organism, which can indicate information about the health effects associated with different target doses of exogenous chemical substances or their metabolites. Biomarkers of effect includes three categories: early biological effects, structural and/or functional changes, and disease markers. Biomarkers of effect can provide a link between toxicant exposure and adverse effects, and can be used to determine dose-response relationships.

Biomarkers of Susceptibility

Biomarkers of susceptibility refer to indicators that can reflect the body's innate or acquired ability to respond to external substances. For example, the genetic polymorphisms of metabolic enzymes and target molecules in the body after exposure to environmental chemicals can be determined. Additionally, when environmental factors act as stressors, the state of response and adaptability of the body's nervous, endocrine, and immune systems can also reflect susceptibility. Identifying biomarkers of susceptibility can help determine susceptible individuals and populations, and they should be given full consideration in risk assessment and management.

Biomarkers of exposure, effect, or individual susceptibility can link the presence of a chemical in various environmental compartments to specific sites of action in target organs and to host responses. A biomarker must be sensitive, specific, relevant, and measurable in the population. The presence of biomarkers provides information about the correlation and mechanisms between exposure and effects. By detecting changes in biomarkers, one can evaluate the extent to which a chemical can impact an organism, thus gaining a better understanding of its potential toxicity or pathogenicity.

Common Indices of Toxicity

Median Lethal Dose

Determination of the median lethal dose ($\boldsymbol{LD_{50}}$) is usually the first experiment performed with a new chemical and LD_{50} is the most commonly used measure of chemical toxicity. The LD_{50} is the experimentally derived single dose of a substance that can be expected to cause death in 50 percent of the animals tested. The LD_{50} is a statistically obtained virtual value. It is a calculated value always accompanied by some means of estimation of the error of the value, such as the probability range of the value. The LD_{50} values are usually given in milligrams of chemical per kilogram of body weight (from the viewpoint of chemistry and for comparison of relative potencies of different chemicals, giving the LD_{50} in moles of chemical per kilogram body weight would be desirable).

When using LD_{50} values for toxicity characterization, the limitations of LD_{50} values should be explicitly noted. The most serious limitations on the use of LD_{50} values for hazard characterization include the lack of information on dose-response and chronic effects of a chemical. Chemicals with low acute toxicity may have carcinogenic or teratogenic effects at doses that do not induce acute toxic responses. Other limitations include insufficient information on toxic effects other than lethality, the cause of death, and the time to toxic effect. Moreover, LD_{50} values are not constant, but are influenced by many factors (e. g. age, sex, strain, ambient temperature, type of feed, caging, method of administration, and other environmental conditions) and may differ by almost one order of magnitude when determined in different laboratories.

When animals are exposed to chemicals in the air they breathe or the water they live in, the dose the animals receive is usually unknown. For these situations, the median lethal concentration (***LC_{50}***) is usually determined, that is, the concentration of chemical in the air or water that causes death to 50 percent of the animals. In reporting a LC_{50}, it is imperative that the time of exposure be indicated.

NOAEL and LOAEL

NOEL, no observable effect level, is the highest dose level of a chemical that produces no effect in the organisms or population under known specified conditions (as in a test or controlled experiment). Operationally, a determination of "no effect" simply means that the results of the test or experiment are not statistically significantly different from those of controls. Toxicologists often use the NOEL interchangeably with the "no observed adverse effect level" (***NOAEL***). The NOAEL specifies that the effect (s) for observation or measurement may be only adverse or deleterious. ***LOAEL***, lowest observed adverse effect level, is the lowest dose that results in the appearance of a mild, but deleterious effect. The NOAEL and LOAEL may be expressed as milligram (or gram) of a chemical per kilogram body weight of the animal, or as mg/L of water, or as ppm(mg/kg) in food.

It is important that when using the NOAEL or LOAEL, it should be specified which effect is being measured, in what population, and what the route of administration is since they vary with the conditions of the exposure and the nature of the adverse effect (i. e. the indicator of toxicity) considered for a given chemical. The NOAEL is not an absolute, no effect level, and it often requires modification as new information becomes available. The NOAEL for the most sensitive indicator of toxicity in the most sensitive test species is usually employed for regulatory purposes and for setting an exposure limit or a "safe" dose value, e. g. ***PEL*** (permissible exposure level), ***RfD/RfC*** (reference dose/concentration), or ***ADI*** (acceptable daily intake). All of these various safety indicators use NOAEL or NOEL values as part of the calculation.

Threshold Dose

A ***threshold dose*** is a dose at which toxicity is first observed; at doses below this level, the probability of an individual responding approaches zero.

Another important aspect of dose-response relationship at low doses is the concept of the threshold dose. Extrapolation of the shape of monotonic dose responses at low doses can be performed by assessing thresholds and or using linear, non-threshold extrapolation (Figure 2-7). For most compounds and types of toxic effect there certainly exists a threshold dose. For chemical carcinogens acting by a genotoxic mechanism, this is a controversial issue and for regulatory purposes their effect is assumed to be a no-threshold phenomenon.

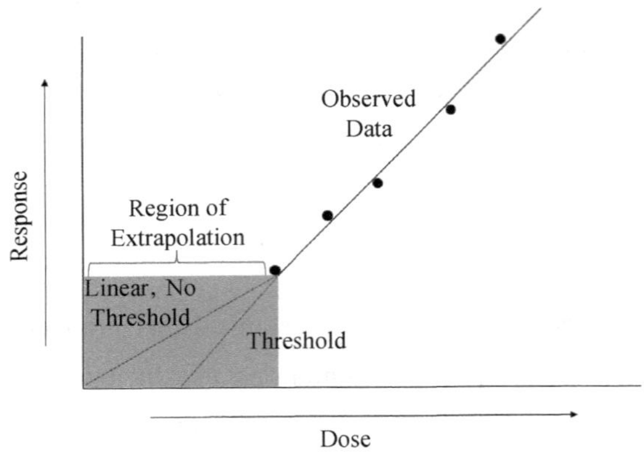

Figure 2-7 Extrapolation of dose responses at low doses

Experimental data are shown as individual dots. The gray box represents the region where empirical data are lacking and the shape of the curve needs to be extrapolated. Two approaches, threshold and linear, no threshold are shown. The threshold approach continues the linear regression of the experimental data, maintaining the same slope. The linear, no threshold approach extrapolates the curve using the lowest data point and regresses back to the zero-response intercept. This extrapolation is typically performed for genotoxic carcinogens.

For a given chemical there can be multiple sites or mechanisms of toxicity, each with its own adverse effect and corresponding threshold doses. For a given effect there may be different threshold doses in different individuals. Further, the threshold dose in the same individual may vary from time to time for any effect.

Obviously, the identification of a threshold depends on the particular response that is measured, the sensitivity of the measurement, and the number of subjects studied. It is difficult to establish a true "no effects" threshold experimentally for any chemical since there are the interindividual variability in response and qualitative changes in response pattern with dose. The threshold dose will fall between the experimentally determined NOAEL and LOAEL. The actual threshold is not available, therefore the NOAEL, or LOAEL are commonly used as a surrogate measure for the threshold dose.

The concept of threshold dose is important in toxicology because it implies that there is a "no effect level" or "safe" doses of exposure, which helps to establish safe levels of exposure for chemicals and to identify potential hazards.

Benchmark Dose (BMD)

The NOAEL approach for estimating maximum safe exposure levels (e. g. RfD) faces two main criticisms. First, its accuracy in approximating the threshold dose depends heavily on dose selection and spacing in studies, potentially leading to overly conservative estimates due to poor experimental design. Second, it fails to consider the overall dose-response curve shape, focusing solely on one or two low doses.

To address these limitations, the benchmark dose (BMD) method was proposed. The BMD is a statistically derived point estimate of the dose causing a specific adverse effect, calculated from dose-response data. It also offers a more quantitative analysis of dose-response relationships and aids in setting regulatory limits.

The BMD approach utilizes computer modeling of the entire dose-response curve and calculates the lower confidence bound for a dose at a specified benchmark response (BMR), typically set at 5% - 10% above background for animal data. The dose at which the BMR occurs is called the effective dose (ED). For regulatory purposes, the lower confidence limit of the ED (BMDL) is often used.

This method overcomes the shortcomings of the NOAEL approach by considering all response data, measuring data variability, and providing more consistent results between experiments. The BMDL, using the lower bound of a 95% confidence limit, increases estimate reliability. Consequently, the BMD approach offers a more robust and comprehensive method for determining safe exposure levels in toxicology (Figure 2-8).

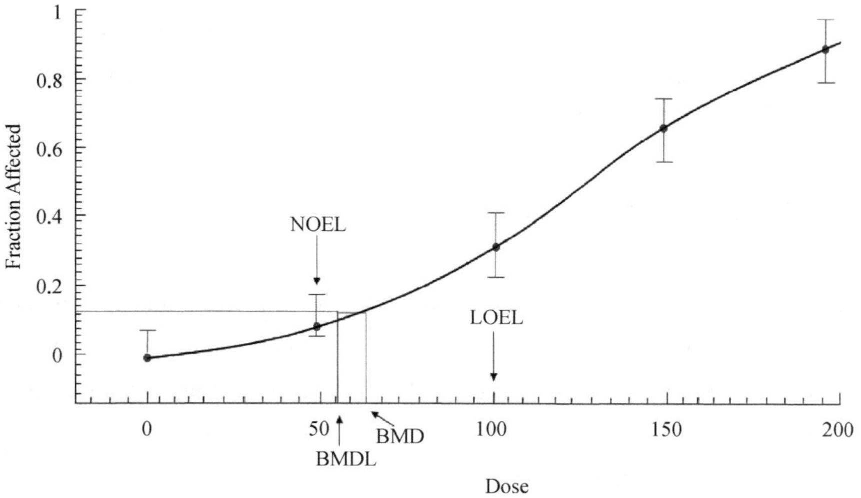

Figure 2-8 **Derivation of the benchmark dose**

Evaluating the Dose-Response Relationship

Comparison of Dose-Responses

Figure 2-9 illustrates a hypothetical quantal dose-response curve for a desirable effect of a chemical (effective dose, ***ED***) such as anesthesia, a toxic effect (toxic dose, ***TD***) and the lethal dose (***LD***). Even though the curves for the effective dose and the lethal dose are nearly parallel, the mechanism by which the drug works is not necessarily the one by which the lethal effects are caused. The same admonition applies to any pair of "effect" curves or any other pair of toxicity or lethality curves.

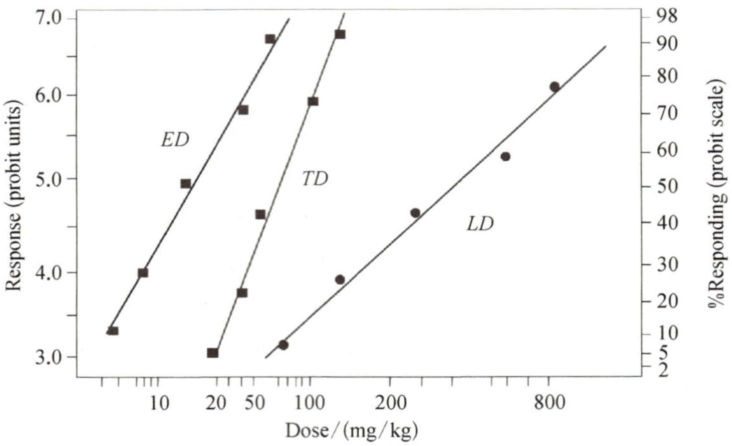

Figure 2-9 Comparison of several dose-response curves for a chemical

The effective dose (*ED*), toxic dose (*TD*), and lethal dose (*LD*) curves plotted on a log dose-probit scale.

Margins of Safety and Exposure

Margin of safety

Margin of safety (MOS) is the ratio of NOAEL obtained from animal toxicology studies to the predicted, or estimated human exposure level or dose. It is often used to assess the safety of cosmetic ingredients. For example, China Food and Drug Administration (CFDA) uses this approach.

- MOS = NOAEL/Estimated Exposure Dose

For a chemical substance with health thresholds (i.e. not genotoxic and not carcinogenic), **a MOS >= 100** is generally considered to be protective.

MOS is also defined as the ratio of **derived reference dose (i.e. ADI, RfD, DNEL)** to the predicted, or estimated human exposure level or dose.

MOS = Derived Reference Dose/Estimated Exposure Dose. Bigger is better. Minimum requirement is >1.

Margin of exposure

Margin of exposure (MOE) is the ratio of NOAEL obtained from animal toxicology studies to the predicted, or estimated human exposure level or dose. It is commonly used in human health risk assessment (i. e. assessing the safety of a cosmetic ingredient or a food impurity).

- MOE = NOAEL/Estimated Exposure Dose

For a chemical substance with health thresholds (i. e. not genotoxic and not carcinogenic), **a MOE >= 100** is generally considered to be protective.

Toxic Effect Zone

The effect zone is a parameter used to describe the characteristics of toxic effects of chemical substances in biological systems, and is further divided into acute toxic effect zone (Z_{ac}) and chronic toxic effect zone (Z_{ch}).

Acute toxic effect zone (Z_{ac})

Z_{ac} is defined as the ratio of LD_{50} to the acute threshold dose (Lim_{ac}): $Z_{ac} = LD_{50}/LimV_{ac}$. A smaller Z_{ac} value indicates a narrow range of doses between causing mild harm and acute death, indicating a higher risk of mortality. Conversely, a larger Z_{ac} value suggests a lower risk of acute toxicity-related death.

Chronic toxic effect zone (Z_{ch})

Z_{ch} represents the ratio of acute threshold dose (Lim_{ac}) to chronic threshold dose (Lim_{ch}), indicating the range of doses between Lim_{ac} and Lim_{ch}: $Z_{ch} = Lim_{ac}/Lim_{ch}$. A higher Z_{ch} value suggests a larger range of doses, from mild chronic toxic effects to more pronounced acute toxicity, making it easier to overlook and increasing the risk of chronic poisoning. Conversely, a lower Z_{ch} value indicates a lower risk of chronic poisoning.

Safety Limit Value

The study and designation of safety limit values is one of the important aspects of toxicology. With the continuous development of toxicology, the study and designation of safety limit values is also constantly improving. The advancement of scientific technology and the accumulation of a large amount of experimental data make the development of safety limit values more accurate and reliable. This helps to guide the management and decision-making in various fields such as workplace safety, environmental monitoring, and food safety, to ensure the health and safety of the public.

Safety and Safety Evaluation

In toxicology research, ***safety*** refers to a chemical that, under prescribed conditions of use and quantity, does not cause harm to humans or animals, neither causing acute or chronic toxicity nor potential harm to the exposed individuals and their offspring.

Safety evaluation refers to the process of assessing potential risks associated with a product, substance, or activity. It involves identifying and evaluating the hazards that may occur and determining whether they pose an acceptable level of risk to human or animal health. Safety evaluation may include various types of testing, such as toxicity testing, environmental testing, and efficacy testing, to determine the safety and effectiveness of the product, substance, or activity. The results of safety evaluation are used to make informed decisions about the use, regulation, and management of the product, substance, or activity to protect human, animal health and the environment.

Risk and Risk Assessment

Risk refers to the probability of a specific factor exerting a potentially harmful effect on an organism, system, or population under specific exposure conditions. In relation to safety, risk is an important new concept proposed in toxicological evaluation research. Safety emphasizes the conditions and regulations that "do not produce" health hazards, while risk focuses on studying the probability of "producing" health hazards under specific conditions.

Risk assessment is the process of identifying and analyzing potential hazards and their associated risks in order to determine the likelihood and severity of adverse effects. It involves evaluating the probability of an event occurring and the magnitude of its consequences. Risk assessment is typically conducted to inform decision-making and develop strategies for risk management and mitigation.

The process of risk assessment generally involves several steps, including hazard identification, exposure assessment, dose-response assessment, and risk characterization. Hazard identification involves identifying potential hazards and their adverse effects. Exposure assessment determines the extent of exposure to the hazard, in which the concentration of the agent in the relevant medium and time of exposure are evaluated. Dose-response assessment examines the relationship between the dose of a hazardous agent and the likelihood and severity of health effects, including information on the concentration above which the agent induces toxic effects to identify NOEL. Finally, risk characterization combines the previous assessments to estimate the overall risk level and communicate the findings with relevant stakeholders.

Safety Limit Value and Virtual Safety Dose

Through toxicological safety evaluation tests, the LOAEL and NOAEL of the toxicity of the test substance can be obtained as approximate values for the threshold. Based on this, a safe limit can be calculated as Safe Limit Value = NOAEL/Safety Factor. The ***Safety Factor*** (also known as the uncertainty factor) is usually set at 100. It is generally believed that the safety factor of 100 is set to take into account the differences between species (×10) and between individuals (× 10). There are three basic methods for extrapolating animal experimental results to humans: ① the Safety Factor method, the specific value of which is often obtained by expert consultation and weighted average method; ② pharmacokinetics extrapolation, which is widely used in drug safety evaluation and taking into account differences in receptor susceptibility; ③ mathematical models. However, toxicologists have no unified opinion on the best model and the biological significance of the model.

For chemicals with a threshold of toxic effects, the ***safe limit value*** refers to the restrictive value of the concentration and exposure time specified for various factors (physical, chemical, and biological) related to human health in the living and production environment and various media (air, water, food, soil, etc.) in order to protect public health. Below this concentration and exposure time, based on existing knowledge, no direct and/or indirect harmful effects can be observed.

For chemicals without a determinable threshold of toxic effects, any dose of exogenous chemicals above "0" is considered unsafe, such as genotoxic carcinogens and mutagens. Therefore, for these types of chemicals, it is not applicable to establish safe limit values. Instead, the concept of the virtual safe dose is introduced. The ***virtual safe dose (VSD)*** of a chemical carcinogen refers to a dose below which the excess cancer incidence rate is below one in a million (10^{-6}) at a 99% confidence level.

In fact, the principles that governments generally follow when setting safety limit values for various substances are usually based on ensuring health while also considering economic and technical feasibility. Because of this, even for the same chemical, government agencies or organizations in different countries may propose or establish different types and/or values of safety limit. Safety limit values can generally be divided into two categories: ① Health-based safety limit values which are established solely to protect human health, including ***ADI*** (the maximum amount of a certain chemical substance that the human body can safely consume in a day), ***TDI*** (tolerable daily intake, the maximum amount of a toxic substance that the human body can be exposed to on a daily basis over the long term without experiencing significant health risks), ***RfD/RfC*** (the maximum daily dosage/concentration of a chemical substance that can be consumed on a daily basis without causing significant health effects over the long term), and occupational exposure limit values proposed by the World Health Organization (WHO). ② Safety limit values related to specific exposure conditions and media which are established to ensure health protection while considering economic and technological factors, including occupational health standards, ambient air quality standards, water environment quality standards, limits for hazardous substances in soil, and limits for hazardous substances in food.

At sufficiently high doses, any substance may be described as toxic. Among chemicals there is a wide spectrum of doses needed to produce toxic effects. The toxicant is the chemical capable of causing a deleterious effect on a living organism in small amount. Xenobiotics are referred to as active substances that are exogenous in origin and may enter and interact with an organism.

Adverse effects are defined as pathological lesions, or biochemical, metabolic or genetic changes that affect the performance of the organism, impair the ability to adapt to environmental changes, or cause mutations in the genetic information transmitted to offspring. The spectrum of toxic effects of chemicals is broad, and they can be grouped in different ways based on timescale (acute and chronic), general site of action (local and systemic), basic mechanisms of toxicity (reversible versus irreversible), or certain specific states of response (hypersensitivity and idiosyncratic reactions).

Pathological changes to certain species, organs or tissues by a chemical are termed selective toxicity. Most chemicals do not cause a similar degree of toxicity in all organs; instead, they usually elicit their major toxicity in only one or two organs. The organs damaged are referred to as target organs of toxicity of the particular chemical.

"Dose" usually implies the exposure dose, the total amount of chemical administered to an organism or incorporated into a test system. The concept of dose can be furtherly defined in terms of internal dose, delivered dose, and biologically effective dose.

The dose-response (effect) relationship is the quantitative relationship between the amount of a toxicant administered (under a particular set of conditions) and the incidence or intensity of a specified adverse effect on living systems. The dose-response relationship is the most classic and fundamental concept in toxicology. There are two different types of dose-response relationships: individual "graded" and "quantal" (all-or-none) dose-response relationships. The graded dose-response describes the response of an individual to varying doses of a chemical. A quantal dose-response relationship characterizes the distribution of responses to different doses in a population of individual organisms. In plotting dose versus response (effect), a bell-shaped frequency-response curve known as a normal frequency distribution is observed. The reason for this normal distribution is that there are differences in susceptibility to chemicals among individuals. In toxicology, frequency-response curves are not commonly used to illustrate the dose-response relationship; instead, cumulative dose-response curves are generally used. The typical dose-response curve is usually sigmoidal in shape. By the probit transformation the cumulative sigmoidal dose-response curve is transformed into a straight line. Converting the data to straight lines is essential for comparison between toxic effects of different chemicals.

Some xenobiotics, while toxic at high doses, produce beneficial or stimulatory effects at low doses and this is what the concept of "hormesis" means.

Several important parameters can be obtained from the dose-response curve. These are the doses affecting 50 percent of the animals such as pharmacological effect (ED_{50}), toxic effect (TD_{50}), lethal effect (LD_{50}), and LOAEL and NOAEL. The threshold dose is defined as the dose at which a chemical agent firstly demonstrates an effect. Generally, systemic toxicity and teratogenicity are considered as threshold phenomena, whereas genotoxic carcinogenicity and mutagenicity are non-threshold phenomena. The NOAEL/LOAEL, or

BMD, commonly used as surrogate measures for the threshold dose, is usually employed for setting an exposure limit or a "safe" dose value.

Several indices can be used to evaluate the dose-response relationships. These are therapeutic index (TI) for drugs, margin of exposure (MOE), maximal efficacy and potency.

(An Yan)

CHAPTER 3

Biological Transportation of Toxicants

Introduction

Toxic effects are generally dose-dependent, as the severity of a chemical's adverse effects is primarily determined by its concentration at the target site. However, there are significant variations in toxicity across different target organs, owing in part to differences in organ-specific microenvironments (such as pH and receptors) and distinct toxicokinetic handling of chemicals. The disposition of chemical toxicants is typically divided into four sequential phases: absorption, distribution, metabolism (biotransformation), and excretion, collectively referred to as the ADME process. This chapter primarily focuses on absorption, distribution, and excretion, which are collectively essential for determining the extent and dynamics of chemical transport within the body. Figure 3 - 1 illustrates the major organ systems and factors influencing the disposition of toxicants.

Biomembranes and Biological Transportation

Toxicants typically cross structurally similar biomembranes during their transport through biological systems. These membranes, approximately 7-9 nm thick, are primarily composed of a phospholipid bilayer, mainly phosphatidylcholine and phosphatidylethanolamine. Phospholipids are amphiphilic molecules, possessing a hydrophilic polar head and a hydrophobic lipid tail. The bilayer also contains various proteins, including transmembrane

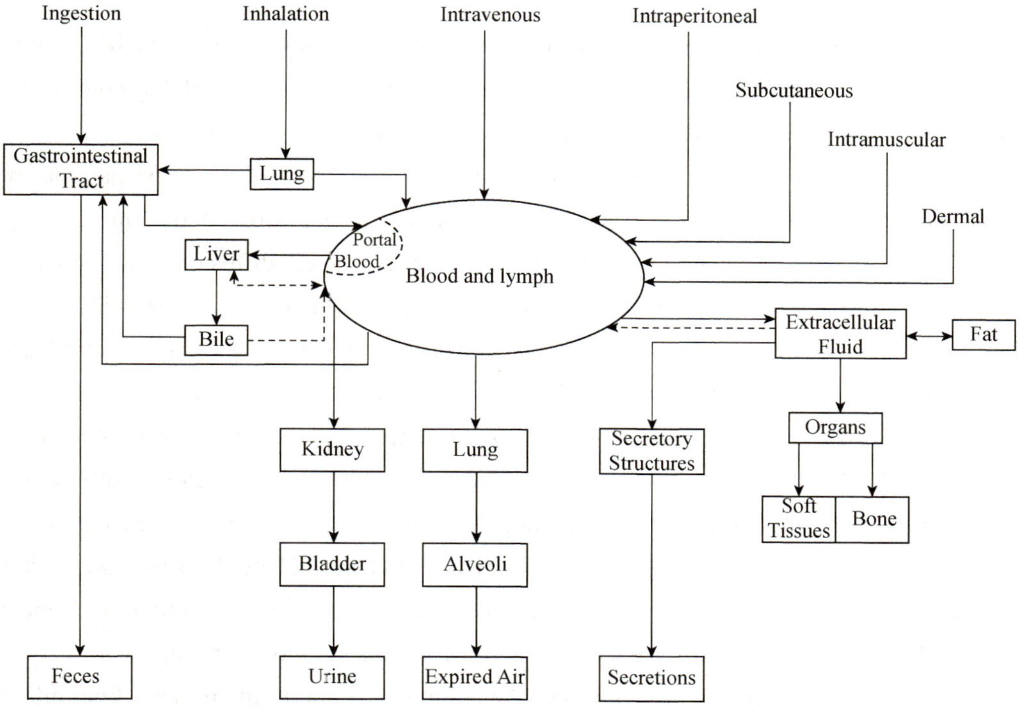

Figure 3-1 Diagram of the disposition of toxicants

proteins that span the entire lipid bilayer. These proteins function as crucial receptors, transporters, or forming aqueous pores and ion channels. Only substances with specific physicochemical properties, such as lipid solubility and polarity/charge, can pass through the bilayer. To reach their target sites, toxicants may need to cross multiple cellular membranes from the external environment.

The primary modes of toxicant passage through biomembranes include simple diffusion, filtration, active transport, facilitated diffusion, and endocytosis.

Simple Diffusion

Simple diffusion, also known as lipid-soluble diffusion, is the primary mechanism by which most toxicants passively cross biomembranes. It is an energy-independent process that does not require carriers and is unaffected by saturation or competitive inhibition. The rate of simple diffusion is primarily influenced by the concentration gradient and the thickness of the membrane.

Lipid-soluble substances, such as alcohol, benzene, and steroid hormones, diffuse more readily through the membrane because they can dissolve in the lipid bilayer. The rate of diffusion is determined by Fick's law:

$$R = K \times A \times (c_1 - c_2)/d \tag{3-1}$$

Here, R is the diffusion rate, K denotes the diffusion constant of a specific chemical substance, A is the surface area of the biomembrane, c_1 and c_2 represent the concentration gradient on either side of the biomembrane, and d is the membrane thickness.

Among these factors, the concentration gradient across the biomembrane has the most significant impact on the diffusion rate. A higher lipid/water partition coefficient ($K_{lipid/water}$) indicates a higher lipid solubility, which generally enhances diffusion rate across the membrane. Substances with higher lipid solubility, such as alcohols and steroids, diffuse more efficiently. However, substances with extremely high $K_{lipid/water}$ may face difficulty crossing the membrane, as they must navigate both lipid and aqueous phases.

The efficiency of simple diffusion is also influenced by the dissociation state of the compound. Nonionized molecules, which are less polar and more lipophilic, diffuse more readily than their ionized counterparts. The degree of dissociation depends on the compound's pK_a (the pH at which the compound is 50% ionized) and the pH of the surrounding fluid. Generally, weak organic acids are more likely to remain nonionized in acidic environments, while weak organic bases tend to remain nonionized in alkaline environments.

This nonionized, neutral form enhances the compound's ability to cross the lipid bilayer. The ratio of ionized or nonionized forms can be calculated using the Henderson-Hasselbalch equation:

For acids:

$$pK_a - pH = \log \frac{[\text{nonionized}]}{[\text{ionized}]}$$

For bases:

$$pK_a - pH = \log \frac{[\text{ionized}]}{[\text{nonionized}]}$$

At low pH, weak acids such as benzoic acid predominantly exist in their nonionized form, enhancing membrane permeability, while weak bases such as aniline are mostly ionized, reducing diffusion. As pH increases, weak acids dissociate and become more ionized, while bases become nonionized, increasing their ability to diffuse. Nonionized forms of weak acids and bases are more readily absorbed across membranes due to their higher lipid solubility.

Filtration

Filtration refers to the passive movement of water and small solutes through porous membrane, driven by hydrostatic or osmotic pressure gradients. The ability of molecules to pass through the membrane depends on the size of the pores. For instance, in the kidneys, the glomerular capillaries feature relatively large pores (approximately 70 nm), allowing small molecules and ions to filter through, while larger molecules like albumin (approximately 60 kDa) are retained. In contrast, cellular tight junctions have much smaller pores (3 to 6 Å), permitting the passage of only very small molecules, typically those with molecular weights of a few hundred Daltons or less.

Active Transport

Active transport is a crucial process that facilitates the movement of toxicants across biological membranes against their concentration gradients, utilizing specific carrier proteins. This ATP-dependent process is essential for the absorption, distribution, and excretion of many xenobiotics.

Key characteristics of active transport include:

Selective Specificity: Carrier proteins exhibit high selectivity for certain chemical toxicants, allowing only substances with specific structural features to be transported. For instance, P-glycoprotein, a well-known efflux transporter, selectively exports a variety of drugs and toxicants, influencing their bioavailability and tissue distribution.

Saturation Capacity: Active transport systems have a finite transport capacity. When the concentration of the substrate exceeds a certain threshold, the system reaches saturation, meaning no further increase in transport rate can occur, regardless of the concentration increase. This concept is critical in understanding the pharmacokinetics of both therapeutic agents and toxic substances.

Competitive Inhibition: Chemical toxicants sharing the same carrier proteins can interfere with each other's transport. This competition can lead to altered distribution and toxic effects, which is particularly relevant in polypharmacy or exposure to environmental pollutants.

Energy Dependence: Active transport requires energy, typically derived from ATP, to move toxicants against their concentration gradient. This makes the process vulnerable to metabolic inhibitors, such as certain drugs that can block the transport of toxicants or drugs themselves, altering their pharmacological or toxicological effects.

Facilitated Diffusion

Facilitated diffusion is a carrier-mediated but energy-independent process in which substances move along their concentration gradient across biomembranes. However, unlike active transport, facilitated diffusion occurs along the concentration gradient and does not require energy input. This passive transport mechanism is distinguished from simple diffusion by the involvement of specific carrier proteins, which endow facilitated diffusion with several key features: ① Substrate specificity, meaning that carriers recognize and transport only certain molecules; ② Saturability, indicating a transport limit when the carriers reach maximum capacity; ③ Competitive inhibition, showcasing molecules with similar structures can compete for transport via the same carrier.

Facilitated diffusion is crucial for the efficient transport of certain substances, including many drugs and toxins, and plays a significant role in how toxicants distribute throughout the body. While it shares similarities with simple diffusion, its reliance on carriers adds a level of specificity and regulation that influences the pharmacokinetics of toxicants.

Endocytosis (Phagocytosis and Pinocytosis)

Endocytosis refers to the energy-dependent process by which cells internalize extracellular material via vesicle formation. When solid particles are engulfed, the process is termed phagocytosis; for liquid, it is known as pinocytosis. Although endocytosis is not a major route for small toxicants, it plays an important role in the cellular uptake of particulate matter, nanoparticles, and certain macromolecular toxicants.

Absorption of Toxicants

Absorption refers to the process by which chemical toxicants traverse biological membranes at the site of exposure to enter the systemic circulation. The primary sites of absorption are the gastrointestinal tract, respiratory tract, and skin. In toxicological studies, additional routes of administration are sometimes used, such as intraperitoneal injection, intravenous injection, subcutaneous injection, and intramuscular injection.

Absorption Through the Gastrointestinal Tract

The gastrointestinal tract is one of the primary routes for the absorption of chemical toxicants. Toxicants may enter the food chain through environmental media such as air, water, or soil. Upon ingestion, either accidental or intentional, they are subject to gastrointestinal absorption. This pathway is also responsible for the absorption of orally ingested drugs and accidentally consumed toxins.

The main mechanism for the absorption of chemical toxicants in the gastrointestinal tract is simple diffusion. However, some toxicants, resembling nutrients or endogenous compounds, utilize the tract's specific active transport systems to enter the bloodstream, showcasing the complexity and specificity of absorption processes. In specific instances, especially for macromolecular or particulate toxicants, absorption may also occur via filtration, phagocytosis, or pinocytosis.

While the entire gastrointestinal tract, including the oral cavity and rectum, has the potential to absorb toxicants. The absorption is minimal in these areas due to short residence times and limited surface area. The small intestine is the primary site of absorption due to its vast surface area, enhanced by villi and microvilli. The stomach also plays a significant role in the absorption of certain substances.

For weak organic acids and weak organic bases, absorption depends largely on their dissociation state. In the acidic environment of the stomach (pH ~ 2), weak acids such as benzoic acid predominantly exist in a non-ionized, lipophilic form, facilitating their absorption. In contrast, weak basic substances mostly exist in the dissociated state in the stomach, hindering their absorption. In the small intestine, with a pH close to 7, weak basic substances (like aniline) exist in their non-dissociated form and are absorbed more efficiently, while weakly acidic substances are less readily absorbed. However, the large surface area of the small intestine and the continuous removal of absorbed substances via blood flow allow for the absorption of a considerable amount of weak organic acids.

Beyond simple diffusion, active transport also plays a role in the absorption of certain toxicants in the gastrointestinal tract. Some toxicants mimic essential nutrients or endogenous compounds, allowing them to use the transport systems of these substances. This structural mimicry enables toxicants to hijack endogenous transport systems, leading to selective but sometimes enhanced absorption. For example, 5-fluorouracil can be absorbed via the uracil transport system; thallium, cobalt, and manganese can use the iron transport system; and lead can be absorbed through the calcium transport system. Additionally, certain particles, such as azo dyes and polystyrene latex particles, can be absorbed through phagocytosis and pinocytosis.

Several factors influence the absorption of toxicants in the gastrointestinal tract, including the pH, lipid solubility, and dissociation constant of the chemicals. Other contributing factors include the quantity and nature of gastrointestinal contents, peristalsis, emptying rate, and the presence of intestinal microbiota. Active transport proteins, such as MDR1, MRP2, and BCRP, located on the brush border membrane of intestinal epithelial cells, can efflux their substrates (e. g. cyclosporine, paclitaxel, vinblastine, and colchicine) back into the intestinal lumen, making their absorption difficult. Inhibiting MDR1 activity can enhance the effectiveness of certain antitumor drugs.

Chemical toxicants absorbed through the gastrointestinal tract may undergo metabolism within gastrointestinal cells or be transported to the liver via the portal vein system for biotransformation. Some toxicants may be excreted into bile without undergoing prior biotransformation. This should not be confused with the first-pass effect, a form of presystemic metabolism that primarily occurs in the liver (and to some extent in the intestine). The first-pass effect reduces the amount of toxicant reaching the systemic circulation, thereby decreasing its potential toxic effects. In contrast, certain lipophilic compounds such as benzo(a)pyrene, 3-methylcholanthrene, promethazine, and DDT, can bypass hepatic metabolism by being absorbed via the lymphatic system, thereby entering the systemic circulation directly and achieving broad tissue distribution. Moreover, corrosive or highly irritant substances can damage the gastrointestinal mucosa, facilitating direct entry of toxicants into the bloodstream through disrupted epithelial barriers.

Absorption Through the Respiratory Tract

Respiratory absorption refers to the uptake of toxicants from the air, which may be present as gases, vapors, or particulate matter such as smoke, fog, or dust. This process occurs primarily in the lungs. The extensive alveolar network, large surface area, short gas exchange distance, dense capillary network, and high blood perfusion in the lungs make them highly efficient at absorbing airborne toxins, making the lungs one of the most efficient non-invasive routes of systemic absorption.

The mechanisms of absorption differ between gases, vapors, and aerosols; each will be discussed separately.

The absorption of gases and vapors in the respiratory system is primarily influenced by their lipophilicity and concentration, which determine the rate of absorption and the extent of their effects at the site of action. The mucous glands in the nasopharynx, upper respiratory tract, including the trachea and bronchial mucosa, secrete watery mucus to moisten the mucosal surface. This mucus plays a critical role in trapping inhaled irritants and reducing their penetration into the lower respiratory tract. For water-soluble irritant gases, such as hydrochloric acid and ammonia, absorption occurs mainly in the upper respiratory tract, where they can cause local congestion and discomfort if their concentration is moderate. However, at high concentrations, these gases may bypass the upper respiratory tract's natural defenses and reach the alveolus, where they can induce direct chemical injury, including alveolar epithelial damage, chemical pneumonitis, or pulmonary edema. In contrast, gaseous substances with higher lipid solubility, such as nitrogen dioxide, sulfur dioxide, and chloroform, typically cause less irritation in the upper respiratory tract. Although these gases are not readily absorbed in the upper airway, they can easily penetrate deeper into the respiratory tract and be absorbed into the blood through the alveoli, primarily via simple diffusion. The partial pressure gradient between the toxicant in alveolar air and pulmonary capillary blood primarily governs the rate of absorption. A greater partial pressure difference facilitates faster absorption. During the initial phase of absorption, the concentration of the gaseous substance in the alveolar air is high, and the gas continuously dissolves into the blood, being carried away by the bloodstream. As absorption continues, the concentration of the gas in the blood increases, and the rate of absorption slows. Eventually, dynamic equilibrium is reached when the rate at which the gas enters the blood equals to the rate at which it returns to the alveolar gas. At this point, the partial pressure difference becomes zero, and absorption ceases. The ratio of the concentration of the gaseous substance in the blood (mg/L) to its concentration in the alveolar gas (mg/L) at equilibrium is known as the blood/gas partition coefficient. This coefficient is a constant value for each specific gaseous substance. For example, the blood/gas partition coefficient of ethylene is 0. 14, that of carbon disulfide is 5, that of benzene is 6. 85, that of chloroform is 20, that of ethanol is 1, 300, and that of methanol is 1, 700. A higher blood/gas partition coefficient indicates greater solubility in blood, leading to delayed equilibration and prolonged absorption duration. This is particularly important for toxic gases that may accumulate in the blood and have prolonged toxic effects.

Both pulmonary ventilation and pulmonary blood flow are critical in maintaining the partial pressure difference of gaseous substances between the alveolar gas and the blood. For substances with a high blood/gas partition coefficient, the rate of absorption is primarily influenced by ventilation. This is because the concentration of these substances in the alveolar gas is more easily adjusted by changes in the frequency and depth of breathing (i. e. ventilation limitation). Therefore, increased pulmonary ventilation enhances absorption of these gases. However, for substances with a low blood/gas partition coefficient, the rate at which the gas is removed after absorption depends on pulmonary blood flow (i. e. perfusion limitation). In this case, a higher pulmonary blood flow rate facilitates more efficient absorption, as it helps carry the absorbed gas into the systemic circulation more quickly.

The absorption of aerosolized particles is similar to that of gases, but it is primarily influenced by liposolubility and inhalation concentration. The size of the particles plays a crucial role in determining where they deposit in the respiratory tract. Larger particles ($\geqslant 5\ \mu m$) typically deposit in the nasopharyngeal region (upper respiratory tract). These particles are typically cleared through mucociliary transport and sneezing. On the one hand, insoluble particles deposited on the ciliated mucous layer of the nasal surface are moved downwards by cilia, eventually being swallowed within minutes. Soluble particles, on the other hand, dissolve in the mucus and are either absorbed into the blood via nasal epithelial cells or transferred to the pharynx. Fine particles (approximately $2.5\ \mu m$) primarily deposit in the trachea and bronchi. These particles are moved backward by the mucociliary escalator and are either coughed up or swallowed into the gastrointestinal tract. Clearance can be accelerated by reflex mechanisms such as coughing and sneezing. Very fine particles ($\leqslant 1\ \mu m$) can reach the alveoli and be absorbed into the bloodstream. Alternatively, they may travel further into the distal bronchioles and are cleared by alveolar macrophages through processes such as phagocytosis. These particles may then enter the lymphatic system, where they may persist for prolonged periods. Particles with a diameter $\leqslant 0.1\ \mu m$ (100 nm) are classified as ultrafine particles or nanoparticles. Among these, particles sized between 10 to 20 nm are most likely to deposit in the alveoli and either be absorbed into the blood or engulfed by macrophages. Once phagocytosed, they can be transported through the lymphatic system.

Particles often act as carriers for gases, vapours, and smoke, thereby prolonging their residence time and enhancing their toxicity within the respiratory tract. PM2.5 refers to the particulate matter in the atmosphere with a diameter smaller than or equal to 2.5 μm. Compared to larger particles, PM2.5 has a smaller diameter, allowing it to adsorb a large number of toxicants. Additionally, PM2.5 particles remain in the atmosphere for longer periods and travel greater distances, thus exerting greater impacts on human health and atmospheric environmental quality. Furthermore, nanoparticles also tend to adsorb a greater quantity of chemical toxicants, reaching deeper into the alveoli, thereby increasing their toxicity. Accumulating evidence indicates that nanoparticle toxicity is determined more by the physicochemical nature of surface-adsorbed substances than by particle size alone.

Absorption Through the Skin

Dermal absorption is the process by which chemical toxicants traverse the skin, the body's primary barrier against environmental agents, and enter the systemic circulation. The skin is composed mainly of the epidermis and dermis. The stratum corneum, the outermost layer of the epidermis, consists of densely packed, non-viable corneocytes and serves as the primary rate-limiting barrier to transdermal absorption. Toxicants first diffuse through the stratum corneum, then permeate viable epidermal layers (granular, spinous, basal), and ultimately access the dermal capillaries and lymphatics for systemic uptake. Skin appendages, such as hair follicles, sweat and sebaceous glands, may facilitate localized uptake of toxicant, yet contribute $<1\%$ to total transdermal absorption due to limited surface area.

Transdermal absorption comprises two phases. ①Penetration, passive diffusion of the toxicant through the stratum corneum. ②Absorption, subsequent movement of the compound through the viable epidermis and dermis into dermal capillaries or lymphatic vessels.

The penetration stage refers to the passive diffusion of chemical toxicants through the stratum corneum. Dermal permeability increases with lipophilicity and decreases with molecular weight; compounds >400 Da generally have limited penetration. Regional permeability correlates with stratum corneum thickness: scrotum>arm>back>leg>abdomen>hands/feet. This variability is due to differences in the thickness of the stratum corneum: the thicker the stratum corneum, the more difficult it is for chemical toxicants to penetrate. However, no area of the body is completely impermeable to penetration. Hydrophilic compounds penetrate poorly via the stratum corneum but may access systemic circulation via skin appendages like hair follicles or sweat glands.

The absorption stage refers to the process by which chemical toxicants pass through the deeper layers of the epidermis (including the granular, spinous, and basal layers) and the dermis, ultimately entering the systemic circulation via capillaries or lymphatic vessels. These cellular layers contain nonselective, porous aqueous diffusion media, and their barrier function is much weaker than that of the stratum corneum. Factors influencing absorption include blood flow, the movement of interstitial fluid, and interactions between dermal components.

In addition to the physicochemical properties of toxicants and anatomical characteristics of the skin, several other factors can significantly influence percutaneous absorption. The integrity of the stratum corneum plays a critical role; it can be compromised by agents such as dimethyl sulfoxide (DMSO), acids, and organic solvents, which increase its permeability by disrupting the tightly packed corneocytes. Hydration also affects skin permeability—when the stratum corneum absorbs moisture, its water content may increase by 3-fold to 5-fold, leading to a 2-fold to 3-fold increase in permeability. Elevated skin temperature enhances molecular diffusion across the dermal layers, accelerating absorption. Moreover, inflammatory conditions such as vasodilation and edema can increase blood flow and tissue permeability, furtherly promoting dermal uptake of toxicants.

Absorption Through Other Routes

Beyond the commonly studied oral, respiratory, and dermal routes, toxicological investigations frequently employ parenteral administration methods—including intravenous (IV), intraperitoneal (IP), subcutaneous (SC), and intramuscular (IM) injections—particularly in experimental animal models. The selection of administration route depends on the desired onset of action, dosing accuracy, and specific experimental objectives, as each route modulates the compound's pharmacokinetic behavior and toxicological profile.

Intravenous injection introduces substances directly into the bloodstream, achieving 100% bioavailability and rapid systemic exposure while bypassing absorption barriers and hepatic first-pass metabolism.

Intraperitoneal injection, widely used in rodent studies, delivers compounds into the peritoneal cavity, where they are absorbed through the peritoneal vasculature. Substances often enter the portal circulation and may be subject to hepatic first-pass metabolism before reaching systemic circulation.

Subcutaneous and intramuscular injections produce slower and more controllable absorption profiles. SC injections, administered into less vascular adipose tissue, typically form depots that release compounds gradually. IM injections, administered into more vascular muscle tissue, offer faster absorption. In both cases, the absorption rate is modulated by local blood flow and the physicochemical characteristics of the substance.

Distribution of Toxicants

After absorption, toxicants are rapidly distributed throughout the body via the bloodstream and, to a lesser extent, the lymphatic system. Although systemic distribution may occur from minutes to hours, it is typically heterogeneous among different organs and tissues. Initially, regional blood perfusion plays the predominant role in determining the extent of tissue exposure. Organs with high perfusion rates, such as the heart, liver, kidneys, adrenal glands, thyroid, lungs, and small intestine, tend to accumulate higher concentrations of toxicants during the initial distribution phase. In contrast, poorly perfused tissues, including skin, adipose tissue, connective tissue, and skeletal muscle, exhibit delayed onset and reduced extent of toxicant uptake.

Over time, the distribution becomes increasingly influenced by the toxicant's physicochemical properties and its tissue-specific binding affinities, in addition to blood perfusion. This leads to a secondary phase of redistribution, often involving sequestration in storage sites. For example, after absorption, lead initially accumulates in red blood cells and soft tissues such as the liver and kidneys. However, within several weeks, approximately 90% of the total body burden of lead is redistributed to and sequestered in bones, where it may persist for decades.

Volume of Distribution (V_d)

The volume of distribution (V_d) is a theoretical pharmacokinetic parameter that describes the apparent volume in which a toxicant would need to be evenly distributed to produce the observed plasma concentration. It reflects the extent to which a substance distributes beyond the vascular compartment and is inversely proportional to its concentration in plasma.

Body water is functionally divided into two main compartments: intracellular fluid and extracellular fluid. The extracellular fluid comprises plasma and interstitial fluid. If a toxicant is predominantly confined to the plasma compartment, its plasma concentration will be relatively high, resulting in a low volume of distribution. Conversely, if the toxicant extensively distributes into total body water or is sequestered within peripheral tissues, the plasma concentration will be low, resulting in a high V_d. However, the distribution of toxicants is not solely determined by aqueous compartments. Tissue-specific accumulation and binding significantly affect V_d. Lipophilic substances, for instance, may accumulate in adipose tissue, acting as long-term reservoirs. Other toxicants may preferentially bind to proteins or structural components in organs such as the liver, bones, or kidneys, thereby altering their distribution profile and toxicokinetic behavior. Redistribution from these storage sites can lead to prolonged biological half-lives and delayed toxicity.

Therefore, V_d not only serves as an index of distribution extent but also provides insight into tissue-specific toxic potential and the persistence of toxicants within the body. Table 3-1 summarizes the estimated sizes of major physiological compartments relevant to toxicant distribution.

Table 3-1 Estimates of the Size of the Major Compartments That Contribute to Volume of Distribution

Compartment	Percentage OF Total	Liter in 70-kg Human	Plasma Concentration After 1 G OF Chemical/(mg/L)
Plasma water	4.5	3	333
Total extracellular water	20	14	1
Total body water	55	38	26
Tissue binding	—	—	0-25

Chemical Toxicants Storage in Tissues and Organs

Tissue accumulation of toxicants takes place when their rate of absorption exceeds the rates of biotransformation and excretion, resulting in elevated concentrations in specific organs. Different toxicants show affinity for different tissues depending on their physicochemical properties. For example, carbon monoxide (CO) preferentially binds to hemoglobin, while lead accumulates in bones. Such patterns of selective accumulation have direct implications for both acute and chronic toxicity. Accumulated toxicants can impair the function of specific organs, either by exerting effects locally on target organs or remotely through redistribution. For example, paraquat preferentially accumulates in the lungs, causing pulmonary congestion, edema, inflammation, necrosis, and ultimately progressive fibrosis. In contrast, lipophilic compounds such as DDT tend to accumulate in adipose tissue without causing direct local toxicity, but may later redistribute and exert harmful effects on other organs, including the nervous system. Any site where toxicants accumulate can serve as a storage depot. These storage depots maintain a dynamic equilibrium with the free toxicants in the plasma. When free toxicants in the bloodstream are metabolized or excreted, toxicants in storage depots dissociate and re-enter circulation to restore equilibrium. If the accumulation site is not the target organ, this storage may reduce the toxicant levels reaching critical organs, potentially mitigating acute toxic effects. While such storage may initially buffer toxic effects, it also poses risks. As circulating toxicants decline due to clearance, storage depots may act as continuous source, releasing toxicants over time and contributing to chronic toxicity. Under conditions of physiological stress, such as illness, fasting, or exposure to additional chemicals, stored toxicants may be mobilized rapidly, increasing systemic exposure and potentially triggering a toxic response.

Plasma Proteins as a Storage Depot: Chemical toxicants absorbed into the bloodstream can reversibly bind to various plasma proteins, primarily albumin. Acidic toxicants typically bind to albumin, while basic substances often bind to α1-acid glycoprotein. Neutral compounds may exhibit minimal protein binding or bind depending on their lipophilicity. Other important plasma binding proteins include transferrin, which binds iron; ceruloplasmin, which binds copper; α- and β-lipoproteins, which bind lipophilic substances; and α1-acid glycoprotein, which binds basic substances.

The binding of chemical toxicants to plasma proteins is typically transient and reversible, establishing a dynamic equilibrium between the bound and unbound fractions. As free toxicants are eliminated or redistributed, bound toxicants dissociate from the plasma proteins to restore equilibrium. Given the limited binding capacity of plasma proteins, saturation results in elevated levels of unbound toxicants in circulation, thereby increasing systemic toxicity. Competitive displacement may occur when multiple toxicants vie for the same protein-binding sites. In such cases, toxicants with lower binding affinity dissociate more readily, increasing the concentration of free compounds and potentially enhancing toxicity. For instance, DDE, a metabolite of DDT, can displace bilirubin from albumin, increasing the concentration of free bilirubin in the blood and contributing to jaundice. Environmental factors, including pH, ionic strength, and temperature, can modulate protein-toxicant binding affinity. Alterations in these conditions may affect the ionization state of toxicants or alter protein conformation, thereby influencing binding dynamics and systemic distribution.

Liver and Kidney as a Storage Depots: The liver and kidneys serve as major sites of toxicant accumulation because they continuously metabolize and eliminate a wide range of endogenous and exogenous compounds. In hepatocytes, organic anion transporting polypeptides (OATPs) mediate uptake of various organic acids and anions from the bloodstream, contributing significantly to hepatic clearance. The liver and kidneys also contain high levels of metallothionein (MT), a thiol-rich protein with a high binding affinity for metals such as cadmium, mercury, zinc, and lead. This binding serves a cytoprotective role by sequestering metal toxicants and limiting their bioavailability and cellular toxicity. In the liver, cadmium bounded to MT is retained within hepatocytes and is less likely to be excreted via the bile, contributing to its hepatic accumulation. In contrast, cadmium-MT complexes are particularly nephrotoxic because they are filtered through the glomeruli and reabsorbed by proximal tubular cells. Accumulation within renal tubular cells disrupts normal cellular functions, leading to structural damage and ultimately impairing renal function.

Fat as Storage Depot: Many environmental toxicants, including organochlorine pesticides (e. g. chlordane and DDT), dioxins, furans, polychlorinated biphenyls (PCBs), and polybrominated biphenyls (PBBs), are characterized by a high degree of lipophilicity. After systemic absorption, these compounds tend to accumulate in adipose tissue due to their affinity for lipid-rich environments. In this storage compartment, toxicants are often sequestered in a biologically inactive form, thereby reducing their circulating concentrations and acute toxicity to critical target organs. Adipose tissue may thus act as a temporary protective reservoir, modulating the systemic bioavailability of lipophilic toxicants. Individuals with higher levels of adiposity, such as individuals with obesity, tend to have an increased capacity to sequester lipophilic toxicants. For such individuals, adipose tissue can constitute up to 50% of total body mass, whereas it typically accounts for approximately 20% in lean individuals. However, during periods of increased lipolysis, such as fasting, weight loss, or metabolic stress, previously sequestered toxicants can rapidly be mobilized into the bloodstream. This sudden release can overwhelm detoxification pathways and lead to re-exposure of vulnerable target organs.

Bones as Storage Depot: Bones serve as a significant long-term storage depot for several inorganic toxicants, particularly those that can substitute for calcium or other mineral constituents of the bone matrix. Lead (Pb), strontium (Sr), and fluoride (F^-) are classic examples of such toxicants. Historically, lead was considered to exert minimal direct toxicity on bone. However, recent evidence suggests that chronic skeletal lead burden may contribute to reduced bone mineral density and increased risk of osteoporosis. These toxicants can be released back into the bloodstream via bone resorption processes during physiological conditions such as aging, pregnancy, and lactation, or under pathological conditions such as bone loss. This process increases systemic bioavailability and may pose toxicity risks to other organs.

Biological Barriers

Certain organs and tissues are protected by specialized biological barriers that selectively restrict or delay the entry of chemical toxicants. These barriers are essential for protecting highly sensitive regions from toxic insult. Among the most significant are the blood-brain barrier and the blood-cerebrospinal fluid barrier in the central nervous system, as well as the placental barrier, which separates maternal and fetal circulations.

Blood-Brain and Blood-Cerebrospinal Fluid Barrier: The blood-brain barrier (BBB) is a dynamic and highly selective interface between the blood and the central nervous system

(CNS). It consists of tightly joined capillary endothelial cells, which restrict paracellular diffusion of polar and hydrophilic toxicants. The main anatomical and physiological features of the BBB include: ① Tight junctions between endothelial cells that restrict the paracellular diffusion of hydrophilic, water-soluble and ionized compounds. ② Astrocytic end-feet, which envelop the capillaries and secrete regulatory molecules that maintain the structural and functional integrity of the barrier. ③ Efflux transport proteins—such as P-glycoprotein (P-gp), breast cancer resistance protein (BCRP), and multidrug resistance-associated proteins (MRPs)—which actively expel a wide range of xenobiotics, including anions, cations, neutral molecules, and conjugated compounds, from the endothelial cells back into the bloodstream. ④ Low protein content in cerebrospinal fluid (CSF), which limits the transport of protein-bound toxicants into the brain. As a result, only toxicants that are both lipophilic and non-ionized—and not substrates for efflux transporters—can effectively cross the BBB and exert neurotoxic effects.

The blood-cerebrospinal fluid barrier (BCSFB), located primarily at the choroid plexus and arachnoid membrane, also plays a critical role in protecting the CNS. Like the BBB, it features tight junctions and active transport systems that prevent xenobiotics from entering the CSF. Furthermore, the low protein content of the CSF limits the transport of protein-bound or water-soluble toxicants. Only the free (unbound) fraction of a toxicant in blood is available for distribution to the brain. The ability of a toxicant to cross the BBB is primarily influenced by its lipid solubility and ionization status. While increased lipid solubility facilitates entry into the CNS by enabling diffusion across lipid bilayers, ionized or highly polar compounds are poorly absorbed due to limited membrane permeability. In contrast, methylmercury, a highly lipophilic form, easily crosses the BBB and accumulates in the brain, causing significant central neurotoxicity. Additionally, the BBB is immature in neonates, making newborns more susceptible to the neurotoxic effects of substances like morphine and lead.

Placental Barriers: The placenta acts as a selective semi-permeable barrier that regulates the bidirectional exchange of nutrients, gases, and xenobiotics between the maternal and fetal circulations. The effectiveness of the placental barrier in preventing fetal exposure to chemical toxicants depends on its structural complexity, which varies across species. In general, placentas with fewer cellular layers separating the maternal and fetal blood supply are more permeable to xenobiotics, increasing the likelihood of fetal exposure.

Most chemical toxicants cross the placenta by passive diffusion, driven by concentration gradients. The rate of transfer depends on the compound's molecular weight, lipid solubility, degree of ionization, and protein binding. Lipophilic toxicants readily penetrate the placental membrane and may reach a dynamic equilibrium between the maternal and fetal compartments. However, fetal accumulation varies by tissue type. Due to the limited metabolic capacity of the fetal liver and the sparse development of fetal adipose tissue, the accumulation of lipophilic toxicants such as TCDD is restricted. In contrast, the fetal brain—protected by an immature blood-brain barrier—is particularly vulnerable to neurotoxicants such as lead and methylmercury, which can easily cross the placental barrier and accumulate in high concentrations.

In addition to passive diffusion, the placenta contains active transport systems that help regulate the movement of substances. Transporters such as P-glycoprotein (P-gp), BCRP, and MRPs are expressed in placental tissue and can actively export toxicants from the fetal to the maternal circulation. The placenta also possesses enzymatic activity capable of biotransforming certain xenobiotics, thereby reducing their potential fetal toxicity.

Several other specialized barriers in the body also serve to protect vital tissues from chemical injury. The blood-testis barrier in the male reproductive system and the blood-ocular barrier in the eye function similarly to the BBB by limiting the entry of circulating toxicants into sensitive compartments. These barriers play essential roles in preserving tissue function and integrity by regulating the selective permeability of toxicants and endogenous compounds.

Excretion of Toxicants

Excretion refers to the physiological process through which the body eliminates chemical toxicants via multiple routes. The primary site of excretion is the kidney, where toxicants are removed from the bloodstream through glomerular filtration, tubular secretion, and reabsorption, and ultimately excreted in the urine. The gastrointestinal tract contributes to the elimination of toxicants that are metabolized by the liver and secreted into bile, eventually being expelled in feces. Volatile and gaseous toxicants are mainly eliminated through pulmonary exhalation. In addition, minor excretory routes—such as cerebrospinal fluid, breast milk, sweat, saliva, hair, and nails—may also contribute to the elimination of specific compounds.

Renal Excretion

The kidneys are the principal excretory organs responsible for removing chemical toxicants from the blood through three main processes: glomerular filtration, tubular secretion, and tubular reabsorption. These mechanisms closely resemble those used in the elimination of endogenous waste products.

Glomerular Filtration: The kidneys receive approximately 25% of the cardiac output, and about 80% of this blood flow is directed to the glomeruli. The glomerular capillaries possess fenestrated endothelium (~70 nm), which permits the filtration of low-molecular-weight solutes, provided they are not bound to plasma proteins, which typically remain in circulation. Molecules with molecular weights below that of albumin (~60 kDa) may be filtered, provided they are in free form.

Toxicants filtered into the tubular lumen may either be excreted in urine or reabsorbed, depending on their physicochemical properties. Compounds with high lipid solubility (logP) readily diffuse across tubular epithelial cells and are reabsorbed into the bloodstream, whereas water-soluble toxicants tend to remain in the tubular fluid and be excreted. Additionally, only unbound toxicants are freely filtered; those bound to plasma proteins are generally excluded from filtration. The urinary excretion of weak acids and weak bases is heavily influenced by urine pH. Weak acids are predominantly dissociated in alkaline urine, increasing their water solubility and enhancing excretion. Conversely, weak bases are more ionized in acidic urine, promoting their elimination. This principle is clinically relevant: for instance, urine alkalinization using sodium bicarbonate is employed to treat phenobarbital poisoning, enhancing the drug's ionization and urinary clearance.

Tubular Secretion: Tubular secretion involves the active transport of chemical toxicants, particularly those that are not protein-bound. Specific transporter families—such as organic anion transporters (OATs), organic cation transporters (OCTs), and organic anion transporting polypeptides (OATPs)—facilitate the movement of toxicants from the bloodstream into renal tubular cells. Efflux transporters such as multidrug resistance proteins (MDRs), multidrug resistance-associated proteins (MRPs), and breast cancer resistance protein (BCRP) then export these substances into the tubular lumen for elimination. Competition among substrates may affect secretion rates. For instance, probenecid can inhibit the OAT system and decrease penicillin excretion. Active tubular secretion involves saturable transport systems—including OATs, OCTs, and OATPs for uptake into renal tubular cells, and MDRs, MRPs, and BCRP for efflux into the lumen—that can be competitively inhibited by drugs such as probenecid, which reduces the excretion of organic acids like penicillin.

Tubular Reabsorption: Tubular reabsorption is strongly influenced by the physicochemical properties of toxicants, particularly their lipid solubility. Compounds with high lipid solubility (e. g. high LogP values) are more likely to passively diffuse across tubular epithelial membranes and be reabsorbed into the bloodstream. In contrast, hydrophilic substances with low lipid solubility remain in the tubular lumen and are excreted. Reabsorption is also influenced by urinary pH and volume, which can alter the concentration gradient across the tubular epithelium and thereby modulate the extent of passive transport. Urinary pH can be manipulated pharmacologically to increase the excretion rate of specific toxicants. Agents like ammonium chloride (to acidify urine) and sodium bicarbonate (to alkalinize urine) are commonly used. The manipulation of urine pH modifies the electrochemical gradient across the renal tubule, thereby influencing passive reabsorption.

In neonates, renal function is immature, leading to delayed excretion and prolonged half-lives of many toxicants, thereby increasing their vulnerability to toxic effects. Additionally, reabsorption of low molecular weight proteins such as cadmium-metallothionein (Cd-MT) complexes may cause nephrotoxicity by accumulating in the proximal tubules. The urinary concentration of toxicants typically reflects blood levels and can serve as a non-invasive biomarker for exposure and systemic burden.

Biliary Excretion and Enterohepatic Circulation

The liver plays a pivotal role in eliminating lipophilic exogenous and endogenous compounds. These substances undergo biotransformation into more polar, less toxic metabolites, which are then actively secreted into the bile. Bile flows through the bile ducts to the gallbladder, where it is stored and subsequently released into the intestine, facilitating fecal excretion. While low molecular weight compounds are typically excreted via the kidneys, compounds with a molecular weight exceeding 300 Da are preferentially eliminated through the bile. Thus, biliary excretion is a major route for eliminating conjugated metabolites, such as glucuronides and glutathione conjugates. This process is energy-dependent and subject to saturation. Experimental evidence indicates that bile duct ligation in animals significantly increases the risk of acute toxicity, underscoring the importance of this excretion route.

Enterohepatic Circulation: Enterohepatic circulation describes the recycling of substances between the liver and the intestine. After being secreted into bile and transported to the small intestine, certain drugs and their metabolites can be reabsorbed and returned to the liver via the portal vein. For instance, highly polar compounds like trichothecene G are excreted into bile but undergo minimal intestinal reabsorption, resulting in their elimination via feces. In contrast, compounds like chloramphenicol are conjugated with glucuronic acid in the liver, secreted into bile, reabsorbed in the intestine, and recycled to the liver, prolonging their systemic presence. The significance of enterohepatic circulation depends on factors such as bile flow rate, reabsorption efficiency, and intestinal microbial activity. Disruption of this cycle, for example, by using antibiotics to suppress gut flora or administering bile acid sequestrants like colesevelam, can reduce reabsorption and enhance elimination, lowering systemic toxicity.

Excretion through the lungs

Gaseous and volatile toxicants are eliminated primarily through the lungs by passive diffusion. The rate of exhalation depends on the solubility of the compound in blood.

Compounds that are poorly soluble in blood, such as ethylene, are rapidly exhaled, whereas highly soluble anesthetics like halothane and methoxyflurane are eliminated more slowly. Elimination of low-solubility gases is perfusion-limited, whereas that of highly soluble substances is ventilation-limited.

Other Excretion Pathways

Milk: Certain toxicants are excreted into breast milk through passive diffusion, posing potential health risks to nursing infants. Lipophilic substances—including arsenic compounds, organochlorine pesticides (e. g. aldrin, DDT), PCBs, PBBs, dioxins, and furans—readily diffuse into milk fat and are concentrated in breast milk. Metals that mimic calcium, such as lead, and compounds that form calcium-chelating complexes can also be excreted into milk, potentially increasing infant exposure.

Skin: The skin, the body's largest organ, plays a minor role in toxicant excretion. Approximately 0. 7 liters of water are lost daily via sweat, providing a limited route for the elimination of water-soluble substances. In some cases, excretion through sweat can lead to local irritation or dermatitis.

Hair: Hair serves as a slow but stable route for the excretion and long-term deposition of certain toxicants. Elements like mercury and drugs such as cocaine can become incorporated into hair shafts during growth. Hair analysis is widely used as a non-invasive method for monitoring chronic exposure to toxicants.

(Wu Jing)

CHAPTER 4

Biotransformation of Toxicants

Introduction

Biotransformation refers to the process by which endogenous or exogenous chemical substances undergo structural modifications in the body through enzymatic reactions or, occasionally, non-enzymatic reactions. The primary goal of biotransformation is to convert lipophilic compounds into hydrophilic metabolites, facilitating their excretion via urine or bile. During this process, the toxicity of the substance may be reduced, a phenomenon known as detoxification. However, certain metabolic pathways can produce reactive intermediates or more toxic metabolites, a phenomenon referred to as metabolic activation. In toxicology, biotransformation is a critical component of the ADME (Absorption, Distribution, Metabolism, and Excretion) process, particularly in the metabolism phase. Through biotransformation, chemicals may be converted into water-soluble metabolites that are easier to excrete, or they may generate more toxic metabolites that increase their toxic effects. For example, some drugs and environmental pollutants, during their metabolic processes, can generate reactive intermediates such as epoxides, which may induce cytotoxicity or carcinogenicity. Therefore, while biotransformation generally serves to detoxify substances, it can also result in the activation of toxicity, highlighting the need for thorough metabolic pathway analysis to assess the potential risks of xenobiotics.

The primary site of biotransformation is the hepatocytes within the liver, which contain a high concentration of metabolic enzymes. However, other tissues such as the kidneys, lungs, gastrointestinal tract, and skin also contribute to the process, although to a lesser extent. These tissues play a role in local toxicity or tissue-specific metabolism.

Biotransformation can be categorized into two sequential phases based on the types of reactions involved. Phase Ⅰ reactions introduce or unmask polar functional groups, such as hydroxyl, carboxyl, amino, or thiol groups, through oxidation, reduction, or hydrolysis. These reactions increase the reactivity of the compound, making it more amenable to subsequent processing. Phase Ⅱ reactions involve conjugation with endogenous molecules such as glucuronic acid, sulfate, glutathione, or amino acids, resulting in highly water-soluble conjugates that can be easily excreted via urine or bile.

Although biotransformation is traditionally divided into two phase reactions—Phase Ⅰ and Phase Ⅱ reactions—the sequence is not always strictly followed. In most cases, Phase Ⅰ reactions, such as oxidation or hydrolysis, occur firstly to introduce or expose functional groups that facilitate Phase Ⅱ conjugation. However, there are exceptions. For example, morphine undergoes direct conjugation with glucuronic acid in Phase Ⅱ metabolism without requiring prior Phase Ⅰ reactions. Conversely, certain steroids are first conjugated in Phase Ⅱ and subsequently undergo oxidation in Phase Ⅰ. These exceptions highlight the flexibility and complexity of biotransformation pathways.

The toxicological significance of biotransformation lies in its dual roles of detoxification and activation. Phase Ⅰ reactions often produce reactive intermediates that can bind to cellular macromolecules, causing mutagenesis or carcinogenesis. In contrast, Phase Ⅱ reactions typically reduce the reactivity of metabolites and enhance their excretion. Together, these phases balance activation and detoxification, ultimately determining the toxicological outcome of xenobiotics. Understanding these processes is crucial for drug development and assessing toxicological risks.

Factors Influencing Biotransformation

The efficiency of biotransformation processes is influenced by various intrinsic and extrinsic factors, including genetic polymorphisms, age, sex, diet, and exposure to enzyme inducers or inhibitors.

Genetic Variability

Genetic differences in key metabolic enzymes, such as cytochrome P450 isoforms, UDP-glucuronosyltransferases, and N-acetyltransferases, lead to significant interindividual variability in the metabolism of xenobiotics. For example, polymorphisms in CYP2D6 and NAT2 can impact the efficacy and toxicity of numerous drugs and environmental chemicals.

Individuals classified as "slow metabolizers" due to genetic variations may experience toxic accumulation of certain drugs that are otherwise safely processed in "rapid metabolizers". For instance, polymorphisms in CYP2D6 can affect the metabolism of drugs like codeine and certain antidepressants, leading to either subtherapeutic effects or increased adverse reactions in individuals with specific genetic profiles.

Age and Sex

Neonates, due to their immature enzyme systems, exhibit reduced metabolic capacity, increasing their sensitivity to toxicants. For example, infants are particularly vulnerable to acetaminophen (paracetamol) toxicity because their liver enzymes are not fully developed, which can lead to a higher risk of hepatotoxicity even with doses considered safe for elder children or adults. In severe cases, this may result in acute liver failure, requiring liver transplantation. Similarly, age-related declines in hepatic enzyme activity may impair biotransformation in elderly individuals, necessitating careful adjustments in drug dosages. For instance, in elder adults, cytochrome P450 enzyme activity often decreased, which can result in prolonged half-lives of medications such as warfarin or digoxin. This increased sensitivity can lead to adverse effects or toxicity if dosages are not appropriately managed.

Sex differences also influence biotransformation rates due to hormonal variations. For example, studies have shown that women metabolize certain drugs, such as the sedative midazolam, more rapidly than men, potentially requiring different dosing strategies based on sex. Hormonal fluctuations, particularly estrogen and testosterone, can modulate the activity of various metabolic enzymes, affecting the processing of xenobiotics.

Dietary Influences

Dietary components play a crucial role in modulating biotransformation. Certain compounds, such as indoles and isothiocyanates found in cruciferous vegetables, can induce Phase Ⅱ enzymes, promoting detoxification. Conversely, pollutants like heavy metals (e. g. lead and mercury) and persistent organic pollutants (e. g. dioxins) can inhibit metabolic enzymes, impairing detoxification pathways and increasing susceptibility to toxicity. For instance, exposure to lead can interfere with cytochrome P450 enzyme function, which is essential for the metabolism of various drugs and environmental chemicals, potentially resulting in the accumulation of toxic substances in the body.

Nutritional deficiencies—particularly inadequate intake of protein, vitamins, and essential minerals—can reduce the synthesis of biotransforming enzymes. For example, a deficiency in vitamin B6 has been shown to impair drug metabolism due to its role as a cofactor in enzymatic reactions. Similarly, inadequate zinc intake can impair the function of metallothioneins, proteins that regulate the levels of heavy metals in the body. Certain dietary habits can also influence the activity of enzymes involved in biotransformation. High-fat diets, for instance, may alter the expression of metabolic enzymes, potentially leading to increased toxicity from xenobiotics. Studies indicate that a diet rich in saturated fats can downregulate the expression of cytochrome P450 enzymes, affecting the body's ability to metabolize medications.

Biotransformation Enzymes

Fundamental Characteristics of Biotransformation Enzymes

The human body encounters a wide range of xenobiotics, making it evolutionarily impractical to maintain dedicated enzymes for each compound. Instead, biotransformation enzymes have evolved to exhibit broad substrate specificity, enabling individual enzymes to metabolize multiple xenobiotics efficiently. A prime example of this is the cytochrome P450 (CYP) enzyme family, which plays a crucial role in the metabolism of various substances, including drugs, environmental pollutants, and endogenous compounds.

Biotransformation enzymes can be classified into two main categories: constitutive enzymes and inducible enzymes. Constitutive enzymes are continuously expressed at a constant level, whereas inducible enzymes are synthesized in response to exposure to xenobiotics or specific chemical inducers. Genetic polymorphisms also exist within these enzymes, leading to variations in their amino acid sequences among individuals. This genetic diversity significantly contributes to inter-individual differences in the rates of xenobiotic metabolism. For example, polymorphisms in enzymes like CYP2D6 and NAT2 influence the efficacy and toxicity of various drugs and environmental chemicals, with individuals categorized as "slow metabolizers" at risk for toxic accumulation when processing drugs that are otherwise safe in "rapid metabolizers".

The stereochemical aspects of biotransformation are particularly significant. Many xenobiotics contain chiral centers, existing as stereoisomers that undergo stereoselective metabolism. For instance, methsuximide, an anti-epileptic drug, is administered as a racemic mixture. Its S-stereoisomer is rapidly hydroxylated and cleared via the CYP2C19 enzyme, whereas the R-stereoisomer is metabolized much more slowly. This stereoselective metabolism also extends to enzyme inhibition. Quinidine, a CYP2D6 inhibitor, strongly inhibits CYP2D6 activity, while its stereoisomer quinine exhibits much weaker inhibition. Furthermore, achiral molecules can be metabolized to produce stereoisomeric metabolites, often with preferential formation of one specific isomer.

Distribution of Biotransformation Enzymes

Biotransformation enzymes are widely distributed throughout vertebrate organisms. The liver serves as the primary metabolic organ, containing the highest concentration and most diverse array of biotransformation enzymes. The small intestine also plays a significant role in xenobiotic metabolism, particularly in the first-pass metabolism of orally administered substances. Other tissues at key sites of xenobiotic exposure, such as the skin, lungs, nasal mucosa, and eyes, also contribute to biotransformation processes. Additionally, organs like the kidneys, adrenal glands, pancreas, spleen, heart, brain, reproductive organs (testes and ovaries), and placenta exhibit varying degrees of metabolic activity. The gut microbiota also plays a crucial role in xenobiotic metabolism, influencing both drug efficacy and toxicity.

At the subcellular level, biotransformation enzymes are primarily localized in the endoplasmic reticulum (microsomes) and cytosol, with lesser activity in mitochondria, nuclei, and lysosomes. This distribution pattern correlates with the lipophilicity of the xenobiotics. Enzymes that metabolize highly lipophilic compounds are typically membrane-bound, while those responsible for the metabolism of water-soluble compounds are predominantly found in the cytosol.

Enzyme Induction and Inhibition

Xenobiotics can modulate biotransformation processes by inducing or inhibiting metabolic enzymes. Induction involves the increased expression or stabilization of enzymes, resulting in enhanced metabolic capacity. For example, compounds such as phenobarbital and polycyclic aromatic hydrocarbons induce cytochrome P450 enzymes, thereby accelerating the metabolism of various substances. Although enzyme induction typically facilitates detoxification, it can also increase the production of reactive intermediates, amplifying toxicity.

On the other hand, enzyme inhibition reduces metabolic activity, often resulting in prolonged systemic exposure and heightened toxicity. Inhibitors can act through competitive binding, interference with cofactors, or direct inactivation of enzymes. For example, the antifungal drug ketoconazole inhibits CYP3A4 by occupying its active site, leading to decreased clearance of drugs metabolized by this enzyme, which can increase the risk of adverse effects.

Many xenobiotics exhibit dual effects, acting as both enzyme inducers and inhibitors depending on the dose and duration of exposure. Piperonyl butoxide is an example of such compounds. Initially, it inhibits cytochrome P450 activity, but with prolonged exposure, it induces enzyme expression, resulting in a biphasic response.

Phase Ⅰ Reactions

Phase Ⅰ reactions include oxidation, reduction, and hydrolysis. Among these, oxidation is furtherly subdivided into microsomal monooxygenation, cytoplasmic and mitochondrial oxidation, and cooxidation catalyzed by prostaglandin synthetase. Aside from reduction reactions, most Phase Ⅰ reactions introduce polar groups into molecules, facilitating their subsequent catalysis by Phase Ⅱ enzymes. These reactions are primarily mediated by specific metabolic enzymes.

Oxidation Reactions

Cytochrome P450

The cytochrome P450 enzyme system plays a central role in oxidation reactions and is highly versatile in its catalytic capabilities (Figure 4-1). It is characterized by the binding of carbon monoxide (CO) to the reduced heme iron in the enzyme, which results in a distinct spectral absorption peak at 450 nm. This system, also referred to as a mixed-function oxidase or monooxygenase, is crucial for detoxifying a wide range of chemical toxicants while occasionally activating certain compounds into reactive intermediates. Widely distributed across various tissues, the cytochrome P450 enzyme system is most concentrated in the smooth endoplasmic reticulum of liver cells.

Structurally, the cytochrome P450 enzyme system comprises three main components: hemoproteins, flavoproteins, and phospholipids. Cytochrome P450 and cytochrome b5 are the primary hemoproteins, with cytochrome P450 serving as the active catalytic center. Flavoproteins, such as NADPH-cytochrome P450 reductase, facilitate electron transfer from NADPH to cytochrome P450, while phospholipids stabilize the protein components and enable efficient coupling between cytochrome P450 and NADPH-cytochrome P450 reductase. Additionally, cytochrome b5 can enhance the substrate affinity of cytochrome P450, optimizing its catalytic activity.

The cytochrome P450 enzyme system is highly diverse, with numerous isoforms exhibiting unique metabolic activities. This diversity is evident in experimental models where compounds such as 3-methylcholanthrene (3-MC) and phenobarbital (PB) induce different cytochrome P450 isoforms, illustrating the system's capacity for selective induction. Advances in isolation and purification techniques have facilitated the discovery of novel cytochrome P450 enzymes, leading to the establishment of an extensive superfamily.

The classification of the cytochrome P450 superfamily is based on amino acid sequence similarities, as determined by recombinant DNA technology. Sequences with less than 40%

similarity are assigned to different gene families, those with 40% – 55% similarity are categorized into subfamilies within the same gene family, and sequences exceeding 55% similarity are grouped within the same subfamily. The standardized naming convention for cytochrome P450 genes begins with the italicized prefix "CYP," representing cytochrome P450 genes existin all species except for mice and fruit flies. This prefix is followed by an Arabic numeral indicating the gene family, an uppercase letter representing the subfamily (lowercase for mice and fruit flies), and another Arabic numeral specifying the gene within the subfamily. For example, "CYP1A1" designates the first gene in the A subfamily of the first cytochrome P450 gene family. When referring to gene products such as enzymes, mRNA, cDNA, or proteins, the naming format remains the same, but italicization is replaced with regular font, and lowercase letters are converted to uppercase, as in "CYP1A1" or "CYP1A2".

It is widely accepted that cytochrome P450 enzymes involved in the metabolism of chemical toxicants primarily belong to three gene families: CYP1, CYP2, and CYP3. The fundamental reaction catalyzed by the cytochrome P450 enzyme system is monooxygenation. In this reaction, molecular oxygen (O_2) plays a dual role: one oxygen atom is incorporated into the substrate (RH), while the other combines with protons from NADPH to form water. The overall catalytic reaction can be expressed as follows:

$$\text{Substrate (RH)} + O_2 + \text{NADPH} + H^+ \rightarrow \text{Product (ROH)} + H_2O + \text{NADP}^+$$

The catalytic cycle of CYP involves eight steps (A→H), as shown in Figure 4-1, for the oxidation of a substrate (RH) to its hydroxylated metabolite (ROH). In this scheme, iron is shown bound to its fifth ligand, a heme thiolate provided by a highly conserved cysteine (Cys) residue. The former part of the cycle (A→G) involve the activation of oxygen to compound I, and the latter part involves substrate oxidation by compound I (G→H) followed by release of the metabolite (ROH) to restore the enzyme to its resting (ferric) state (H→A).

Major Reaction Types Catalyzed by Cytochrome P450 include:

(1) Aliphatic Hydroxylation: Aliphatic hydrocarbons are hydroxylated at the ω-position (the terminal carbon) or ω-1 position (the penultimate carbon) to form the corresponding alcohol or ketone.

$$R{-}CH_2{-}CH_3 + [O] \longrightarrow R{-}CH_2{-}CH_2OH$$

(2) Aromatic Hydroxylation: Hydroxylation occurs on the aromatic ring, forming phenols.

$$C_6H_6 + [O] \longrightarrow C_6H_5OH$$

(3) Epoxidation: In aliphatic and aromatic compounds, oxygen is inserted into a double bond between two carbon atoms, forming an epoxide. This reaction is an important step in the bioactivation of certain compounds, such as aflatoxin B_1 and benzopyrene, which can

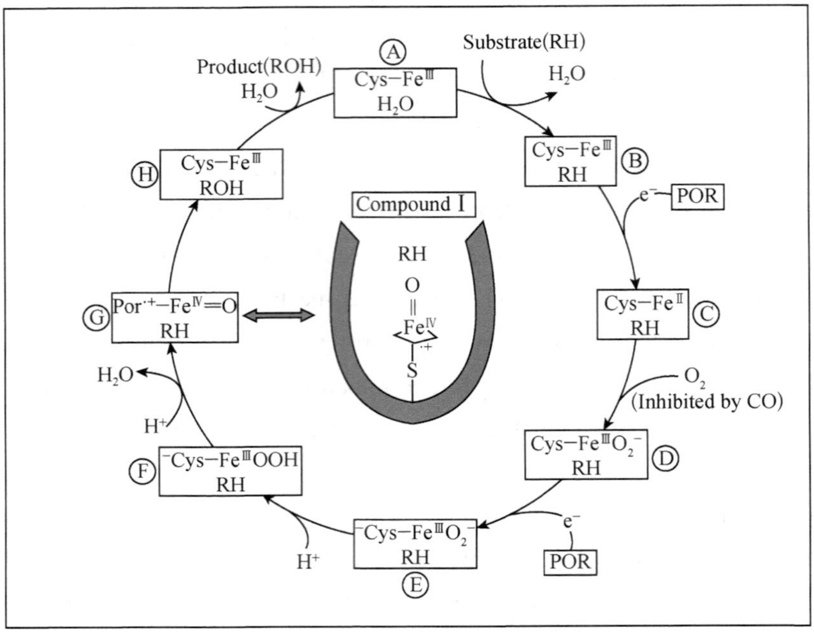

Other reactions

One−electron reduction	C(Cys−Fe^{II}RH)	→ A(Cys−Fe^{III}+$RH^{\cdot-}$)
Superoxid anion production	D(Cys−$Fe^{III}O_2^-$RH)	→ B(Cys−$Fe^{III\,III}$RH)+$O_2^{\cdot-}$
Hydrogen peroxide production	E($^-$Cys−$Fe^{III}O_2^-$RH)+$2H^+$	→ B(Cys−Fe^{III}RH)+H_2O_2
Hydrogen peroxide shunt	B(Cys−Fe^{III}RH)+H_2O_2	→ F($^-$Cys−Fe^{III}OOH RH)+H^+
Peroxide shunt to form Compound I	B(Cys−Fe^{III}RH)+XOOH	→ G($Por^{\cdot+}$−Fe^{IV}=O RH)+XOH

Figure 4-1 Catalytic cycle of cytochrome P450

form highly toxic intermediates.

$$R-CH=CH-R'+[O] \longrightarrow R-\overset{O}{\widehat{CH-CH}}-R'$$

(4) Heteroatom Oxidation and N-Hydroxylation: Chemicals containing heteroatoms (S, N, I) are oxidized, often leading to increased toxicity, such as the formation of sulfoxides, sulfones, N-oxides, and hydroxylamine derivatives.

$$R-S-R'+[O] \longrightarrow R-SOR'+[O] \longrightarrow R-SO_2-R'$$

$$C_6H_5-NH_3+[O] \longrightarrow C_6H_5-NH_2OH$$

(5) Dealkylation of Heteroatoms (O, S, N): Alkyl groups attached to heteroatoms undergo oxidation, followed by cleavage and rearrangement, forming aldehydes or ketones. For example, dimethylnitrosamine undergoes N-dealkylation, generating a free methyl radical capable of alkylating DNA.

$$R-(NH \cdot O \cdot S)-CH_3+[O] \longrightarrow R-(NH_2 \cdot OH \cdot SH)+HCHO$$

(6) Oxidative Group Transfer Reactions: Cytochrome P450 enzymes catalyze various oxidative reactions, including oxidative deamination, desulfuration, and dehalogenation. For example, organophosphorus pesticides like parathion undergo oxidative desulfuration to form more toxic metabolites like paraoxon.

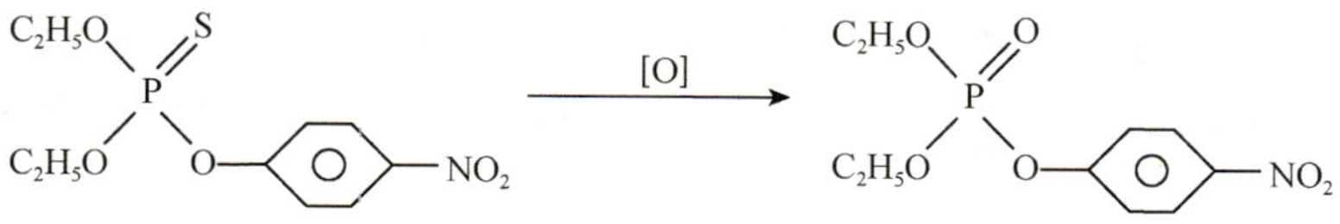

(7) Ester Hydrolysis: Ester groups are cleaved, with oxygen atoms from the FeO^{3+} complex being incorporated, leading to the formation of carboxylic acids and aldehydes.

$$R_1COOCH_2R_2+[O] \longrightarrow R_1COOH+R_2CHO$$

(8) Dehydrogenation: Cytochrome P450 enzymes also catalyze dehydrogenation, such as the formation of N-acetyl-p-benzoquinone imine from acetaminophen, a hepatotoxic intermediate.

Flavin-containing Monooxygenase (FMO)

Flavin-containing monooxygenases (FMOs) represent a crucial enzyme system localized in the microsomes of multiple tissues, including the liver, kidneys, small intestine, brain, and lungs. This enzyme system utilizes flavin adenine dinucleotide (FAD) as its essential cofactor and requires both NADPH and molecular oxygen (O_2) for catalytic function. FMOs oxidize a diverse range of substrates containing nitrogen (N), sulfur (S), and phosphorus (P) heteroatoms. These include amines, hydrazine, thiols, thioethers, thioketones, thiocarbamides, and phosphines, converting them into their corresponding N-oxides, sulfoxides, and phosphine oxides.

FMOs play a critical role in detoxifying alkaloids like pyrrolizidine and senecionine. These compounds undergo FMO-mediated oxidation to form relatively non-toxic N-oxides, which are safer than the highly reactive pyrrole derivatives formed by cytochrome P450 enzymes. However, FMOs are unable to catalyze oxidation reactions at carbon centers or perform O-, S-, or N-heteroatom dealkylation, distinguishing them from cytochrome P450 enzymes in their functional capacities (Figure 4-2).

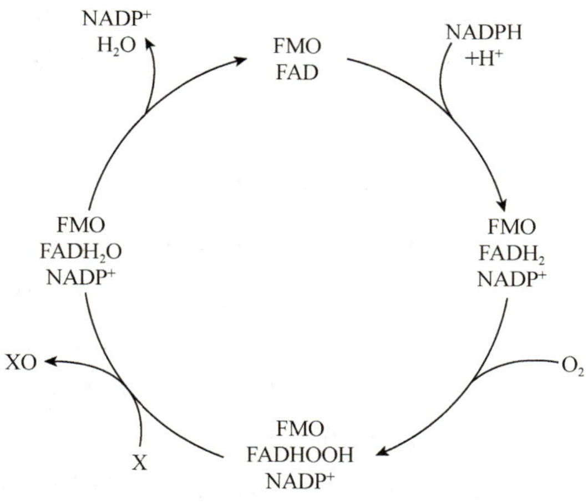

Figure 4-2 Catalytic cycle of flavin monooxygenase (FMO)

Monoamine Oxidase

Monoamine oxidase (MAO) is a crucial enzyme in the oxidative deamination of amines, including serotonin and various xenobiotics. MAO catalyzes the transformation of primary amines into aldehydes with the concurrent release of ammonia. Secondary amines are converted into primary amines and aldehydes. The aldehyde intermediates are furtherly oxidized to carboxylic acids. While MAO is most concentrated in the brain, it is also present in the liver, kidneys, intestines, and platelets.

Alcohol Dehydrogenase and Aldehyde Dehydrogenase

Alcohol dehydrogenase (ADH) is a family of cytosolic enzymes primarily found in the liver, but also present in significant amount in the kidneys, lungs, and gastric mucosa. The ADH system consists of five distinct classes, each with unique substrate specificities and tissue distribution patterns. Class Ⅰ ADH (α-ADH, β-ADH, γ-ADH) predominantly catalyze the oxidation of ethanol and other low-molecular-weight fatty alcohols. Class Ⅱ ADH (π-ADH), primarily expressed in the liver, specializes in the oxidation of higher molecular weight fatty and aromatic alcohols. Class Ⅲ ADH (χ-ADH) is involved in the oxidation of long-chain alcohols, such as amyl alcohols and their higher homologs, as well as aromatic alcohols. Class Ⅳ ADH (σ- or μ-ADH) is notably absent in liver tissue and is most active in metabolizing vitamin A and medium-chain alcohols. Class Ⅴ ADH, though identified, lacks a designated subunit nomenclature.

Aldehyde dehydrogenase (ALDH) is a NAD^+-dependent enzyme system that catalyzes the oxidation of aldehydes into their corresponding carboxylic acids. ALDH also exhibits esterase activity. There are 19 distinct ALDH isoforms, each with unique structural and functional characteristics. Genetic polymorphisms affecting ALDH can result in variations in the enzyme's ability to metabolize aldehydes, leading to differences in individual responses to alcohol and other substances.

Other Important Enzymes

In addition to the cytochrome P450 enzyme system, several other important enzymes play crucial roles in the metabolism of xenobiotics. These include Aldo-Keto Reductases (AKRs), Xanthine Oxidoreductase (XOR), Aldehyde Oxidase (AO), and Peroxidases, which participate in oxidation-reduction reactions and play key roles in the metabolism of a wide range of xenobiotics.

Aldo-Keto Reductases are NADPH-dependent enzymes found in the cytoplasm, responsible for the reduction of polycyclic aromatic hydrocarbons (PAHs) and other potentially toxic compounds. They play a significant role in both detoxifying certain chemicals and activating others into more reactive metabolites.

Peroxidase enzymes, such as Prostaglandin H Synthase (PHS), catalyze reactions that involve the oxidation of xenobiotics while simultaneously reducing hydrogen peroxide or hydroxy lipids. PHS has dual catalytic functions: cyclooxygenase and non-oxidase activities. The cyclooxygenase function converts arachidonic acid into prostaglandin intermediates, while the non-oxidase function reduces these intermediates to prostaglandin H_2. PHS is especially important in extrahepatic tissues, where cytochrome P450 enzymes are less abundant. In these tissues, PHS can generate metabolites that may be more toxic or carcinogenic, contributing to the potential harmful effects of certain xenobiotics.

Reduction Reactions

Reduction reactions are essential for the biotransformation of xenobiotics, with key contributions from cytochrome P450 enzymes, flavoproteins, and the intestinal microbiota. These reactions help metabolize a wide range of substances, including metals, aldehydes, ketones, sulfur compounds, and halogenated hydrocarbons. These processes play a crucial role in modulating the toxicity of foreign compounds.

Azo- and Nitro- Reduction

Cytochrome P450 enzymes, aldehyde oxidase, and NAD(P)H quinone oxidoreductase-1 (NQO1) are involved in the reduction of azo and nitro compounds. NQO1, also known as DT-diaphorase, is a cytosolic enzyme found mainly in liver cells. The reduction of 2, 6-dinitrotoluene by intestinal bacteria is a key step in liver tumor development in male rats. After the initial metabolism in the liver, the compound is excreted as a glucuronide conjugate and later reduced by intestinal bacterial nitroreductases. These products are then hydrolyzed in the liver, releasing reactive metabolites that can bind to DNA and potentially cause mutations, leading to liver cancer.

Carbonyl Reduction

Carbonyl reductase is an NADPH-dependent enzyme found in various tissues, including the liver, kidneys, and brain. It reduces aldehydes to primary alcohols and ketones to secondary alcohols. This enzyme plays an important role in the detoxification of a variety of xenobiotics, including drugs like flupirtine, roxithromycin, and itraconazole. The wide tissue distribution of carbonyl reductase makes it an essential component in the metabolism of many substances.

Quinone Reduction

Quinones undergo two types of reduction: a two-electron reduction catalyzed by NQO1, which forms non-toxic hydroquinones, and a one-electron reduction catalyzed by NQO2, which leads to the formation of reactive semiquinone radicals. These semiquinones can undergo autoxidation, generating reactive oxygen species (ROS) such as superoxide and hydroxyl radicals, contributing to oxidative stress and subsequent tissue damage. This mechanism is associated with the toxicity of compounds like doxorubicin (cardiotoxicity), paraquat (pulmonary toxicity), and 6-hydroxydopamine (neurotoxicity).

Other Important Reduction Reactions

Reduction is also involved in several other metabolic processes, including the reduction of disulfides, sulfur oxides, nitrogen oxides, as well as dehalogenation reactions. Dehalogenation involves the removal of halogen atoms (e. g. F, Cl, Br, I) from aliphatic molecules. This process can occur through reductive or oxidative mechanisms, including β-elimination, where halogen atoms are removed alongside hydrogen atoms from adjacent carbon atoms, forming carbon-carbon double bonds.

Hydrolysis Reaction

Hydrolysis reactions, catalyzed by a variety of enzymes found in tissues such as plasma, liver, kidneys, intestine, and nervous tissues, are essential in the biotransformation of chemical toxicants. These enzymes include esterases, amidases, peptidases, and epoxide hydrolases. The hydrolysis of toxicants is crucial in detoxifying harmful compounds and, in some cases, activating prodrugs to their active forms.

Carboxylesterases, Cholinesterases and Paraoxonases

The hydrolysis of esters, amides, and thioesters is primarily catalyzed by carboxylesterases and two distinct types of cholinesterases: true acetylcholinesterase (AChE), found in membranes, particularly in red blood cells, and pseudocholinesterase (also known as butyrylcholinesterase or BChE) found in serum. These enzymes are crucial in the breakdown of various esters and amides, affecting the duration and target of action of several toxicants.

Paraoxonases (PONs), another key enzyme, catalyze the hydrolysis of phosphate esters, such as those found in organophosphate pesticides. The combined action of carboxylesterases, cholinesterases, and paraoxonases significantly influences the detoxification of xenobiotics, such as organophosphates and other ester-containing toxicants. Notably, carboxylesterases can both detoxify and bioactivate chemicals by converting them into either less toxic or, in some cases, more toxic metabolites.

Epoxide Hydrolases (EH)

Epoxide hydrolases (EH) are widely distributed across several tissues, including the liver, lungs, kidneys, and brain. It catalyzes the hydrolysis of epoxides into vicinal diols (compounds with hydroxyl groups on adjacent carbon atoms). This reaction plays a critical role in detoxifying electrophilic epoxides, which are highly reactive and can bind to DNA and proteins, causing cellular damage.

There are two main types of epoxide hydrolases: microsomal epoxide hydrolase (mEH) and soluble epoxide hydrolase (sEH). Both types are involved in the detoxification of xenobiotics, particularly those formed by cytochrome P450 enzymes. However, some dihydrodiol metabolites, such as benzo(a)pyrene-7, 8-dihydrodiol-9, 10-epoxide, are resistant to EH hydrolysis due to their unique chemical structure. These metabolites can evade detoxification, leading to mutagenic and carcinogenic effects. Understanding these metabolic pathways is crucial in assessing the risks posed by environmental carcinogens.

Phase Ⅱ Reactions

Phase Ⅱ reactions, also known as conjugation reactions, are essential biochemical processes that enhance the elimination of xenobiotics by increasing their water solubility and reducing their biological activity. These reactions involve the enzymatic attachment of endogenous hydrophilic molecules to functional groups such as hydroxyl (−OH), amino ($-NH_2$), carboxyl (−COOH), thiol (−SH), carbonyl (−C=O), and epoxide (−O−), which may be intrinsic to the toxicant or introduced during Phase Ⅰ metabolism. Conjugation reactions generally detoxify xenobiotics, facilitating their excretion via urine or bile. However, in certain cases, conjugation can lead to metabolic activation, resulting in more toxic or carcinogenic metabolites. For example, 2-acetylaminofluorene (2-AAF), after undergoing N-hydroxylation, can be converted into an electrophilic ultimate carcinogen through conjugation with sulfate, glucuronic acid, or acetylation. Although the liver is the primary site for Phase Ⅱ metabolism, other organs, including the kidneys, intestines, lungs, spleen, and brain, also contribute to xenobiotic conjugation.

Glucuronidation

Glucuronidation is the predominant Phase Ⅱ conjugation reaction, responsible for detoxifying a broad range of xenobiotics. It is catalyzed by UDP-glucuronosyltransferases (UGTs), which transfers a glucuronic acid moiety from uridine diphosphate glucuronic acid (UDPGA) to toxicants containing hydroxyl (−OH), carboxyl (−COOH), amino ($-NH_2$), or thiol (−SH) functional groups (Figure 4−3). This reaction significantly enhances the hydrophilicity of xenobiotics, facilitating renal or biliary excretion. While smaller glucuronides are excreted in urine, larger conjugates are transported via bile into the intestines for elimination. However, some β-glucuronides excreted in bile can be hydrolyzed by β-glucuronidase, an enzyme produced by intestinal microbiota. This hydrolysis releases the parent toxicant, allowing it to be reabsorbed into circulation, a process known as enterohepatic recirculation. This phenomenon prolongs the biological half-life of certain xenobiotics, such as morphine and specific carcinogens, potentially increasing toxicity.

$$\text{UDPGA}+\text{ROH}\xrightarrow{\text{UGTs}}\text{R-O-GA}+\text{UDP}$$

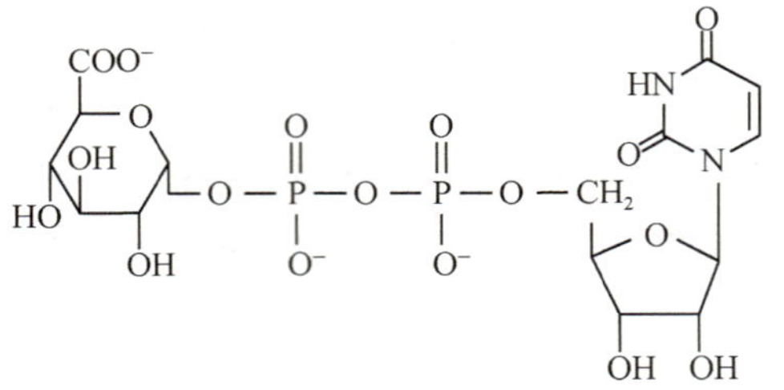

Figure 4-3 Uridine diphosphate glucuronic acid (UDPGA)

Sulfation

Sulfation is another major Phase Ⅱ conjugation pathway, primarily targeting phenolic (-OH), amino ($-NH_2$), and thiol (-SH) functional groups. It is catalyzed by sulfotransferase (SULT), which transfers a sulfate group (SO_4^{2-}) from 3'-phosphoadenosine-5'-phosphosulfate (PAPS) to xenobiotics, resulting in the formation of sulfate esters (Figure 4-4). These conjugates are highly water-soluble, allowing for rapid urinary excretion, with a minor fraction eliminated via biliary secretion. A key limitation of sulfation is that the availability of PAPS is limited, typically ranging from 4 to 80 μmol/L, in contrast to UDPGA concentrations of 200 to 350 μmol/L. This difference means that at low xenobiotic concentrations, sulfation is the dominant conjugation pathway, whereas at higher

$$\text{PAPS}+\text{ROH}\xrightarrow{\text{SULT}}\text{R-O-SO}_3\text{H}+\text{PAP}$$

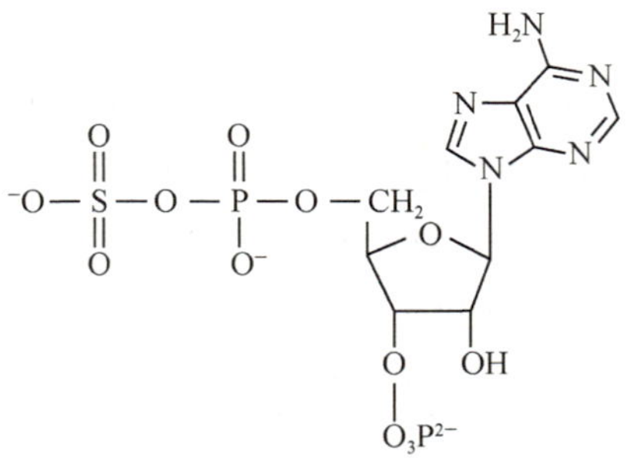

Figure 4-4 3'-Phosphoadenosine-5'-phosphosulfate (PAPS)

concentrations, glucuronidation predominates. This concentration-dependent metabolic shift illustrates the complementary nature of these two conjugation pathways. Although sulfation generally enhances detoxification, in some cases, it may contribute to toxicity by forming reactive electrophilic intermediates that can bind to DNA and proteins, potentially leading to carcinogenesis.

Glutathione Conjugation

Glutathione (GSH) is a tripeptide (γ-glutamyl-cysteinyl-glycine) that plays a central role in detoxifying electrophilic xenobiotics and scavenging reactive oxygen species (ROS) (Figure 4-5). This conjugation is catalyzed by glutathione S-transferase (GST), which facilitates the reaction between the nucleophilic thiol (-SH) group of GSH and electrophilic atoms (C, N, S, O) in toxicants. The resulting GSH conjugates are highly polar and readily excreted via urine following their conversion into mercapturic acid derivatives. This reaction serves as a crucial defense mechanism against electrophilic carcinogens, reactive oxygen species, and toxic metabolites. However, GSH depletion due to excessive toxicant exposure can impair cellular detoxification, leading to oxidative stress and tissue damage. Furthermore, overexpression of GST enzymes has been linked to chemotherapy resistance, particularly in cancers treated with cisplatin and other alkylating agents.

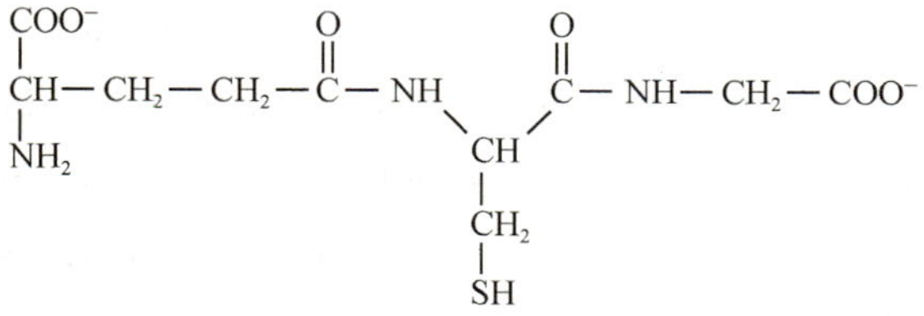

Figure 4-5 **Glutathione**

Acetylation

Acetylation is a Phase Ⅱ reaction that modifies aromatic amines and hydrazine-containing xenobiotics, reducing their reactivity and altering their solubility. It is catalyzed by N-acetyltransferases (NATs), which transfers an acetyl ($-COCH_3$) group from acetyl coenzyme A (Acetyl-CoA) to the toxicant (Figure 4-6). While acetylation often facilitates detoxification, it may also lead to bioactivation. For example, N-hydroxylated aromatic amines can be converted into highly reactive acetoxy metabolites, which may generate DNA-damaging electrophiles, increasing carcinogenic potential. Acetylation exhibits genetic polymorphisms, leading to slow and fast acetylator phenotypes. Slow acetylators have a higher risk of toxicity from aromatic amines, increasing susceptibility to bladder cancer, while fast acetylators may rapidly metabolize certain drugs, affecting therapeutic efficacy.

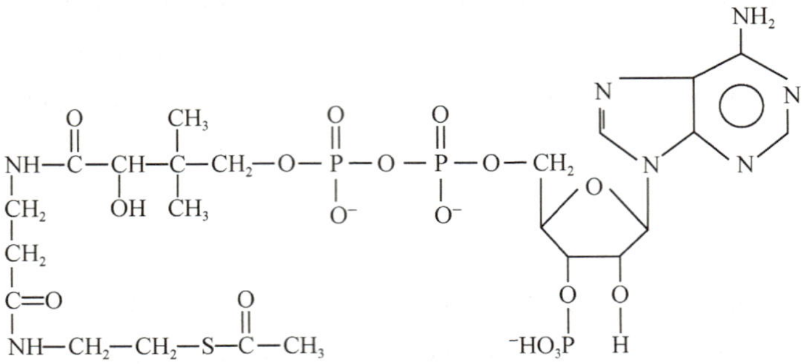

Figure 4-6 Acetyl coenzyme A

Amino Acid Conjugation

Amino acid conjugation plays a significant role in the metabolism of xenobiotics, particularly for those containing carboxyl groups. This process is a two-step biochemical reaction. The first step involves the activation of the xenobiotic by acyl-CoA synthetase, which converts the xenobiotic into an acyl-CoA thioester. The second step involves the transfer of the acyl group to amino acids such as glycine, glutamine, or taurine, via acyl-CoA N-acyltransferase. This conjugation significantly enhances the water solubility of the compound, facilitating its excretion, primarily through the urine.

A well-known example of this process is the conjugation of benzoic acid to form hippuric acid (hippurate), which aids in its detoxification and excretion. Some nonsteroidal anti-inflammatory drugs (NSAIDs), such as salicylic acid, also undergo similar conjugation. In addition, xenobiotics with aromatic hydroxylamine structures may conjugate with serine or proline, forming N-esters. These conjugates may decompose into electrophilic species, which can potentially lead to cellular damage, emphasizing the dual nature of biotransformation reactions.

Phase Ⅱ conjugation reactions generally enhance the water solubility of xenobiotics, facilitating their excretion while often reducing their toxicity. However, in certain cases, these reactions may generate reactive intermediates that can increase toxicity. A thorough understanding of these reactions is essential for predicting drug metabolism, assessing toxicokinetics, and evaluating the risk of chemical exposure on an individual level.

Toxicokinetics

Toxicokinetics is the study of how toxic substances are absorbed, distributed, metabolized, and excreted in the body. It provides insights into the time-dependent behavior of chemicals and helps us understand their movement through biological systems. By examining the concentration of a toxicant in the body over time, toxicokinetics allows us to assess how chemicals interact with the body and predict their toxicological effects.

The primary objective of toxicokinetics is to determine the key pharmacokinetic parameters that describe the absorption, distribution, metabolism, and excretion (ADME) of toxicants. These parameters are crucial for evaluating the potency, effectiveness, and potential risks of chemicals. Understanding the time-concentration relationship for toxicants is essential for making informed decisions about their safety and regulation. In the context of toxicology frameworks like TOX21, toxicokinetics provides critical information about exposure routes, systemic distribution, and potential risks.

Classical Toxicokinetics

Toxicokinetics focuses on measuring toxicant concentrations in biological tissues and correlating them with toxic effects. Since direct measurement in tissues poses technical challenges, blood sampling is commonly used as a surrogate for assessing toxicant levels. This is based on the principle that toxicants often reach dynamic equilibrium between plasma and various tissues, making plasma concentration a reliable indicator of overall distribution.

This concept has led to the development of time-concentration profiling, in which plasma toxicant concentrations are plotted against time to generate pharmacokinetic curves. These curves allow researchers to construct kinetic models that describe the ADME of toxicants. Such models are fundamental to modern toxicokinetics and provide valuable insights into how toxicants move through biological systems.

Basic Concepts

Toxicokinetics is based on two fundamental principles: rate processes and compartmental modeling.

Rate Processes

(1) First-order kinetics: In first-order rate processes, the elimination of a toxicant is directly proportional to its concentration in the body. A key characteristic of this process is that the biological half-life ($t_{1/2}$) remains constant, meaning that a fixed percentage of the toxicant is eliminated per unit of time. This results in a concentration-time curve that shows exponential decay. Most chemicals follow first-order kinetics.

(2) Zero-order kinetics: Zero-order kinetics occurs when metabolic or transport systems become saturated, limiting the elimination rate to a maximum value, independent of the toxicant's concentration. This results in a linear concentration-time curve. Zero-order kinetics

are typically observed when the body's elimination mechanisms, such as those for high-dose ethanol or certain drugs, become overwhelmed.

Compartmental Modeling

Compartmental modeling is used to simplify the complexity of the body by grouping tissues, organs, and fluids into compartments that share similar characteristics in terms of distribution and metabolism. This approach helps in understanding how toxicants move through the body and how they are eliminated over time.

(1) One-compartment Model: The one-compartment model assumes that a toxicant is uniformly distributed throughout the body immediately after administration. This model simplifies the pharmacokinetic description, assuming that the substance reaches equilibrium between plasma and tissues quickly. The time-concentration curve generated by this model follows a first-order exponential decay.

(2) Multi-compartment Model: In the multi-compartment model, the body is divided into a central compartment (blood and highly perfused organs) and peripheral compartments (less perfused tissues such as fat, muscle, and bone). Toxicants initially distribute into the central compartment and later move to peripheral compartments. The distribution and elimination phases of toxicants in this model are reflected in a biexponential curve, where the initial rapid decline represents distribution, and the slower phase represents elimination.

Compartment models in toxicology can be categorized into open and closed systems based on the consideration of toxicant elimination. Open systems incorporate the processes of metabolism and excretion, which facilitate the removal of toxicants from the body through routes such as urine, bile, or other biological pathways. This model is most commonly applied in toxicokinetic studies, as it reflects the natural processes by which chemicals are eliminated from living organisms. In contrast, closed systems assume no external elimination, focusing solely on the distribution and transformation of toxicants within the body. These models are primarily used in experimental settings where the emphasis is on the internal kinetics of toxicants, without considering their metabolism or excretion (Figure 4-7).

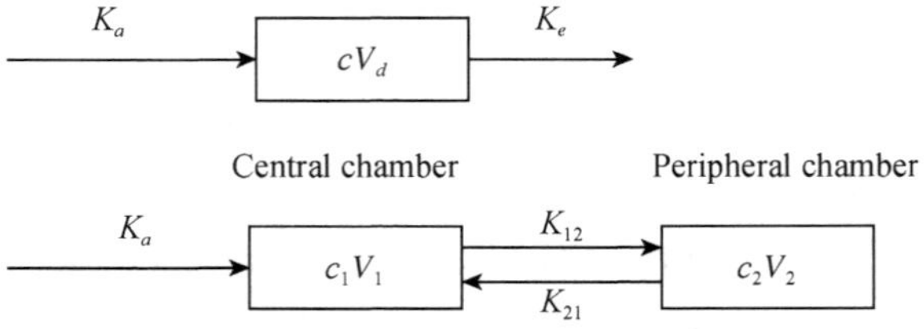

Figure 4-7 One-compartment and two-compartment open models

K_a: Absorption rate constant; K_e: Elimination rate constant; V_d: Volume of distribution; c, c_1, c_2: Compartemt concentrations; K_{12}, K_{21}: Distribution rate constant

Compartmental Model and Time–Concentration Curve

The compartment model is a theoretical approach used to describe how toxicants are distributed and eliminated from different biological compartments. It simplifies the body's complexity by grouping tissues and organs that share similar distribution and transformation characteristics.

One-Compartment Model and Its Time-Concentration Curve

The one-compartment model assumes that a chemical toxicant is immediately and uniformly distributed throughout the body after administration. In this model, the toxicant reaches equilibrium between the bloodstream and tissues quickly, and the rate of its elimination follows first-order kinetics. The concentration-time curve for this model typically shows exponential decay.

The differential equation for a one-compartment model is:

$$\frac{dC}{dt} = -k_e C$$

After integration, this equation yields the following exponential form:

$$C = C_0 e^{-k_e t}$$

Here, C is the concentration toxicant at time t, C_0 is the initial concentration of toxicant at time $t=0$, k_e is the first-order elimination rate constant, and t is time.

The time-concentration curve for intravenous (IV) administration begins at its maximum concentration (C_0) and declines exponentially. For extravascular routes (e. g. oral or intramuscular), the curve will show a slower rise and a delayed peak, followed by a decline as the toxicant is eliminated (Figure 4–8).

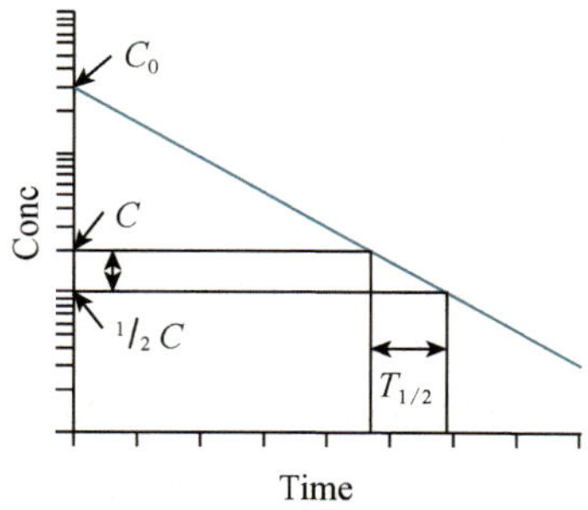

Figure 4–8 Time–concentration curve for a one-compartment single-dose model

The plasma concentration versus time curves of toxicants exhibiting kinetic behavior conforming to a one-compartment modelfollowing intravenous bolus injection.

The solid curve in the figure represents the concentration-time relationship following IV injection, while the dotted curve demonstrates the effect of absorption on the concentration-time curve for extravascular administration. Moreover, in the elimination phase, the slope of the semi-logarithmic plot of concentration versus time is proportional to $-k_e/2.303$. The biological half-life $t_{1/2}$, which is the time required for the concentration to reduce by half, can be determined from this relationship.

▶ Two-Compartment Model and Its Time–Concentration Curve

The two-compartment model divides the body into a central compartment (blood and highly perfused organs such as the liver, kidneys, heart, and lungs) and a peripheral compartment (less perfused tissues like fat, skin, and muscle). After administration, the toxicant initially enters the central compartment and then distributes to the peripheral compartment, while also being eliminated. This process takes time, and the two-compartment model reflects this with a biexponential decay in the time-concentration curve (Figure 4–9).

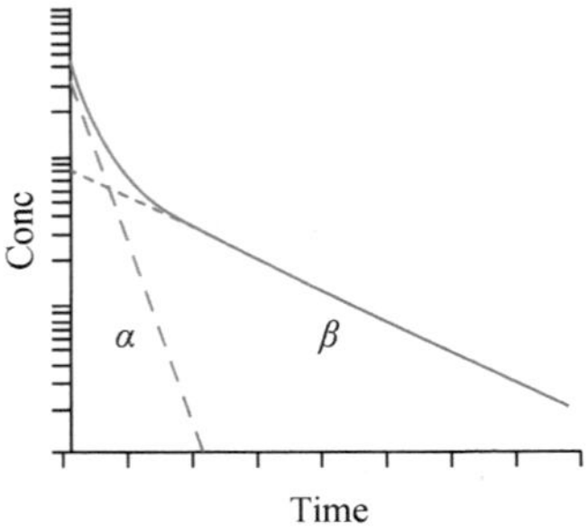

Figure 4–9 **Time-concentration curve for a two-compartment model following a single intravenous dose**

The equations for the central compartments in a two-compartment model are:

$$\frac{dC_1}{dt} = k_{21}C_2 - k_{12}C_1 - k_{10}C_1$$

For the peripheral compartment:

$$\frac{dC_2}{dt} = k_{12}C_1 - k_{21}C_2$$

Here C_1 and C_2 are the concentrations in the central and peripheral compartments, respectively, k_{12} and k_{21} are the rate constants for distribution between the central and peripheral compartments, and k_{10} is the rate constant for elimination from the central compartment.

After applying Laplace transformation, the equations become:

Central compartment: $C_1 = Ae^{-\alpha t} + Be^{-\beta t}$

Peripheral compartment: $C_2 = e^{-\beta t} - e^{-\alpha t}$

Here, α and β represent the rate constants for distribution and elimination processes, respectively, and are related to k_{12}, k_{21}, and k_{10}. The parameters A and B represent the contributions from the distribution and elimination phases.

The time-concentration curve for a two-compartment model shows an initial rapid decline during the distribution phase, followed by a slower decline in the elimination phase. This biexponential pattern reflects both the distribution of the toxicant from the central compartment to the peripheral compartment and its elimination.

It's important to note that when chemicals are administered via nonintravenous routes, the absorption phase may obscure the distribution phase, making the curve resemble a one-compartment model. This can lead to potential misinterpretation of the toxicokinetic processes.

Fundamental Toxicokinetic Parameters

Several fundamental parameters are used in toxicokinetics to describe the absorption, distribution, and elimination of toxicants:

Apparent Volume of Distribution (V_d)

The apparent volume of distribution represents the theoretical volume that would be required for a toxicant to be distributed at the same concentration as in the plasma. It provides insight into the distribution of the toxicant throughout the body. The formula for calculating V_d in a one-compartment model is:

$$V_d = X_0 / C_0$$

Here, X_0 represents the dose of the toxicant (mg/kg), C_0 represents the plasma concentration of the toxicant at $t=0$ (mg/L), and V_d is expressed in unit of L/kg.

Elimination Rate Constant (K_e)

The elimination rate constant (K_e) represents the proportion of the total body content of a chemical toxicant eliminated from the body per unit time and is expressed in units of reciprocal time (h^{-1}). For example, if the K_e value of a chemical toxicant is 0.1 h^{-1}, approximately 10% of the total body content of the substance is eliminated per hour. A higher K_e value indicates a faster rate at which the chemical toxicant is eliminated from the body.

Area Under the Curve (AUC)

The area under the curve (AUC) refers to the total area covered by the time-concentration curve from the onset of the appearance of a chemical toxicant in the plasma to complete elimination. For intravenous injection of the toxicant, the formula for calculating the AUC in a one-compartment model is as follows:

$$\text{AUC} = X_0 / V_d K_e = C_0 / K_e$$

The formula for calculating the AUC in the two-compartment model is as follows:

$$AUC = A/\alpha + B/\beta$$

The AUC is expressed in mg/(L · h). A larger AUC indicates a slower rate of elimination of the chemical toxicant from the body.

Half-life ($t_{1/2}$)

The half-life ($t_{1/2}$) refers to the time required for the plasma concentration of a chemical toxicant to decrease by half. It is another important parameter for measuring the body's ability to eliminate chemical toxicants. The calculation formula for the half-life in a one-compartment model is as follows:

$$t_{1/2} = 0.693/K_e$$

The formulas for calculating the distribution phase and elimination phase half-life in a two-compartment model are as follows:

Distribution phase: $t_{1/2}\alpha = 0.693/\alpha$

Elimination phase: $t_{1/2}\beta = 0.693/\beta$

The unit of $t_{1/2}$ can be minutes (min), hours (h), or days (d). A larger $t_{1/2}$ value indicates a slower rate of elimination of the chemical toxicant from the body.

Clearance (CL)

Clearance (CL) is the volume of plasma from which a chemical toxicant is completely removed through all elimination pathways per unit time. It serves as a key parameter reflecting the body's efficiency in eliminating chemical toxicants.

The formula for calculating the CL in a one-compartment model is as follows:

$$CL = K_e \cdot V_d = X_0/AUC$$

The formula for calculating the CL in a two-compartment model is as follows:

$$CL = V_d \cdot \beta = V_1 \cdot k_{10} = X_0/AUC$$

The unit of CL is mL/min. A larger CL indicates a faster rate of elimination of the chemical toxicant from the body.

Bioavailability (F)

Bioavailability (F), also known as biological availability, refers to the rate and extent at which a chemical toxicant is absorbed into the systemic circulation when administered. This parameter is commonly used to compare the absorption efficiency of toxicants administered through different routes. In general, a higher F value indicates greater systemic exposure and potentially stronger toxic effects on the body. The calculation formula for bioavailability is as follows:

$$F = \frac{(AUC_{non\text{-}IV}/Dose_{non\text{-}IV})}{(AUC_{IV}/Dose_{IV})}$$

where $AUC_{non\text{-}IV}$, AUC_{IV}, $Dose_{non\text{-}IV}$, and $Dose_{IV}$ are the respective areas under the blood concentration versus time curves and doses for non-IV and IV administrations.

Nonlinear Pharmacokinetics

Nonlinear pharmacokinetics occurs when the elimination of a toxicant no longer follows a simple first-order rate process and transits to a zero-order process. This shift happens when the body's metabolic, transport, or protein binding capacities become saturated, limiting the rate of elimination.

Nonlinear pharmacokinetics can be identified by several key observations. First, the plasma concentration of the toxicant does not decrease exponentially, indicating a non-exponential decline. Second, AUC does not increase proportionally with the dose, suggesting a dose-response discrepancy. Third, pharmacokinetic parameters such as V_d, CL, K_e, and $t_{1/2}$ vary with increasing doses. Additionally, competitive inhibition may occur when toxicants metabolized by the same enzyme system or actively transported compete with each other, affecting their elimination rates. Finally, once the body's elimination capacity becomes saturated, the dose-response curve no longer shows proportional changes with increasing doses, reflecting the saturation effects of elimination processes.

The Michaelis-Menten equation represents the underlying kinetics of nonlinear elimination:

$$CL_{int} = \frac{V_{max}}{K_m + [S]}$$

In the equation, CL_{int} is the intrinsic clearance. V_{max} is the theoretical maximum rate of metabolism. K_m is the Michaelis constant, which represents the concentration of the toxicant at which the metabolism rate is half of V_{max}. [S] is the unbound concentration of the substrate.

When the concentration of the toxicant is much lower than K_m, the rate of elimination is approximately proportional to concentration, following first-order kinetics. In contrast, when the concentration is much higher than K_m, the elimination rate becomes constant and independent of concentration, resulting in zero-order kinetics.

Toxicological Implications

Nonlinear pharmacokinetics has significant implications for toxicology. Toxicants that exhibit nonlinear kinetics are eliminated more slowly from the body, leading to higher concentrations in target organs over longer periods. This can intensify their toxic effects. Under chronic exposure or high doses, the body burden of the toxicant can accumulate, leading to a situation where the body is unable to eliminate the substance at a rate sufficient to maintain a steady-state. As a result, the dose-response relationship becomes unpredictable, and the toxicological effects may become more intense and dangerous.

Physiologically Based Toxicokinetic (PBTK) Model

Although classical toxicokinetic models are commonly used in toxicology, they have certain limitations. These models divide the body into compartments based on kinetic characteristics, which, while useful, do not fully reflect the anatomical and physiological nuances of how chemicals interact with the body's organs and tissues. Classical models may not effectively account for the complex biological processes of ADME in different organ systems.

In contrast, Physiologically Based Toxicokinetic (PBTK) models offer a more sophisticated and biologically realistic approach. They integrate anatomical and physiological features into the model, providing a more accurate representation of how toxicants move through the body. Here are some advantages of PBTK models:

(1) Quantification of Toxicant Distribution: PBTK models help to quantify how toxicants are distributed across different organs and tissues, offering a temporal understanding of the process.

(2) Impact of Physiological Parameters: These models take into account physiological factors, such as blood flow rates and tissue characteristics, that affect the absorption and distribution of toxicants.

(3) Extrapolation from Animal Data to Humans: PBTK models utilize biological scaling methods to extrapolate animal data to human scenarios, offering more reliable predictions of human exposure to toxicants.

(4) Complex Chemical Interactions: These models are especially useful for studying interactions between multiple pollutants, particularly when exposure occurs through multiple routes.

The rapid development of PBTK models in recent years has provided researchers with powerful tools to better understand the dynamics of toxicant distribution and elimination, enhancing risk assessments and improving environmental health studies.

Physiological Compartments in PBTK Models

A key feature of PBTK models is their ability to represent the body through interconnected compartments (Figure 4 - 10). Each compartment represents a specific anatomical or physiological space where a toxicant can be distributed. These compartments include organs, tissues, and other areas in the body, and each is characterized by distinct properties such as volume and blood perfusion rates.

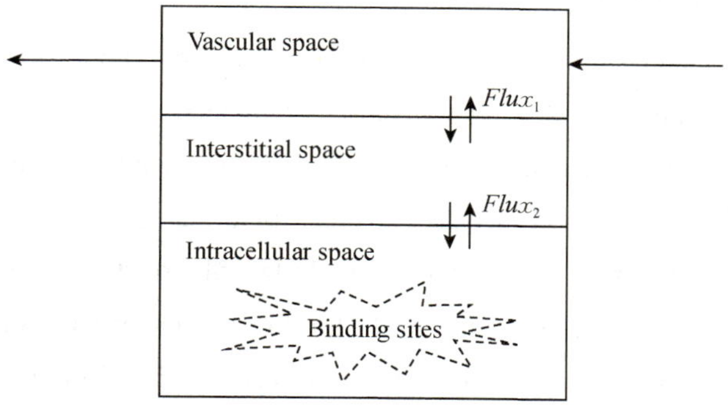

Figure 4-10 **Basic structure of compartments in a physiological model**

In a PBTK model, the body is represented by interconnected compartments, each reflecting specific anatomical or physiological spaces. These compartments include the vascular space, which represents the blood perfusion system; the interstitial space, which is the extracellular matrix surrounding cells; and the intracellular space, which is the fluid within cells. This compartmental structure enables PBTK models to track the movement of toxicants as they transit through different regions of the body, offering a detailed and dynamic understanding of how these substances are distributed, transformed, and eliminated.

Chemical toxicants enter the vascular subcompartment at a specific rate, which is determined by the blood flow rate (Q_t, L/h) to the subcompartment and the concentration of the toxicant in the blood (C_{in}, mg/L). Within the compartment, toxicants move from the vascular space to the interstitial space at a net rate ($Flux_1$), then transition from the interstitial space to the intracellular fluid at a different net rate ($Flux_2$). $Flux_1$ represents the transfer rate between vascular lumen and interstitial space, and $Flux_2$ represents the transfer rate between interstitial space and intracellular environment. Additionally, some toxicants may bind to cellular components, resulting in both free and bound states coexisting within the compartment. Toxicants exit the vascular space with a venous blood concentration (C_{out}), completing the flow dynamics within the compartment.

When developing a physiological model, it is crucial to determine which compartments to include and how they should be interconnected. These decisions depend on the characteristics of both the organism and the chemical toxicant. For example, a model studying the distribution of a chemical toxicant in fish would include the gills, whereas a model for mammals would incorporate the lungs. The structure of the model may also vary based on the chemical's properties. Since no single physiological model is universally applicable to all toxicants, an ideal model should include all significant organs and tissues relevant to the specific toxicant under study.

Key Parameters in PBTK Models

Several key parameters are essential for the accurate functioning of PBTK models. These include anatomical, physiological, and transport parameters:

Anatomical Parameters: These parameters describe the volume of each compartment and any subcompartments (e. g. blood vessels, tissues, or organs).

Physiological Parameters: This category includes blood flow rates (Q_t, expressed in volume per unit time, such as mL/min or L/h) to various organs and tissues, and other biological factors that govern how toxicants are absorbed, distributed, and eliminated from the body.

Transport Parameters: Transport parameters describe how substances cross biological membranes via diffusion or other mechanisms. For simple diffusion, the net transport rate (*Flux*, expressed in mg/h) of the chemical toxicant from one side of the membrane to the other is given by:

$$Flux = PA \times (C_1 - C_2)$$

Here, *PA* is the permeability coefficient (L/h), which is the product of the membrane permeability constant (P, μm/h) and the total membrane area (A, μm^2). C_1 and C_2 represent the free concentrations of the toxicant on either side of the membrane. The magnitude of *PA* is influenced by the diffusion rate of the toxicant and the thickness of the cell membrane. In general, a thinner membrane, larger surface area, and higher concentration difference favor diffusion.

Thermodynamic Parameters

These parameters primarily include the total concentration of the chemical toxicant in tissues (C), the free concentration (C_f), and the ratio between them. If the chemical toxicant does not bind to any molecules within the body, its free concentration equals the total concentration ($C = C_f$). However, this scenario is rare, most chemical toxicants bind to tissue components to varying degrees, and their distribution in tissues depends mainly on the composition of the tissue rather than its own concentration. Thus, there is a proportional relationship between the free concentration and the total concentration: $C = C_f \times P_t$. Here, P_t represents the tissue partition coefficient.

Factors Limiting the Transmembrane Transport of Chemical Toxicants

The movement of chemical toxicants across biological membranes can be limited by two primary factors, perfusion limitation and diffusion limitation.

Perfusion-limited compartments

These occur when the ability of a tissue to take up a toxicant is limited by the blood flow reaching the tissue. In such cases, the rate of toxicant uptake depends on the blood perfusion rate, rather than the rate at which the toxicant crosses the cell membrane. This type of limitation is seen in tissues where blood flow is the primary factor controlling the rate of delivery of the toxicant to the tissue.

Diffusion-limited compartments

In contrast, diffusion-limited compartments occur when the uptake of toxicants into the tissue is primarily restricted by the permeability of the cell membrane and the surface area available for diffusion (Figure 4-11). This is typically observed when the blood flow is sufficiently fast, and the movement of toxicants is controlled by how easily they can cross the cellular membranes.

Both perfusion-limited and diffusion-limited compartments influence how a toxicant is distributed and eliminated in the body. Understanding these factors helps us predict the behavior of toxicants in different tissues and under varying conditions of exposure.

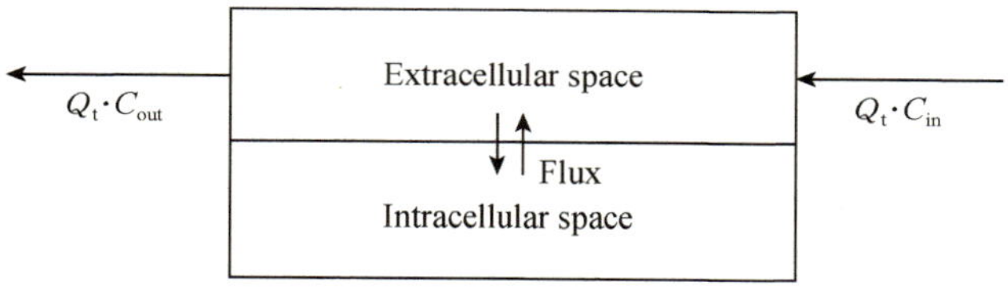

Figure 4-11 Perfusion-limited compartment (top diagram) and diffusion-limited compartment (bottom diagram)

The Application of Physiologically Based Toxicokinetic Models

PBTK models are essential tools in toxicology, offering a comprehensive approach to understanding the movement and effects of toxicants within the body. By incorporating physiological parameters and compartmental structures, these models provide deeper insights into how toxicants are absorbed, distributed, metabolized, and excreted across various tissues and organs. As such, PBTK models play a crucial role in several key areas of toxicology:

Risk Assessment

PBTK models help establish dose-response relationships by providing more accurate estimates of the tissue concentrations of toxicants. This helps in predicting the health risks associated with specific exposures and in setting safety standards.

Development and Revision of Exposure Limits

Traditional methods of monitoring toxicant concentrations, especially in occupational settings, focus on airborne concentrations. However, these methods do not directly reflect the actual dose absorbed into the body. PBTK models provide a more accurate measure of internal exposure by estimating toxicant concentrations in various body compartments, including blood and tissues, helping to revise exposure limits based on actual risk.

Experimental Design and Toxicity Testing

In toxicity studies, PBTK models allow for the accurate simulation of the body's response to different exposure scenarios, reducing the number of animals required for experiments and improving the quality of the data obtained. These models are particularly useful in carcinogenicity and chronic toxicity testing.

Despite their advantages, PBTK models have certain uncertainties, especially in terms of model selection and parameter estimation. However, with advancements in computational tools and modeling software, it has become possible to apply PBTK models to predict human responses based on animal data and in vitro studies. This integration of in vitro models with PBTK offers exciting prospects for improving the accuracy and reliability of toxicology predictions, making it a promising area for future research.

(Wu Jing)

CHAPTER 5

Mechanisms of Toxicity

Introduction

Elucidating the mechanisms underlying toxicity and understanding potential hazards associated with specific chemicals is paramount in toxicology. This understanding is crucial for estimating, evaluating, interpreting, and preventing toxic effects through both qualitative and quantitative characterization. Given the vast number of potential toxicants and the multitude of biological structures and processes that can be impaired, there exists an extensive array of possible toxic effects. Consequently, numerous pathways may lead to toxicity, necessitating a comprehensive approach to toxicological research and risk assessment.

In the intricate landscape of toxicology, a common sequence of events unfolds when a toxicant, such as tetrodotoxin, interacts with its target, resulting in cellular dysfunction and the manifestation of toxicity. This direct interaction represents one pathway to toxicity. Alternatively, xenobiotics, like 2, 4-dinitrophenol, can adversely influence the broader biological environment, causing dysfunction at multiple levels of biological organization, molecular, organellar, cellular, or organ, ultimately leading to deleterious effects. These diverse mechanisms highlight the complexity of toxicological processes and the importance of understanding toxicant-specific pathways.

The path to toxicity is a complex, multi-step process that involves several key stages. Initially, the ultimate toxicant is formed and delivered to its target site within the body. This step is crucial as the toxic agent may differ from the originally administered compound due to metabolic processes. Once at the target site, the toxicant interacts with specific endogenous molecules, such as proteins or DNA, potentially disrupting normal cellular functions or structures.

In response to these disruptions, the organism activates repair mechanisms at various levels—molecular, cellular, and tissue. These protective responses aim to mitigate damage and restore normal function. However, toxicity can occur if the induced perturbations exceed the organism's repair capacity or if the repair processes themselves become dysfunctional.

This multi-step paradigm, as illustrated in Figure 5-1, underscores the importance of considering both toxicokinetics and toxicodynamics when evaluating potential toxicity. Toxicokinetics deals with how the body processes the toxicant, including its absorption, distribution, metabolism, and excretion. Toxicodynamics, on the other hand, focuses on the toxicant's interactions with biological targets and the resulting cascade of events leading to toxic effects.

Furthermore, the body's compensatory mechanisms play a significant role in modulating the toxic response. These can include the up-regulation of detoxification enzymes or the activation of stress response pathways, as depicted in Figure 5-1. The effectiveness of these compensatory responses can greatly influence the threshold at which toxicity occurs and the

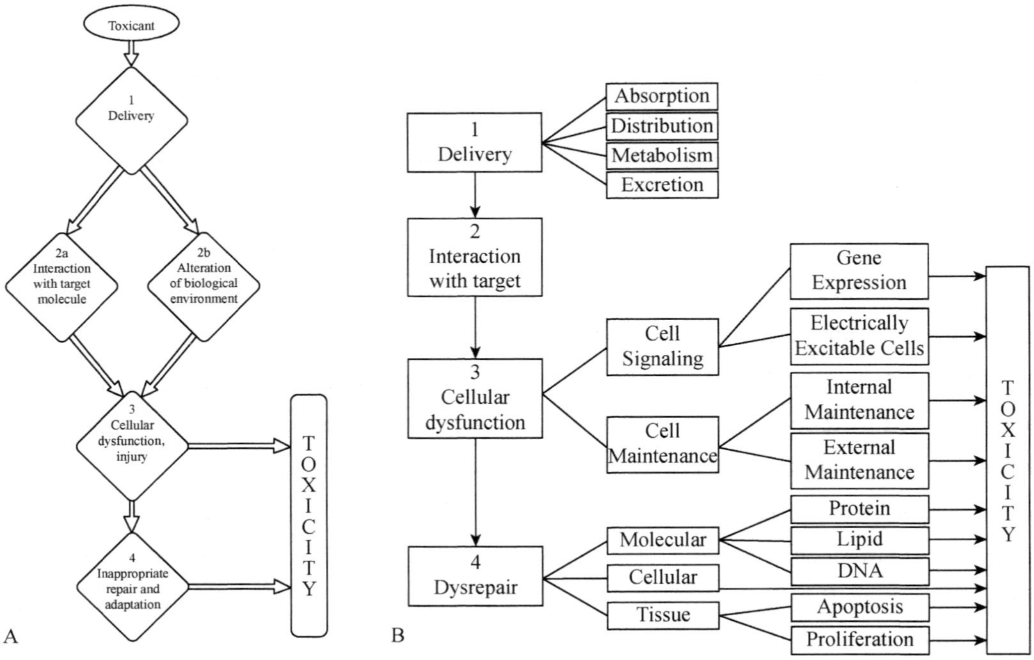

Figure 5-1 Overview of critical events that contribute to the development of toxicity after chemical exposure

These fundamental processes serve as the basis for the organization. Panel A shows more details of critical events underlying the four major processes outlined. Panel B shows more details of the mechanistic events involved in toxic outcomes.

severity of the resulting effects. This chapter delves into the cellular mechanisms that contribute to the manifestation of toxicities, as identified through rigorous research in humans and animal models. Some of these mechanisms have been definitively established, while others remain under investigation. By exploring these intricate processes, we aim to deepen our understanding of toxic effects, enhance our ability to assess and interpret toxicological data, improve our capacity to predict potential toxicities of new compounds, and develop more effective strategies for preventing and mitigating toxic effects. This comprehensive exploration of toxicity mechanisms serves as a foundation for advancing both the theoretical understanding and practical applications of toxicology in public health, environmental protection, and drug development.

Formation of Ultimate Toxicant

The primary determinant of toxicity is the ultimate toxicant, defined as the chemical species that directly interacts with endogenous target molecule such as receptors, enzymes, DNA, microfilament proteins, or lipids. This interaction typically leads to significant structural and/or functional changes in the target molecule, thereby initiating toxicity within the biological system.

The potency of a toxic effect is theoretically correlated with two key factors: the concentration of the ultimate toxicant at its specific site of action, and the persistence of the ultimate toxicant at this site. The local concentration of the toxicant at the target molecule is influenced by a complex interplay of processes that either increase or decrease its presence at the target site. These processes may include: absorption and distribution of the parent compound, metabolic activation or deactivation, binding to plasma proteins or other cellular components, active transport mechanisms, and elimination pathways. Understanding these toxicokinetic and toxicodynamic processes is crucial for accurately assessing and predicting the intensity of toxic effects. These knowledge form the basis for risk assessment, the development of antidotes, and the design of safer chemicals.

Ultimate Toxicants: Types and Examples

The concept of the ultimate toxicant encompasses a spectrum of chemical entities that directly induce toxicity in biological systems. While the parent compound—the initial xenobiotic to which an organism is exposed may act as the ultimate toxicant in certain cases, this is not a universal paradigm in toxicology. Frequently, biotransformation processes generate metabolites that possess greater toxicological potency than their precursor molecules, thus assuming the role of the ultimate toxicant. Moreover, the metabolic fate of some xenobiotics involves the production of reactive oxygen species (ROS) or reactive nitrogen species (RNS), which can function themselves as ultimate toxicants, initiating oxidative stress and subsequent cellular damage. In some instances, the cascade of toxicological events may culminate in the production or accumulation of endogenous molecules that serve as the ultimate mediators of toxicity. This diverse array of ultimate toxicants, spanning parent compounds, metabolites, reactive species, and endogenous molecules, underscores the complexity of toxicological mechanisms and highlights the importance of comprehensive toxicokinetic and toxicodynamic analyses. Table 5-1 provides a detailed illustration of these various types of ultimate toxicants, offering insights into the multifaceted nature of toxicological processes and their implications for risk assessment and therapeutic interventions.

Table 5-1 Types and Examples of Ultimate Toxicants

Types of Ultimate Toxicants	Examples of Ultimate Toxicants
Parent xenobiotics	①lead ions (Pb^{2+}), ② tetrodotoxin, ③ 2, 3, 7, 8 - tetrachlorodibenzo-p-dioxin (TCDD), ④ methylisocyanate, ⑤ hydrocyanic acid (HCN), ⑥ carbon monoxide (CO)
Xenobiotic metabolites	①amygdalin→HCN, ②arsenate→arsenite, ③fluoroacetate→fluorocitrate, ④ethylene glycol→oxalic acid, ⑤hexane→2, 5-hexanedione, ⑥acetaminophen→N-acetyl-*p*-benzoquinoneimine, ⑦CCl_4→CCl_3OO·, ⑧benzo[*a*]pyrene (BP)→BP-7, 8-diol-9, 10-epoxide (BPDE), ⑨benzo[*a*]pyrene (BP)→BP-radical cation
Reactive oxygen species or reactive nitrogen species	①hydrogen peroxide (H_2O_2), diquat, doxorubicin, nitrofurantoin, Cr(Ⅴ), Fe(Ⅱ), Mn(Ⅱ), Ni(Ⅱ)→hydroxyl radical (HO·), ②→Peroxynitrite ($ONOO^-$), ③ paraquat→$O_2^{\cdot-}$ —+NO·
Endogenous compounds	①sulfonamides→albumin-bound bilirubin→bilirubin, ② CCl_3OO·→unsaturated fatty acids→lipid peroxyl radicals or lipid alkoxyl radicals or 4-Hydroxynonenal, ③HO·→proteins→protein carbonyls

Formation of Ultimate Toxicant

Many xenobiotics exhibit direct toxicity due to their inherent chemical properties. Examples include strong acids and bases, nicotine, aminoglycosides, ethylene oxide, methylisocyanate, heavy-metal ions, hydrogen cyanide (HCN), and carbon monoxide (CO). However, for numerous other compounds, toxicity primarily arises from their metabolites. This process of biotransformation resulting in harmful products, is termed toxication or metabolic activation.

With some xenobiotics (such as oxalic acid), toxication confers physicochemical properties that adversely alter the microenvironment of biological processes or structures. Occasionally, chemicals undergo biotransformation, acquiring structural features and reactivity that enhance their interaction with specific receptors or enzymes. For example, the organophosphate insecticide parathion, the rodenticide fluoroacetate, and the antiviral drug fialuridine. Most often, toxication renders xenobiotics and occasionally other molecules in the body, such as oxygen and nitric oxide (· NO), indiscriminately reactive toward endogenous molecules with susceptible functional groups. This heightened reactivity often results from the conversion of xenobiotics into metabolites, such as electrophiles, free radicals, nucleophiles, or redox-active reactants.

Formation of Electrophiles

Electrophiles, molecules possessing an electron-deficient atom with partial or complete positive charge, are generated through various mechanisms.

(1) Oxygen Insertion: This process leads to the formation of nonionic electrophiles such as aldehydes, ketones, epoxides, arene oxides, sulfoxides, nitroso compounds, phosphonates, and acyl halides.

(2) Conjugated Double Bond Formation: Catalyzed by cytochrome P450, this mechanism results in α, β-unsaturated aldehydes and ketones, quinones, and quinoneimines.

(3) Heterolytic Bond Cleavage: This process generates cationic electrophiles including carbonium ions, nitrenium ions, sulfonium ions, and metal ions.

Formation of Free Radicals

Free radicals, molecules or molecular fragments containing unpaired electrons in their outer orbital, form through various mechanisms.

(1) Redox Cycling: Xenobiotics like paraquat, doxorubicin, and nitrofurantoin generate superoxide anion radicals ($O_2^{\cdot-}$) through electron acceptance from reductases.

(2) Peroxidase-Catalyzed Reactions: Nucleophilic xenobiotics such as phenols, hydroquinones, and aminophenols form free radicals through electron loss.

(3) Homolytic Bond Fission: This mechanism is involved in the conversion of CCl_4 to the trichloromethyl free radical ($Cl_3C\cdot$) and subsequent formation of the trichloromethylperoxy radical ($Cl_3COO\cdot$).

Formation of Nucleophiles

While less common, formation of nucleophiles represents another mechanism of toxicant activation. Examples include: ① cyanide formation from amygdalin, acrylonitrile, and sodium nitroprusside, ② carbon monoxide (CO) formation from dihalomethanes via oxidative dehalogenation, ③ hydrogen selenide formation from selenite through reaction with glutathione or other thiols.

Formation of Redox-Active Reactants

Specific mechanisms exist for the formation of redox-active reactants. For example, the nitrite formation induced from nitrate, dapsone hydroxylamine, and 5-hydroxyprimaquine can produce methemoglobin production by cooxidation.

Detoxication and Detoxication Insufficiency

Detoxication encompasses a series of biotransformation processes aimed at eliminating or preventing the formation of ultimate toxicant. The specific pathways involved in detoxication are largely dependent on the chemical nature of the toxicant.

Detoxication of Toxicants Lacking Functional Groups

For toxicants devoid of functional groups, such as benzene and toluene, detoxication involves a comnbination of phases Ⅰ and Ⅱ reactions. These biotransformations result in the conversion of these lipophilic compounds into inactive, highly hydrophilic organic acids, facilitating their excretion from the body.

Detoxication of Nucleophiles

Nucleophilic toxicants undergo detoxication primarily through conjugation reactions targeting their functional groups. Hydroxylated compounds undergo sulfation, glucuronidation, or occasionally methylation. Thiols are methylated or glucuronidated, while amines and hydrazines are acetylated. Thiols and hydrazines are oxidized by flavin-containing monooxygenases. Some alcohols, like ethanol, undergo detoxication through oxidation to carboxylic acids. A specific mechanism detoxifies cyanide to thiocyanate by rhodanese.

Detoxication of Electrophiles

Electrophilic toxicants are predominantly detoxicated through conjugation with the thiol nucleophile glutathione, a process catalyzed by glutathione S-transferases (GSTs). This mechanism is particularly important for metal ions such as Ag^{+}, Cd^{2+}, Hg^{2+}, and CH_3Hg^{+}, which readily react with glutathione. Specific mechanisms include the biotransformation of epoxides and arene oxides to diols and dihydrodiols, and the hydrolysis of organophosphate ester pesticides by epoxide hydrolase and carboxylesterase, respectively.

Others mechanisms include two-electron reduction of quinones to hydroquinones by DT-diaphorase, reduction of α, β-unsaturated aldehydes to alcohols by alcohol dehydrogenase or oxidation to acids by aldehyde dehydrogenase, and complex formation of thiol-reactive metal ions by metallothionein and the redox-active ferrous iron by ferrin. It is noteworthy that the covalent binding of electrophiles to proteins can also be considered a form of detoxification, albeit one that may lead to altered protein function.

Detoxication of Free Radicals

The detoxication of free radicals is of paramount importance, particularly in the elimination of superoxide anion radicals ($O_2^{\cdot-}$) and the prevention of their conversion into more reactive compounds (Figure 5-2). Superoxide dismutases (SOD) in the cytosol and mitochondria convert $O_2^{\cdot-}$ to HOOH, which is then detoxicated by glutathione peroxidase

(GPx) or catalase (CAT). No enzyme eliminates HO ·, and antioxidants like glutathione, α-tocopherol (vitamin E), or ascorbic acid (vitamin C) are generally ineffective. The most effective protection against HO · is preventing its formation by converting its precursor, HOOH, to water (Figure 5-3).

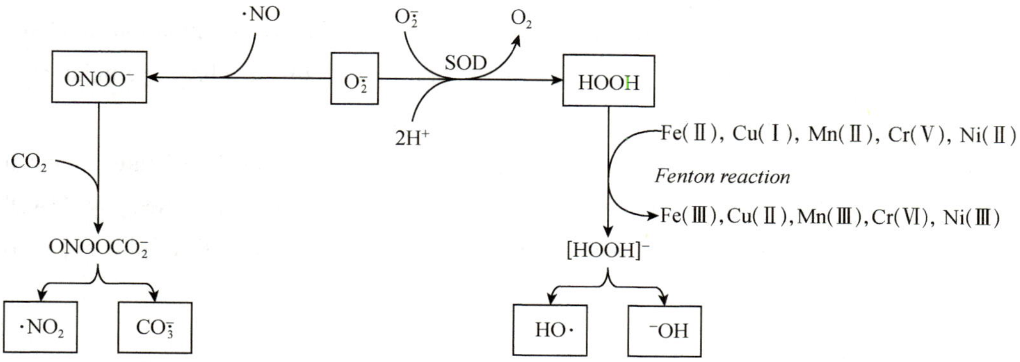

Figure 5-2 Two pathways for toxication of superoxide anion radical ($O_2^{\bar{\cdot}}$) via nonradical products ($ONOO^-$ and HOOH) to radical products ($\cdot NO_2$, $CO_3^{\bar{\cdot}}$ and HO ·)

In one pathway, conversion of $O_2^{\bar{\cdot}}$ to HOOH is spontaneous or is catalyzed by superoxide dismutase (SOD). Homolytic cleavage of HCOH to hydroxyl radical and hydroxyl ion is called the Fenton reaction and is catalyzed by the transition metal ions shown. Hydroxyl radical is the ultimate toxication for xenobiotics that form $O_2^{\bar{\cdot}}$, or for HOOH, the transition metal ions listed, and some chemicals that form complexes with these transition metal ions. In the other pathway, $O_2^{\bar{\cdot}}$ reacts avidly with nitric oxide (·NO), the product of ·NO synthase (NOS), forming peroxynitrite ($ONOO^-$). Spontaneous reaction of $ONOO^-$ with carbon dioxide (CO_2) yields nitrosoperoxy carbonate ($ONOOCO_2^-$), which is homolytically cleaved to nitrogen dioxide ($\cdot NO_2$) and carbonate anion radical ($CO_3^{\bar{\cdot}}$). All three radical products indicated in this figure are oxidants, whereas $\cdot NO_2$ is also a nitrating agent.

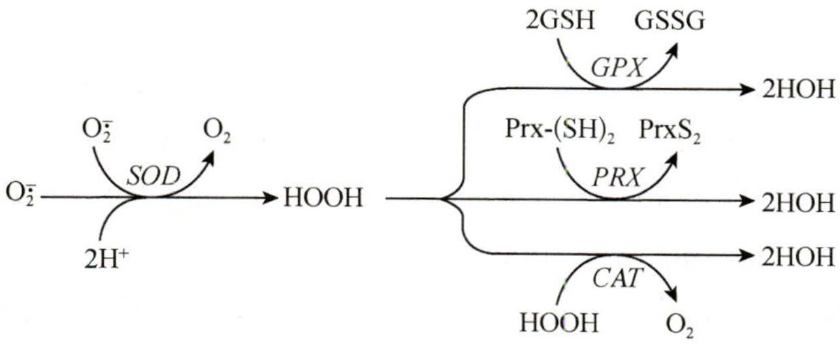

Figure 5-3 Detoxification of superoxide anion radical ($O_2^{\bar{\cdot}}$) and HOOH

Superoxide dismutase (SOD) converts $O_2^{\bar{\cdot}}$ to HOOH, which is further detoxiffed by glutathione peroxidase (GPX), peroxiredoxin (Prx-$(SH)_2$), and catalase (CAT). When GPX reduces HOOH, it forms glutathione disulffde (GSSG), which is reduced back to GSH by glutathione reductase (requires NADPH; see Fig. 4-5). When Prx-$(SH)_2$ reduces HOOH, its catalytic thiol group (-R-S-H) is oxidized to a sulfenic acid group (-R-S-OH), which in turn reacts with another SH group of Prx, forming HOH and Prx disulffde ($PrxS_2$). Finally, catalase converts HOOH into two moles of water. Catalase is a high-capacity system, whereas Prx and GPX can be saturated at high concentrations of HOOH.

Peroxynitrite ($ONOO^-$) exhibits greater stability compared to hydroxyl radicals ($HO\cdot$), rendering it less susceptible to interception by low-molecular-weight biological antioxidant molecules such as glutathione, uric acid, ascorbic acid, and α-tocopherol. However, glutathione peroxidase demonstrates superior efficacy in reducing $ONOO^-$ to nitrite (ONO^-). Notably, $ONOO^-$ interacts with oxyhemoglobin, heme-containing peroxidases, and albumin, which serve as potential sinks for this reactive species. The effective elimination of $ONOO^-$ precursors, namely nitric oxide ($\cdot NO$) and superoxide anion ($O_2^{\cdot -}$), plays a crucial role in preventing $ONOO^-$ accumulation.

Glutathione plays a crucial role in neutralizing peroxidase-generated free radicals through electron transfer. The subsequent oxidation of glutathione is then reversed by NADPH dependent glutathione reductase, contributing to the detoxification of electrophiles and free radicals.

Detoxication Insufficiency

However, when detoxication insufficiency occurs, several factors may impede the process. Firstly, the toxicant might overwhelm the detoxication processes, hindering their effectiveness. Secondly, a reactive toxicant, like $ONOO^-$, can incapacitate detoxicating enzymes such as Mn-SOD. Thirdly, the detoxification process may be reversed upon transfer to other tissues. Lastly, there is a possibility that potentially harmful byproducts are produced during the detoxication process. Detoxication insufficiency poses challenges to the successful elimination of free radicals and electrophiles, emphasizing the importance of understanding and addressing these potential hurdles.

Reaction of the Ultimate Toxicant with the Target Molecule

Toxicity typically arises through the interaction of the ultimate toxicant with a target molecule, leading to subsequent biochemical events. These events result in dysfunction or injury, evident at various biological levels, including the target molecule, cell organelles, cells, tissues, organs, and the entire organism.

Potential targets for toxicants encompass a wide array of endogenous compounds. Macromolecules, particularly nucleic acids (especially DNA) and proteins, are the most prevalent and significant targets. Among smaller molecules, membrane lipids are frequently implicated, while cofactors such as coenzyme A and pyridoxal phosphate are rarely involved. For an endogenous molecule to be considered a target, it must posess suitable reactivity or steric configuration to engage in covalent or noncovalent reactions with the ultimate toxicant. Additionally, the target molecule must be accessible to a sufficiently high concentration of the ultimate toxicant for these reactions to occur. This often involves endogenous molecules located near reactive chemicals or adjacent to their formation sites.

The determinants of interaction of the ultimate toxicant with the target molecule include: ① the attributes of target molecules, ② the types of reactions between ultimate toxicants and target molecules, ③ the effects of toxicants on the target molecules as illustrated in Figure 5-4.

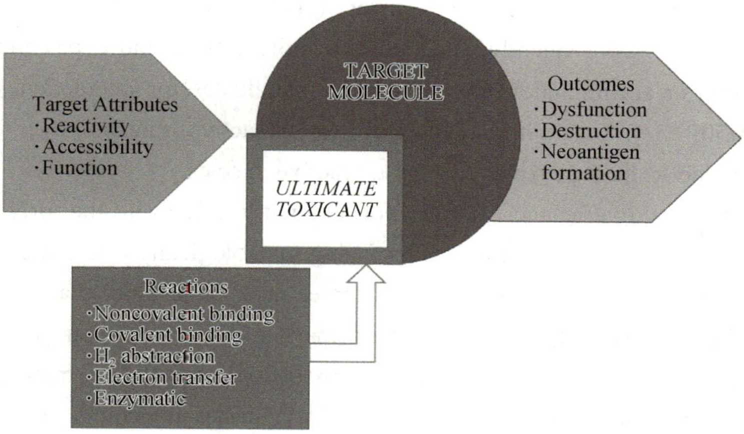

Figure 5-4 Reaction of the ultimate toxicant with the target molecule: the second step in the development of toxicity

The figure illustrates that the properties of the toxic molecule can influence the reaction with its target, the diversity of reactions that can occur with the target, and following the interaction of the toxicant with its target. The types of outcomes that are associated with the toxicity.

Reactive metabolites often initially target the enzyme responsible for their production or nearby intracellular structures. However, it is crucial to recognize that not all chemical-target interactions result in harmful effects. To conclusively identify a target molecule as responsible for toxicity, three key criteria must be met: ① the ultimate toxicant reacts with the target, adversely affecting its function, ② the ultimate toxicant achieves an effective concentration at the target site, ③ the modification of the target is mechanistically linked to the observed toxicity.

Aetributes of Target Molecules

In the study of toxicology, understanding the nature of target molecules is crucial for elucidating mechanisms of toxicity. As for an endogenous molecule, to serve as a viable target for toxicants, it must possess specific characteristics.

(1) Appropriate Reactivity and Steric Configuration: Target molecules must exhibit suitable chemical reactivity and spatial arrangement to engage with ultimate toxicants. This characteristic enables the formation of covalent or noncovalent interactions between the toxicant and the target. The reactivity may involve specific functional groups or structural motifs that are complementary to those of the toxicant's structure. For instance, nucleophilic

centers in proteins or DNA can react with electrophilic toxicants, while hydrophobic pockets in proteins may accommodate lipophilic compounds.

(2) Accessibility to Ultimate Toxicants: The potential target must be physically accessible to a sufficient concentration of the ultimate toxicant. This accessibility is influenced by various factors, including the cellular localization of the target, the distribution of the toxicant within the cell or tissue, and any barriers (such as cell membranes) that may impede the toxicant's access. Consequently, endogenous molecules in close proximity to sites of toxicant formation or accumulation are often prime candidates for interaction. For example, cytochrome P450 enzymes, which generate many reactive metabolites, are themselves frequent targets due to their proximity to these reactive species.

(3) Biological Significance: While not explicitly stated in the original text, this characteristic is implicit in the criteria for identifying toxicologically relevant target molecules. The interaction between the toxicant and the target must have biological consequences that contribute to the observed toxic effects. This may involve disruption of critical cellular functions, alteration of signaling pathways, or induction of cellular stress responses. The biological significance of the interaction is what distinguishes toxicologically relevant targets from molecules that may interact with toxicants but do not contribute significantly to the toxic outcome.

Understanding these characteristics of target molecules is essential for predicting potential toxicities, elucidating mechanisms of action, and developing strategies to mitigate or prevent toxic effects.

Types of Reactions

The ultimate toxicant can interact with target molecules through various mechanisms, primary categorized into two main types of binding: noncovalent and covalent. These interactions can lead to alterations in the target molecules through several processes, including noncovalent binding, covalent binding, hydrogen abstraction, electron transfer, and enzymatic reactions.

Noncovalent Binding

Noncovalent binding, often involving apolar interactions or the formation of hydrogen and ionic bonds, is common in the interaction between toxicants and targets like membrane receptors, intracellular receptors, ion channels, and certain enzymes. This binding is typically reversible due to its relatively low bonding energy.

Covalent Binding

Covalent binding, is practically irreversible and holds significant toxicologic importance as it permanently changes endogenous molecules.

Electrophilic toxicants, including nonionic and cationic electrophiles and radical cations, frequently form covalent adducts with nucleophilic atoms abundant in biological macromolecules like proteins and nucleic acids. Neutral free radicals, such as HO·, ·NO_2, and Cl_3C·, can also covalently bind to biomolecules. Nucleophilic toxicants, although reactive toward electrophilic endogenous compounds, engage in such reactions infrequently due to the rarity of electrophiles among biomolecules.

Hydrogen Abstraction

Hydrogen abstraction is a crucial process in toxicology involving the removal of hydrogen atoms from endogenous compounds by neutral free radicals. These radicals can initiate various reactions, such as forming cross-links with DNA or other proteins. Hydrogen abstraction from different compounds, including amino acids and fatty acids, can result in significant consequences.

Electron Transfer

Electron transfer is a mechanism where chemicals exchange electrons to oxidize or reduce other molecules, producing harmful byproducts. For instance, chemicals can oxidize Fe (Ⅱ) in hemoglobin to Fe (Ⅲ), leading to conditions like methemoglobinemia. N-hydroxyl arylamines, phenolic compounds, and hydrazines can be co-oxidized with oxyhemoglobin, forming methemoglobin and hydrogen peroxide.

Enzymatic Reactions

Enzymatic reactions play a crucial role in the action of certain toxins on specific target proteins. For example, ricin induces hydrolytic fragmentation of ribosomes, blocking protein synthesis. Bacterial toxins, like cholera toxin, catalyze the transfer of ADP-ribose from NAD+ to specific proteins. Snake venoms contain hydrolytic enzymes capable of destroying biomolecules.

Effects of Toxicants on Target Molecules

Dysfunction of Target Molecules

Toxicants can interact with endogenous molecules in various ways, leading to either dysfunction or destruction of these target molecules. Dysfunction may occur when toxicants mimic endogenous ligands, activating protein target molecules. For instance, morphine activates opiate receptors, clofibrate acts on peroxisome proliferator-activated receptor (PPAR), and phorbol esters and lead ions stimulate protein kinase C (PKC). Alternatively, many xenobiotics inhibit the function of target molecules, such as neurotransmitter receptors or ion transporters. Exposure of toxic chemicals can also lead to the opening or closure of membrane ion channels, enzyme inhibition, and impaired assembly or disassembly of cytoskeletal proteins.

Protein function impairment occurs when the toxicant alters the conformation or structure of proteins, particularly those with critical moieties, such as thiol groups, which are essential for catalytic activity. Covalent and oxidative modification of these moieties by xenobiotics can result in aberrant signal transduction, impaired cellular energy and metabolic homeostasis. Additionally, the covalent binding of toxic chemicals to DNA may interfere with DNA's template function, causing nucleotide mispairing during replication. For example, aflatoxin 8, 9-oxide covalent binding leads to the formation of an incorrect codon, while HO · induced mutagenic bases result in mispairing. Doxorubicin causes significant errors in DNA template function by shifting the reading frame.

Destruction of Target Molecules

In addition to adduct formation, toxicants also alter the primary structure of endogenous molecules by means of cross-linking and fragmentation, imposing functional constraints on the linked molecules. For examples, bifunctional electrophiles such as carbon disulfide, acrolein, and nitrogen mustard alkylating agents, as well as hydroxyl radicals can cross-link with protein and/or DNA.

Some target molecules are susceptible to spontaneous degradation after chemical attack. Free radicals such as $Cl_3COO\cdot$ and $HO\cdot$ can initiate peroxidative degradation of lipids by hydrogen abstraction from fatty acids. Apart from hydrolytic degradation by toxins and radiolysis, toxicant-induced fragmentation of proteins is not well documented. However, destruction of the prosthetic group in enzymes is the case. Toxicants can cause various forms of DNA fragmentation. For example, formation of a bulky adduct at guanine N-7 induces depurination, resulting in apurinic sites that are mutagenic. Single-strand breaks typically are caused by hydroxyl radicals via abstraction of H from desoxyribose in DNA, and cleavage of the phosphodiester bond. Multiple hydroxyl radical attacks on a short length of DNA, leads to double-strand breaks that are typically lethal to the affected cell.

Neoantigen Formation

The reaction of the ultimate toxicant with endogenous protein molecules may render them foreign (neoantigen) to the immune system, eliciting an immune response in some individuals. Chemicals like dinitrochlorobenzene, penicillin, and nickel may bind to proteins spontaneously. Others may gain reactivity through autooxidation to quinones (e. g. urushiols) or enzymatic biotransformation.

Toxicity not Initiated by Reaction with Target Molecules

In the field of toxicology, it is crucial to recognize that not all xenobiotics induce toxicity through direct interactions with specific target molecules. While many toxicants do operate via such mechanisms, there exists a significant subset of compounds that exert their harmful effects by altering the biological microenvironment.

One of the primary mechanisms by which xenobiotics can induce toxicity without directly interacting with target molecules is through alteration of hydrogen ion (H^+) concentrations in cellular or extracellular environments. Changes in pH can have profound effects on enzyme activity, protein structure, and various cellular processes. For instance, severe acidosis or alkalosis can disrupt vital physiological functions, leading to systemic toxicity. This mechanism is exemplified by the toxicity of ethylene glycol, a common antifreeze component. Upon metabolism, ethylene glycol produces oxalic acid, which not only causes severe metabolic acidosis but also forms calcium oxalate crystals that can lead to renal damage.

Another important mechanism involves the physicochemical alteration of the lipid phase of cell membranes. Some xenobiotics, particularly those with amphipathic properties, can intercalate into cellular membranes, altering their fluidity, permeability, or structural integrity. These changes can disrupt the function of membrane-bound proteins, including ion channels and receptors, and may compromise the cell's ability to maintain essential electrochemical gradients. This mechanism is particularly relevant for certain classes of anesthetics and some environmental contaminants.

Disruption of transmembrane solute gradients represents yet another critical mechanism of toxicity that does not require direct interaction with specific target molecules. Many cellular processes, including neurotransmission, muscle contraction, and energy production, rely on carefully maintained ion gradients across cell membranes. Xenobiotics that alter these gradients, either by affecting ion channels or by disrupting the energy-dependent processes that maintain these gradients, can have wide-ranging toxic effects.

In some cases, toxicity may result simply from the physical occupation of a site or space by a xenobiotic. This mechanism is particularly relevant in the context of particulate matter toxicity, where the accumulation of particles in the lungs or other tissues can lead to inflammation, fibrosis, or other pathological changes. Similarly, the formation of crystals or precipitates within tissues, as seen with certain drugs or metabolites, can cause mechanical damage and initiate inflammatory responses.

Cellular Dysfunction

Cellular dysfunction is a critical consequence of toxicant interactions with target molecules. The specific type of primary cellular dysfunction caused by toxicants depends on the role of the affected target molecule. In cases where toxicants react with target molecules involved in cellular regulation, the main effects manifest as dysregulation of gene expression and transient cellular function. Conversely, when the target molecule predominantly supports the cell's internal maintenance, the resulting dysfunction poses a threat to the cell's survival. It's essential to note that the ultimate outcome may vary depending on the specific role of the affected target molecule.

Furthermore, if toxicants interact with target molecules serving external functions, the repercussions extend beyond the individual cell. Such interactions can influence the operation of other cells and integrated organ systems, highlighting the interconnected nature of cellular responses to toxicants. Understanding these dynamics is crucial for comprehending the broader impact of toxicant exposure on cellular function and overall organism health. Alteration of cell functions are illustrated in Figure 5-5.

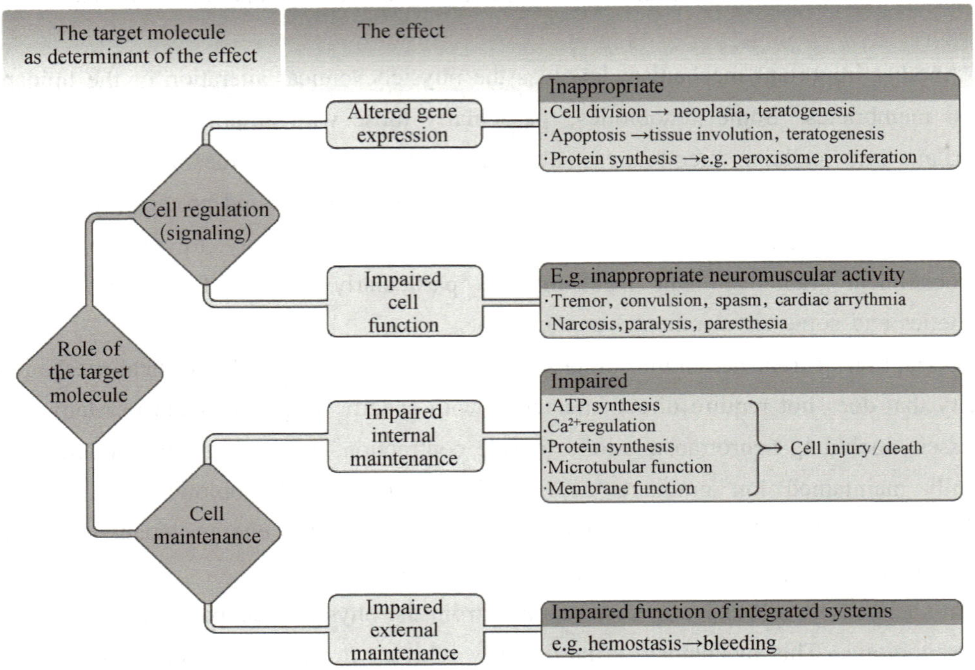

Figure 5-5 Alteration of cell functions

The major effects are manifested as altered regulation of cell signaling or maintenance of cell function, with specific effects including altered gene expression, impaired cell function, impaired intracellular homeostasis, and extracellular homeostasis. Examples of such changes are included on the right side of the figure.

Toxicant-Induced Cellular Dysregulation

Dysregulation of Gene Expression by Toxicants

Gene expression is a tightly regulated process crucial for cellular function and organismal health. Toxicants can disrupt this regulation through various mechanisms, leading to adverse effects.

(1) Dysregulation of Transcription: Toxicants can disrupt transcription through several interconnected mechanisms, significantly impacting gene expression regulation. They may directly interact with transcription elements such as promoters, enhancers, and transcription

factors, altering the binding dynamics between these factors and their target DNA sequences. This can lead to inappropriate gene activation or repression. Additionally, toxicants can bind directly to transcription factors, modifying their structure or function and consequently altering their DNA-binding ability, which can have widespread effects on gene expression patterns. Furthermore, toxicants may induce changes to the DNA itself, either through direct chemical interactions or by influencing epigenetic modifications like DNA methylation or histone modifications. These alterations can affect the accessibility of gene regulatory regions, leading to changes in chromatin structure and gene expression. Epigenetic changes are particularly concerning as they may persist even after the initial exposure has ended, potentially causing long-term alterations in gene expression profiles. Collectively, these mechanisms of transcriptional interference can result in significant disruptions to cellular function and contribute to various pathological conditions, underscoring the importance of understanding toxicant-induced dysregulation of transcription in the field of toxicology. These interactions can lead to inappropriate activation or silencing of genes, potentially affecting cell differentiation and various cellular processes.

(2) Dysregulation of Signal Transduction: Toxicants can significantly disrupt intracellular signaling pathways that play a crucial role in controlling gene activity, leading to dysregulation of signal transduction. This disruption occurs through various mechanisms, with the alteration of protein phosphorylation being the most common. Toxicants can interfere with the delicate balance of kinase and phosphatase activities, leading to abnormal phosphorylation states of key signaling proteins. Additionally, these harmful substances can interfere with G protein activity, a vital component of many signal transduction cascades, potentially altering the transmission of signals from cell surface receptors to intracellular effectors. Toxicants may also disrupt protein-protein interactions, which are essential for the formation of signaling complexes and the proper functioning of signaling pathways. Furthermore, they can modify the synthesis or degradation of signaling proteins, leading to imbalances in the levels of these critical moleculars. These various forms of signaling disruption can have far-reaching consequences on cellular function, particularly affecting cell cycle progression and the ability of tissues to replace damaged cells. Such impairments in cellular renewal and repair processes can ultimately lead to tissue dysfunction, potentially contributing to the development of various pathological conditions. Understanding these mechanisms of signal transduction dysregulation is crucial for comprehending the broad spectrum of toxicant-induced cellular and tissue-level effects.

(3) Dysregulation of Extracellular Signal Production: The dysregulation of extracellular signal production by toxicants is a critical mechanism that can have widespread effects on physiological function, particularly within the endocrine system. Toxicants can interfere with the delicate balance of extracellular signaling molecules in multiple ways. They may affect hormone production or secretion in both the pituitary gland and peripheral endocrine glands,

disrupting the body's hormonal balance. Additionally, toxicants can interfere with autocrine or paracrine signaling pathways, where cells communicate with themselves or nearby cells, respectively. Some toxicants have the ability to mimic natural hormones or act as hormone antagonists, leading to inappropriate activation or inhibition of hormone-responsive pathways. Furthermore, these harmful substances can alter hormone transport mechanisms or affect hormone metabolism, changing the availability and activity of hormones in the body. These various disruptions can result in altered gene expression patterns not only in the cells producing the signaling molecules but also in the cells receiving these signals. Consequently, the effects of toxicant-induced dysregulation of extracellular signal production can ripple through multiple physiological systems, potentially leading to a wide range of adverse health outcomes. This highlights the importance of understanding and addressing the impact of toxicants on extracellular signaling in toxicological research and risk assessment.

Dysregulation of Ongoing Cellular Activity

The dysregulation of ongoing cellular activity is a fundamental mechanism by which toxicants induce adverse effects at the cellular level, leading to organ dysfunction and systemic toxicity. This process involves the interference of toxicants with complex cellular signaling and signal transduction pathways, which are crucial for cells to respond to their environment, communicate, and maintain homeostasis. Toxicants can disrupt any stage of signal coupling, from receptor binding to signal transmission and cellular response, through various mechanisms such as competitive inhibition, allosteric modulation, enzyme inhibition, or interference with second messengers.

The consequences of this disruption can be far-reaching, potentially resulting in altered metabolism, impaired cell growth or division, aberrant differentiation, or cell death. At the tissue and organ level, these effects may manifest as functional impairment, structural changes, or pathological conditions. The insidious nature of toxicant-induced cellular signaling disruption lies in its ability to subtly alter cellular function over time, potentially leading to chronic diseases or increased susceptibility to other stressors.

Electrically excitable cells, such as neurons and muscle cells, are particularly vulnerable to toxicant-induced dysregulation. Xenobiotics can interfere with ion channels, neurotransmitter systems, or other components essential for electrical signaling, leading to altered action potential generation, modified neuronal firing patterns, or disrupted excitation-response coupling. Due to the interconnected nature of the nervous system, toxicant effects on neurons can propagate through neural networks, resulting in complex patterns of neurological dysfunction.

Non-excitable cells, including exocrine secretory cells, pancreatic beta cells, and hepatocytes, are also susceptible to toxicant-induced signaling disruption. While the effects on these cells may appear less immediate or dramatic compared to those on excitable cells, the long-term impacts on health and cellular function can be equally detrimental. Toxicants can interfere with the complex intracellular signaling pathways of non-excitable cells, potentially leading to altered cellular function and contributing to the development of chronic diseases or organ dysfunction.

The interconnected nature of physiological systems means that disruptions in both excitable and non-excitable cells can have ripple effects throughout the body. For example, toxicant-induced alterations in endocrine cell function can lead to hormonal imbalances affecting multiple organ systems, while disruption of immune cell signaling can impact the body's ability to respond to infections and maintain overall health. Understanding these mechanisms is crucial for comprehending the complex effects of toxicants on living organisms and developing strategies to mitigate their impact.

Toxic Alteration of Cellular Maintenance

Impairment of Internal Cellular Maintenance: Toxic Cell Death

In toxic cell death, the impairment of internal cellular maintenance involves complex interactions between multiple biochemical pathways. Cellular survival depends on continuous maintenance of essential functions, including macromolecular synthesis, organelle integrity, and energy production. Toxicants that disrupt these vital processes, particularly those affecting mitochondrial function and protein synthesis, can trigger cell death through three interconnected mechanisms: ATP depletion, calcium dysregulation, and oxidative/nitrative stress.

The agents that impair mitochondrial ATP synthesis can be classified into several types (Table 5-2). When these chemicals interfere with oxidative phosphorylation, they cause ADP accumulation and compromise cellular energy status through several mechanisms, including electron transport chain inhibition, oxidative phosphorylation uncoupling, and direct interference with ATP synthase function. Simultaneously, toxicants alter calcium homeostasis by enhancing Ca^{2+} influx, inhibiting Ca^{2+} efflux, or causing membrane damage. Sustained elevation of intracellular calcium leads to energy depletion, cytoskeletal disruption, enzyme activation, and generation of reactive oxygen and nitrogen species (ROS/RNS).

Oxidative and nitrative stress can arise directly from xenobiotic action or secondarily through calcium-mediated mechanisms. Elevated calcium levels enhance citric acid cycle activity, increase electron transport chain flux, and activate nitric oxide synthase, all contributing to ROS/RNS production. These primary mechanisms create self-amplifying cycles where ATP depletion exacerbates calcium dysregulation, leading to further mitochondrial dysfunction. Similarly, elevated calcium levels facilitate ROS/RNS formation, which in turn inactivates calcium pumps, while ROS/RNS themselves deplete ATP reserves through multiple pathways, including ONOO-induced DNA damage and subsequent PARP activation.

Table 5-2 **Types of Agents Impairing Mitochondrial ATP Synthesis**

Types of Mechanisms of Impairment	Representatives of Agents
A. Class A agents interfere with the delivery of hydrogen to the electron transport chain	fluoroacetate (inhibits the citric acid cycle and the production of reduced cofactors)
B. Class B chemicals inhibit the transfer of electrons along the electron transport chain to oxygen	rotenone, cyanide, paraquat, dinitroaniline, hydrogen sulfide
C. Class C agents interfere with oxygen delivery to the terminal electron transporter, cytochrome oxidase	CO, methemoglobin-forming chemicals (All other chemicals that cause hypoxia)
D. Class D agents inhibit the activity of ATP synthase	
direct inhibition of ATP synthase	DDT, oligomycin
interference with ADP delivery	atractyloside, DDT
interference with inorganic phosphate delivery	benzoquinone
uncouples: deprivation of ATP synthase from its driving force	dinitrophenol, pentachlorophenol, benzonitrile, salicylate
E. Class E agents cause mitochondrial DNA injury and thereby impair synthesis of specific proteins encoded by the mitochondrial genome	zidovudine (dideoxynucleoside antiviral drugs used against AIDS), ethanol (when chronically consumed)

These cascading events ultimately lead to mitochondrial permeability transition (MPT), triggered by the combined effects of calcium overload, ROS/RNS, and metabolic disturbances. MPT results in collapse of membrane potential, cessation of ATP synthesis, matrix swelling, and massive calcium efflux into the cytoplasm. The cellular fate—whether necrosis or apoptosis—depends on the severity of ATP depletion and the extent of mitochondrial damage.

Cell death can proceed through necrosis, occurring with severe ATP depletion and extensive MPT, or through three main apoptotic pathways: the mitochondrial pathway involving cytochrome c release, the DNA damage pathway mediated by p53, and the death receptor pathway involving Fas/TNF signaling. All apoptotic pathways converge on caspase activation. The ultimate mode of cell death is determined by factors including toxicant concentration, exposure duration, ATP availability, and the extent of mitochondrial damage. With lower exposures or early stages typically favoring apoptosis, higher exposures or later stages result in necrosis.

Impairment of External Cellular Maintenance

Toxicants can disrupt the specialized functions of cells that provide critical support to other cells, tissues, and organ systems, leading to widespread physiological dysfunction. This type of toxicity is particularly evident in organs with complex homeostatic functions, such as the liver, kidneys, and endocrine organs. The liver serves as a prime example of how toxicant-induced dysfunction of support cells can have far-reaching consequences throughout the organism.

The liver's parenchymal cells (hepatocytes) perform numerous vital functions that maintain whole-body homeostasis, including plasma protein synthesis, glucose regulation, bile production, xenobiotic biotransformation, and lipid metabolism. Toxicant-induced impairment of these hepatic functions can result in multiple systemic effects. For instance, interference in albumin synthesis leads to reduced plasma osmotic pressure and subsequent edema. Disruption of gluconeogenesis and glycogen storage affects glucose homeostasis, potentially resulting in hypoglycemia. Impaired bile acid synthesis and secretion can cause cholestasis, leading to compromised lipid absorption and accumulation of potentially harmful compounds in the circulation.

Similarly, specialized support cells in other organs can be targeted by toxicants. In the kidneys, damage to podocytes disrupts the glomerular filtration barrier, leading to proteinuria and systemic effects. Toxicant-induced dysfunction of endothelial cells can compromise vascular integrity and tissue perfusion throughout the body. In the nervous system, toxic effects on astrocytes and oligodendrocytes can impair neuronal function through disruption of metabolic support and myelin maintenance.

The mechanisms underlying toxicant effects on support cells frequently involve interference with specific cellular functions, such as protein synthesis and ion transport, disruption of cell-cell communication and signaling pathways, alterations in the extracellular environment, compromise of structural support and tissue architecture, and perturbation of local metabolic networks. The consequences of support cell dysfunction typically extend beyond the directly affected cells, creating cascading effects that can lead to organ failure and systemic toxicity.

Repair or Dysrepair

Repair mechanisms in response to toxicant-induced damage play a crucial role in mitigating the progression of toxic lesions within organisms. These mechanisms operate at molecular, cellular, and tissue levels, encompassing molecular repair, cellular repair, and tissue repair.

Molecular Repair Mechanisms in Response to Toxic Injury

Cellular repair processes at the molecular level represent sophisticated defense mechanisms against toxic injury, involving multiple coordinated pathways that maintain cellular integrity. These repair mechanisms are crucial for preventing the accumulation of damaged biomolecules and maintaining cellular homeostasis.

Protein repair and quality control systems are particularly complex and essential. Proteins with oxidized thiol groups undergo enzymatic reduction through specialized systems, primarily involving thioredoxin and glutaredoxin pathways. These systems utilize NADPH as the ultimate electron donor to maintain their reducing capacity. A specific example is the repair of oxidized hemoglobin (methemoglobin), where electrons are transferred through cytochrome b5 and subsequently regenerated by NADH-dependent cytochrome b5 reductase. This process is critical for maintaining adequate oxygen transport capacity. For irreversibly damaged or misfolded proteins, cells employ the ATP-dependent ubiquitin-proteasome system, which selectively targets and degrades compromised proteins, preventing their potentially toxic accumulation.

Lipid repair mechanisms are equally sophisticated, particularly in addressing peroxidized membrane lipids that can compromise cellular integrity. This process involves a coordinated series of reactions utilizing glutathione peroxidase and glutathione reductase, coupled with NADPH-dependent recycling systems. The repair of oxidized membrane lipids is essential for maintaining membrane fluidity, receptor function, and cellular signaling processes. Additionally, phospholipase A2 can remove oxidized fatty acids from membrane phospholipids, allowing their replacement with intact molecules.

DNA repair mechanisms are perhaps the most elaborate ones, reflecting the critical importance of maintaining genomic integrity. Nuclear DNA is protected by multiple overlapping repair pathways. Direct repair mechanisms, such as O^6-methylguanine-DNA methyltransferase (MGMT), can reverse specific types of DNA damage without breaking the DNA backbone. Base excision repair (BER) addresses oxidized, alkylated, or deaminated bases, while nucleotide excision repair (NER) handles larger DNA lesions, including those caused by UV radiation and chemical adducts. Double-strand break repair utilizes either homologous recombination or non-homologous end joining, depending on the cell cycle phase and the nature of the damage. In contrast, mitochondrial DNA repair capabilities are more limited, primarily relying on BER, making it particularly susceptible to oxidative damage and toxic insult. This vulnerability contributes to the central role of mitochondrial dysfunction in various toxic responses.

Cellular and Tissue Repair Mechanisms in Response to Toxic Injury

Following toxic injury, repair processes occur at both cellular and tissue levels through coordinated mechanisms that restore structural and functional integrity. The nature and efficiency of these repair processes vary significantly among different tissues, reflecting their intrinsic regenerative capacities and specialized functions.

At the cellular level, most tissues respond to injury through the proliferation of surviving cells. This regenerative response is particularly efficient in tissues with high cellular turnover, such as the liver, skin, and gastrointestinal epithelium, where resident stem cells or differentiated cells maintain proliferative capacity. However, this regenerative potential varies markedly among cell types. For instance, mature neurons exhibit limited regenerative capacity, leading to distinct repair mechanisms in the nervous system. In peripheral nerve injury, Schwann cells and macrophages orchestrate repair through myelin debris clearance, axonal guidance, and remyelination support. In contrast, central nervous system repair is more restricted, primarily relying on functional compensation through reserve neurons and synaptic plasticity rather than true regeneration.

The elimination of damaged cells through apoptosis represents a crucial component of the repair process. This programmed cell death pathway serves as a precise mechanism for removing compromised cells while minimizing inflammatory damage to surrounding tissue. Apoptosis is particularly important in tissues with active cell turnover, where it facilitates the orderly replacement of damaged cells. However, in tissues composed primarily of post-mitotic cells, such as cardiac muscle and neurons, the loss of cells through apoptosis can result in permanent functional deficits due to limited regenerative capacity.

Cellular proliferation following injury involves complex signaling cascades initiated by damage-associated molecular patterns (DAMPs) released from injured cells. These signals activate survival pathways in viable cells and stimulate proliferation through growth factors and cytokines. The proliferative response must be precisely regulated to restore tissue architecture while preventing excessive cell growth. This process involves the coordinated action of multiple cell types, including parenchymal cells, stromal cells, and inflammatory cells.

At the tissue level, repair involves not only cellular regeneration but also the restoration of the extracellular matrix and tissue architecture. This process begins with the removal of damaged tissue components and proceeds through stages of cell proliferation, matrix deposition, and tissue remodeling. The inflammatory response, while potentially damaging if excessive, plays a crucial role in initiating and coordinating repair processes. Resident macrophages and activated endothelial cells produce cytokines and growth factors that guide the repair process.

Side reactions accompanying tissue repair include local and systemic responses that support the healing process. Local inflammation helps contain damage and initiates repair mechanisms, while systemic responses, such as acute-phase protein production and fever, create an environment conducive to tissue repair. These responses are mediated by inflammatory mediators and involve complex interactions among multiple cell types and organ systems.

The success of cellular and tissue repair depends on multiple factors, including the extent of initial damage, the tissue's regenerative capacity, and the efficiency of repair mechanisms. Understanding these processes is crucial for developing therapeutic strategies to enhance repair and regeneration following toxic injury.

Mechanisms and Manifestations of Repair Failure in Toxic Injury

Repair failure, or dysrepair, represents a critical component in the progression of toxic injury, occurring at molecular, cellular, and tissue levels. The mechanisms underlying repair failure are complex and multifaceted, often leading to severe pathological outcomes.

Several fundamental mechanisms contribute to repair failure. First, repair processes may exhibit imperfect fidelity, allowing some forms of damage to persist unrepaired. Second, the magnitude of toxic injury may overwhelm existing repair capacity, particularly when critical enzymes or cofactors become depleted. Third, toxicants may directly impair repair mechanisms themselves, creating a vicious cycle of increasing damage. Fourth, certain forms of toxic injury, such as covalent modification of proteins by reactive metabolites, may present intrinsic challenges to repair processes.

The progression of toxic injury in the context of repair failure manifests through several key pathological processes. When molecular repair mechanisms prove insufficient or molecular damage exceeds repair capacity, cellular injury may progress to necrosis. This progression is particularly evident in situations where initial repair mechanisms are overwhelmed or impaired. The efficiency of repair processes emerges as a crucial determinant in dose-response relationships for tissue-damaging toxicants, often establishing threshold effects in toxic responses.

Fibrosis represents a distinctive manifestation of dysrepair at the tissue level. This pathological process develops when the initial reparative response, characterized by increased extracellular matrix production, becomes dysregulated. The resulting excessive accumulation of extracellular matrix components and alterations in matrix composition lead to progressive tissue dysfunction. This process often involves the persistent activation of myofibroblasts and altered expression of matrix-remodeling enzymes, reflecting a fundamental failure in the resolution phase of tissue repair.

Chemical carcinogenesis exemplifies the complex interplay of multiple repair failures. This process typically involves concurrent failures in several protective mechanisms: inadequate DNA repair allowing the persistence of mutagenic lesions, compromised apoptotic responses failing to eliminate damaged cells, and dysregulation of proliferative controls permitting the expansion of transformed cell populations. These repair failures may act synergistically to promote neoplastic transformation and tumor progression.

The role of apoptosis and cell proliferation in repair failure deserves special attention.

These processes normally function as complementary mechanisms to maintain tissue homeostasis and prevent the propagation of toxic injury. When apoptotic mechanisms fail to eliminate irreparably damaged cells, or proliferative responses become dysregulated, the progression of toxic injury may accelerate. The balance between these processes is particularly critical in tissues with high cellular turnover.

Chronic toxic injury often results in complex patterns of repair failure across multiple levels of biological organization. This can create self-perpetuating cycles of damage and inappropriate repair responses. For example, persistent tissue injury may lead to chronic inflammation, which can further promote tissue damage and aberrant repair responses, ultimately contributing to progressive organ dysfunction.

(Li Jianxiang)

CHAPTER 6

Factors Influencing Toxic Effects

Introduction

To manifest the toxic effect within a biological system, the poison, its metabolites, or transformation products must access the pertinent receptor site within the system and attain a sufficient concentration for an adequate duration. Consequently, it is evident that the dosage, route, and duration of exposure significantly influence the biological response of the body to specific poisons. Nevertheless, despite rigorous control over these variables, individuals within a population may still exhibit notable variations in their response to a given poison. Some of these disparities can be attributed to differences in factors influencing the poison's absorption, distribution, metabolism, and excretion. This chapter examines factors that influence toxicological responses, which can be classified into five main categories: ① factors related to the toxic agent, ② factors influencing the subject, ③ factors influencing exposure, ④ external environmental factors, ⑤ interactive toxicity of chemical mixtures.

Factors Related to the Toxic Agent

Chemical Structure

Molecular Structure

Chemical substances produce diverse biological responses that are fundamentally determined by their molecular properties. These effects arise from specific structural recognition and interaction with biological targets, where minor structural modifications can lead to significant changes in biological activity.

This principle is well demonstrated by parathion and its oxidation product parathion-sulfone, both organophosphate insecticides. The oxidative conversion of parathion to paraoxon results in enhanced toxicity (Figure 6-1). Another example is found in fluorinated fatty alcohols and acids, where toxicity correlates with carbon chain length. Compounds with even-numbered carbon chains typically show greater toxicity, while in fluoronitro compounds, odd-numbered carbon chains exhibit higher toxicity within their respective series.

Regarding aflatoxins, AFB_1, AFB_2, AFG_1, and AFG_2 are the four predominant members of this family (Figure 6-2). A notable distinction lies in their structural composition, with B-series aflatoxins possessing a cyclopentanone ring, whereas G-series aflatoxins feature a lactone ring. Despite this, AFB_1 stands out as the most potent carcinogen, followed by AFG_1, AFB_2, and then AFG_2 in terms of their carcinogenic properties.

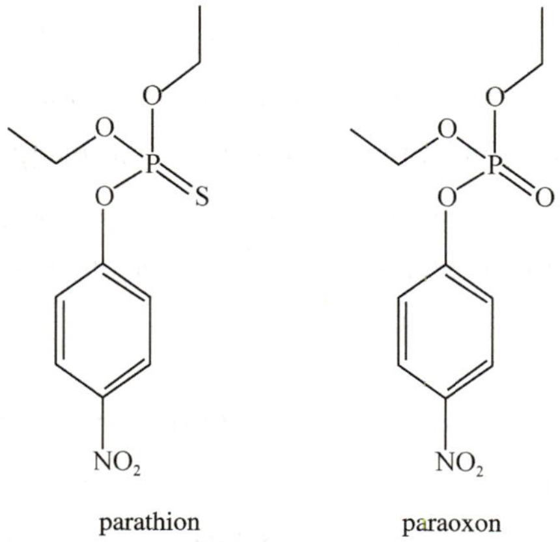

Figure 6-1 **The structure of parathion and paraoxon**

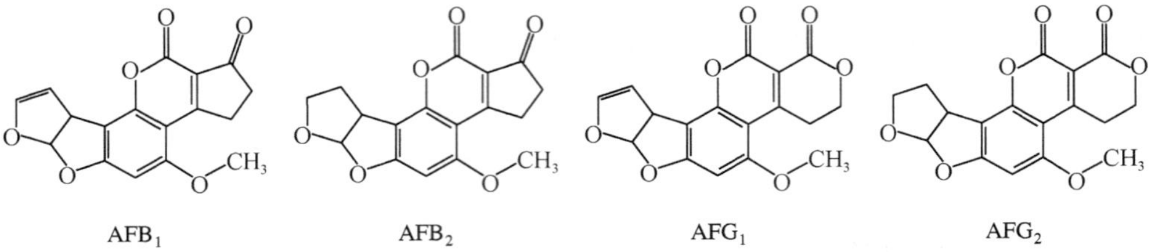

Figure 6-2 **The structure of AFB_1, AFB_2, AFG_1 and AFG_2**

The analysis of molecular structures offers invaluable insights into identifying the potential hazards posed by specific chemicals. The Structure-Activity Relationship (SAR) framework underpins this process, elucidating the intricate connection between the molecular structure of drugs, toxins, and their impact on animals, plants, and the environment. By harnessing advanced intelligent software, particularly neural networks, scientists can delve into vast repositories of toxicological data and systematically establish the link between molecular structures and their corresponding biological activities.

When these relationships are formulated mathematically, they evolve into Quantitative Structure-Activity Relationship (QSAR), which endows researchers with the ability to predict the biological effects of chemicals with a degree of precision.

One of the primary benefits envisioned for QSAR lies in its potential to streamline the drug discovery and safety assessment processes. By predicting the adverse effects of novel compounds in silico, QSAR models can significantly reduce the need for costly and time-consuming biological testing. This not only accelerates the pace of scientific research but also contributes to more efficient use of resources and enhances protection of animal welfare.

As the field of QSAR continues to evolve, it is anticipated that these models will become increasingly sophisticated, enabling more accurate predictions across a broader range of chemical entities and biological endpoints. Ultimately, the integration of QSAR into the drug development pipeline has the potential to revolutionize the way we assess the safety and efficacy of chemicals, leading to safer products and a healthier environment.

Stereoisomers

Stereoisomers, particularly enantiomers, are mirror images of each other that cannot be superimposed, often arising from the presence of chiral centers in molecules. In the context of exogenous chemicals, including drugs, the existence of these stereoisomers can significantly impact their biological behavior and effects.

The stereoselective biotransformation of chiral compounds is a well-documented phenomenon in which one enantiomer is metabolized faster or more efficiently than its counterpart. This is exemplified by the anti-epileptic drug mephenytoin, which exists as a racemic mixture of R- and S-phenytoin enantiomers. In humans, the S-isomer undergoes faster hydroxylation and elimination, highlighting the importance of considering stereochemistry in drug efficacy and pharmacokinetics.

Moreover, the inhibitory effects of chiral compounds on metabolic enzymes, such as the cytochrome P450 enzymes, can also display stereoselectivity. Quinidine, an inhibitor of CYP2D6, illustrates this point, as its enantiomer quinine exhibits much weaker inhibitory activity. This underscores the need to understand the stereochemical basis of drug-enzyme interactions for predicting drug responses and potential adverse effects.

The case of benzo(a)pyrene and its four metabolic products, specifically the benzo(a)pyrene-7, 8-diol-9, 10-epoxides, further emphasizes the importance of stereochemistry in determining biological activity. Despite structural similarities among these stereoisomers, only one, (+)-benzo(a)pyrene 7, 8-diol-9, 10-epoxide-2 (Figure 6-3), possesses significant carcinogenicity. Its ability to preferentially bind to deoxyguanosine residues and form mutagenic N-2 adducts underscores the role of stereochemistry in modulating the carcinogenicity of polycyclic aromatic hydrocarbons (PAHs).

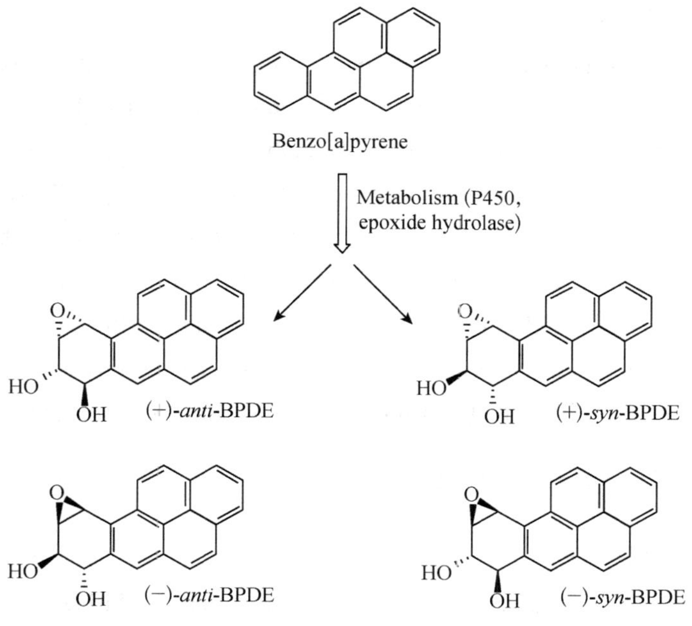

Figure 6-3 Metabolites of Benzo [*a*] pyrene, arrow head represents ultimate carcinogenic species

Structure Similar to Other Chemicals

The molecular structure of a chemical determines not only its toxic potency but also governs its ADME processes within biological systems. A critical aspect of this structure-dependent behavior is evident in the transport mechanisms across biological barriers.

While the gastrointestinal tract employs active transport for specific nutrients and pharmaceuticals, passive diffusion remains the primary mechanism for xenobiotic absorption. However, toxicants structurally resembling endogenous substances may exploit existing transport mechanisms, leading to enhanced absorption and potential toxicity.

A classic example is the transport of methylmercury across biological barriers. Methylmercury forms a complex with cysteine that structurally mimics methionine, enabling its recognition and transport by large neutral amino acid carriers. This molecular mimicry facilitates its passage across the blood-brain barrier, resulting in neurotoxicity.

Transport mechanisms demonstrate remarkable structural specificity in biological systems. The dipeptide and oligopeptide transport system facilitates the absorption of β-lactam antibiotics through specific molecular recognition. Similarly, the stereoselective carrier-mediated transport of chiral compounds becomes particularly evident at low concentrations, where active transport against concentration gradients depends on precise structural compatibility. These structure-dependent transport mechanisms significantly influence a compound's distribution, bioavailability, and ultimately, its toxic potential.

Chemical Valence

Chromium exhibits the ability to form oxides with a diverse range of valence, spanning from Cr^{2+} to Cr^{6+}. However, among these compounds, only those featuring Cr^{3+} and Cr^{6+} valence manifest significant biological effects. Notably, Cr^{6+} compounds display insolubility in water, rendering Cr^{3+} compounds more prone to permeating through cell membranes.

Once within the body, Cr^{6+} undergoes reduction to Cr^{3+}, which subsequently forms complexes with macromolecular entities within cells, triggering toxic reactions. The carcinogenic process associated with lung cancer, specifically attributed to Cr^{6+}, involves its reduction to Cr^{3+} and the generation of an active intermediate product. This intermediate product, in turn, prompts bronchial cell transformation, ultimately leading to carcinogenesis.

Physicochemical Properties

Vapor Pressure

The vapor pressure of a chemical substance significantly influences its potential for respiratory exposure. This physical property is particularly crucial in designing inhalation toxicity studies, as it determines the evaporation rate of test substances under experimental conditions. Volatile organic compounds (VOCs) such as benzene, toluene, and carbon tetrachloride exemplify substances with high vapor pressures that readily form vapors at room temperature.

High vapor pressure substances present unique challenges in oral toxicity studies due to their tendency to volatilize from animal feed. For instance, carbon disulfide (CS_2), with its low boiling point of 46.3 ℃ and high vapor pressure of 297 mmHg (39.5 kPa) at 20 ℃, can rapidly evaporate from feed matrices, leading to significant underestimation of the actual exposure dose.

Solubility

Solubility is a pivotal physical property that significantly influences the absorption and distribution of compounds within the body. The solubility and dispersibility of chemicals in lipids directly affect their uptake in the gastrointestinal (GI) tract. For instance, highly lipophilic compounds like DDT and PCBs demonstrate enhanced absorption due to their ability to readily traverse biological membranes.

In the case of organic acids or bases, absorption patterns are particularly pH-dependent. These toxins exhibit heightened absorption through simple diffusion within specific regions of the GI tract, primarily in their lipid-soluble (non-ionic) state. The gastric environment (pH 1–2) differs markedly from the small intestine (pH 6.8–7.4), creating distinct absorption profiles. Aspirin, a weak organic acid (pKa 3.5), demonstrates enhanced absorption in the acidic stomach environment where it exists predominantly in its non-ionized form. Conversely, weak bases like nicotine show preferential absorption in the small intestine where they become more lipid-soluble.

Solid chemicals with poor solubility, such as lead chromate or mercury sulfide, exhibit limited absorption in the GI tract due to reduced contact with the mucosal lining. This principle explains why metallic mercury poses minimal risk when ingested but presents significant hazards when inhaled as vapor.

The absorption of gases in the lungs depends on their blood/gas partition coefficient. Highly soluble gases like chloroform (blood/gas partition coefficient = 10.3) or hydrogen cyanide rapidly achieve high blood concentrations during each breathing cycle. In contrast, poorly soluble gases such as nitrogen (blood/gas partition coefficient = 0.015) show limited blood uptake, resulting in lower systemic exposure.

Particle Size

The dispersion of particulate matter, specifically its size, is paramount in elucidating the inhalational toxicity of aerosols. This is because particle size significantly influences the deposition location of toxicants within the respiratory system, as well as the underlying mechanisms and efficiency of clearance by the respiratory tract.

The primary determinant of aerosol deposition is the size of the particles. Larger particles, with diameters of 5 μm or larger, tend to be deposited primarily in the nasopharynx. Medium-sized particles, ranging from 1 to 5 μm in diameter, predominantly settle in the bronchial tubes of the lungs. These particles are primarily cleared through the retrograde movement of the mucus layer, facilitated by cilia in the respiratory tract.

Conversely, particles with diameters of 1 μm or smaller have the capability to penetrate deeply into the alveoli. Once there, they can either be absorbed directly into the bloodstream or phagocytosed by alveolar macrophages for subsequent clearance via the lymphatic system.

Ionization

Numerous chemicals are classified as weak organic acids or bases, which can exist in either non-ionized or ionized forms within a solution. Typically, these compounds must adopt an uncharged or non-ionized state to facilitate passive diffusion across biological membranes. Variations in the environmental pH can either elevate the degree of ionization of toxins or diminish the proportion of their non-ionized forms, thereby modulating the transmembrane transport of these toxins.

Weak organic acids and bases in their non-ionized state exhibit lipophilic properties, enabling them to traverse the cell membrane with ease. The rate of this transport is directly proportional to their lipophilicity. The dissociation of these acids and bases in solution is governed by their respective dissociation constants. Consequently, organic acids are more likely to traverse the membrane from acidic environments, whereas organic bases prefer alkaline environments for their membrane permeation.

When a chemical substance is in its dissociated state, it generally exhibits low fat solubility, hindering its passage through the lipid bilayer of the cell membrane. However, some low molecular weight organic anions or cations may still traverse hydrophilic pores, albeit at a relatively slow rate (except for those with extremely small molecular weights). This is because of the fact that hydrophilic pores occupy a smaller area on the cell membrane compared to lipid regions.

Molecular Weight and Membrane Permeability

The majority of chemicals traverse membranes via simple diffusion. Hydrophilic molecules with a molecular weight of approximately 600 or less can permeate the membrane through hydrophilic pores, whereas hydrophobic molecules diffuse through the lipid bilayer. The ease of passage through hydrophilic pores increases with the decreasing size of the hydrophilic molecule, facilitating simple diffusion. Consequently, ethanol is rapidly absorbed from the stomach and small intestine and efficiently diffuses from the bloodstream to various tissues throughout the body.

Impact of Impurities and Contaminants

In assessing the toxicity of a specific chemical, the chemical composition of the samples under investigation is paramount as it significantly influences the overall toxicity. The toxicity of impurities or contaminants present may vastly differ from that of the primary substance being tested and can significantly alter the response of the biological system under examination. For instance, during the production of 2, 4, 5-T, trace amounts of highly toxic impurities like TCDD may be formed. Notably, LD_{50} of 2, 4, 5-T for guinea pigs is 630, 000 times higher than that of TCDD, while the oral LD_{50} of TCDD for female rats is merely 1/10, 000 of that of 2, 4, 5-T's. Hence, even if the TCDD content in 2, 4, 5-T as an impurity is below 0. 5 mg/kg, the observed toxicity is primarily attributed to TCDD rather than 2, 4, 5-T itself. Furthermore, 2, 4, 5-T alone is not carcinogenic when TCDD concentrations are between 0. 12 mg/kg and 0. 033 mg/kg. However, in the presence of 0. 05 ppm TCDD or higher concentrations, 2, 4, 5-T becomes carcinogenic in specific strains of mice and rats. Another study underscores that when TCDD concentrations in 2, 4, 5-T reach 30 mg/kg, its dermal carcinogenicity becomes pronounced.

Factors Influencing the Subject

Toxic effects result from interactions between xenobiotics and living organisms. For toxicity to occur, chemical substances must reach and react with target molecules in the body. Therefore, various biological factors can influence the toxic effects of xenobiotics.

Different animal species may exhibit quantitative and/or qualitative differences in their responses to the same xenobiotic. For example, benzene exposure causes leukopenia in rabbits but leukocytosis in dogs. Furthermore, when humans or animals are exposed to certain xenobiotics under identical dosage and exposure conditions, individual responses can range from no effect to severe injury or death. Such individual variations exist even between identical twins.

Among populations in the same environment, individuals may show significant differences in their risk of illness and severity of damage. Those who demonstrate unusual sensitivity to toxic effects are considered susceptible individuals or high-risk individuals.

The main biological factors affecting xenobiotic toxicity are ① Species and strain variations; ② Genetic variations between individuals; ③ Other physiological factors.

Species and Strain Variations

Anatomical and Morphological Divergences

Due to genomic variations, different species show distinct characteristics in their anatomy, physiology, and transport processes. These differences are evident in organ structure, chromosomal numbers, and physiological parameters. For instance, liver lobulation varies across species, with humans having 5 lobes, dogs 7 lobes, rabbits 5 lobes, mice 4 lobes, and rats 6 lobes (with no gallbladder). Somatic chromosome numbers also differ, being 46 in humans, 78 in dogs, 44 in rabbits, 40 in mice, and 42 in rats. Daily urine output shows marked variation, with rats exhibiting much higher rates than humans, leading to faster xenobiotic excretion. Additionally, pulse rates inversely correlate with body weight across species, with mice having extremely high pulse rates and cardiac output relative to blood volume, resulting in shorter plasma half-lives for xenobiotics.

Variations in anatomical structures constitute a pivotal factor contributing to disparities in absorption rates across different species, particularly through the small intestine. For instance, marked differences exist in the length and functional capabilities of the small intestine between ruminants and omnivores. Since the majority of exogenous compounds undergo absorption via passive diffusion through the intestinal mucosa, this transport mechanism is inherently reliant on both the area and specific location of absorption, thereby underpinning the role of these factors in eliciting species-specific differences in some instances.

Furthermore, anatomical and morphological differences carry significant implications for the selection of experimental animals. In experimental research endeavors focused on emphysema, a comparative analysis was undertaken across multiple animal species to evaluate their pathological and morphological alterations in relation to humans. Notably, horses emerged as the species whose morphological changes most closely resembled those observed in humans, thereby reinforcing their suitability as experimental animals for emphysema research.

Metabolic Variations

Species variations in toxic responses primarily result from differences in metabolic transformation and detoxification mechanisms. This is exemplified by varying responses to cyclohexobarbital across species and mouse strains due to different detoxification enzyme activities. Another notable example is aniline metabolism, which produces more toxic o-aminophenol in pigs and dogs but less toxic p-aminophenol in rabbits. Bioactivation differences also significantly influence toxicity, as demonstrated by β-naphthylamine metabolism, where humans efficiently catalyze N-acetylation, rats are slow acetylators, and dogs lack cytosolic N-acetyltransferase but can still perform activation through alternative pathways. Similarly, 2-acetylaminofluorene (2-AAF) shows species-specific carcinogenicity due to different metabolic pathways.

Since these species differences in anatomy, physiology, and biochemistry stem from genomic variations, comparative studies of structural and functional genomics between humans and animals are essential. Such research helps better understand how species differences influence toxic effects and improves the extrapolation of animal data to humans, ultimately enhancing the reliability of toxicological assessments.

Genetic Variations Among Individuals

Individual variation refers to differences in toxic responses to xenobiotics among members of the same species or strain. Current research suggests that genetic polymorphisms are a major factor contributing to individual differences in toxic responses and disease susceptibility. Additionally, individual repair capabilities and receptor-mediated responses significantly influence toxicity outcomes.

Metabolic Enzyme Polymorphisms

Metabolic enzyme polymorphisms can lead to substantial differences in xenobiotic metabolism. Key polymorphic enzymes include Phase Ⅰ enzymes like Cytochrome P450 (CYP), and Phase Ⅱ enzymes such as Glutathione S-transferases (GST).

Cytochrome P450 enzymes, especially CYP2D6, show significant ethnic variations. For instance, in Chinese populations, CYP2D6 metabolizer phenotypes are distributed as follows: ultra-rapid metabolizers (35.83%), extensive metabolizers (63.33%), and poor metabolizers (0.8%). This contrasts with Caucasian populations, where poor metabolizers comprise 5%–10%. These differences affect drug responses and toxicity profiles.

GST polymorphisms influence detoxification capabilities. GSTM1, GSTT1, and GSTP1 genetic variations are associated with increased susceptibility to various cancers. G-6-PD deficiency, more prevalent in Mediterranean and certain Asian populations, can lead to hemolytic anemia when exposed to specific xenobiotics.

DNA Repair Capacity Variations

Individual differences in repair capabilities significantly impact toxic responses. Different tissues exhibit varying regenerative capacities, liver and kidney show robust regeneration, while neural tissue has limited repair ability. DNA repair enzyme polymorphisms, exemplified by conditions like Xeroderma Pigmentosum (XP), demonstrate how repair deficiencies can dramatically increase sensitivity to environmental toxicants.

O^6-methylguanine-DNA methyltransferase (MGMT) activity varies considerably among tissues and individuals, influencing susceptibility to alkylating agents and certain cancers.

Receptor Variations

Receptors, crucial proteins for xenobiotic interactions, show individual variations in both number and functionality. For example, mutations in calcium release channel receptors can lead to severe reactions to certain anesthetics. The Aryl hydrocarbon receptor (AhR) system, important in dioxin toxicity, exhibits polymorphisms that affect toxic responses and cancer susceptibility.

Recent research has revealed complex receptor-mediated pathways, such as TCDD's interaction with estrogen receptors through AhR-dependent mechanisms, and AhR-independent mitochondrial stress responses. These findings highlight the complexity of receptor-mediated toxic responses and their role in disease development.

Other Physiological Factors

Beyond species, strain, and individual genetic variations, other physiological factors can significantly modulate the toxicity of exogenous chemicals. These factors primarily include health state, immune state, age, gender, nutritional condition, and lifestyle.

Health and Immune State

Health conditions can profoundly impact chemical toxicity. Compromised physiological states often exacerbate the damaging effects of exogenous chemicals. For instance, stress induced by illnesses such as a cold can enhance the hydroxylation of aromatic compounds. Respiratory diseases like asthma may increase sensitivity to air pollutants such as sulfur dioxide (SO_2). Endocrine imbalances can alter toxicity sensitivity. For example, hyperthyroidism and hyperinsulinemia can affect an individual's response to toxins. Hepatic dysfunction significantly impairs the metabolism of xenobiotics, as the liver is the primary organ for xenobiotic metabolism. Liver disease leads to reduced metabolic capacity, extending the plasma half-life of numerous chemicals. Similarly, renal insufficiency or failure prolongs the elimination half-life of many xenobiotics, affecting both efficacy and toxicity.

Low or excessively high immune responses can directly modulate toxicity. Immunocompromised individuals are more vulnerable to chemical insults. Allergic reactions can occur upon exposure to specific drugs or metals, though this is relatively uncommon, primarily affecting sensitive individuals. Furthermore, pregnant or lactating mothers exhibit increased sensitivity to xenobiotic exposure, often with adverse consequences for the developing fetus outweighing any potential benefits.

Age

Age-related differences in organ function significantly affect toxicological responses. Both elderly individuals and infants generally show higher sensitivity to toxic effects due to reduced biotransport and metabolic capabilities compared to healthy adults.

Age impacts biotransport through various mechanisms. Newborns and elderly individuals have lower plasma protein levels, resulting in reduced chemical binding and increased free chemical concentrations. For instance, only 20% of lidocaine binds to plasma proteins in newborns, compared to 70% in adults. Reduced gastric acid secretion in neonates and the elderly alters the absorption of certain xenobiotics and drugs; for example, penicillin absorption increases while acetaminophen absorption decreases. Furthermore, reduced glomerular filtration and tubular secretion in neonates and the elderly diminish the body's clearance of xenobiotics, prolonging exposure and increasing the risk of cumulative toxicity with chronic administration. The higher total body water content in neonates (which decreases with age) significantly influences the distribution of water-soluble drugs. The immature blood-brain barrier in neonates increases their susceptibility to the central nervous system toxicity of substances like morphine. Studies indicate that young children absorb lead 4-5 times and cadmium 20 times more efficiently than adults, possibly due to the interaction of milk proteins with metals, facilitating absorption.

The metabolic capacity of the body varies considerably across different age groups. Fetal and neonatal animals generally exhibit low drug-metabolizing enzyme activity. The time required to reach adult levels varies across species. For instance, the activity of microsomal monooxygenase is low at birth in rats, reaching adult levels only after 30 days, while detectable levels (20%-50% of adult levels) are present in human fetuses at six months gestation. Young animals demonstrate increased sensitivity to many toxins, often 1.5 to 10 times that of adults, primarily due to deficient detoxification enzyme systems. For example, a single dose of 10 mg/kg of hexobarbital induces sleep lasting over 360 minutes in one-day-old mice, but only 27 minutes in 21-day-old mice. Acetaminophen, requiring metabolic activation, shows lower hepatotoxicity in neonatal mice than in adults; carbon tetrachloride exhibits no hepatotoxicity in neonatal rats. Chloramphenicol is primarily excreted as glucuronide conjugates. The deficiency of glucuronidation in neonates leads to sustained high plasma levels of unconjugated chloramphenicol, causing severe cyanosis and even death in infants. Since the developmental deficiency affects not only detoxification enzymes but also activating enzymes, the toxicity of chemicals isn't uniformly higher in infants and children; some exhibit lower toxicity in younger individuals. For example, the LD_{50} of DDT is reported to be more than 20 times higher in neonatal rats than in adults. Elderly animals often exhibit reduced metabolic capacity for certain chemicals compared to adults. Decreased activity of enzymes such as glucose-6-phosphatase, mitochondrial cytochrome reductase, and erythrocyte membrane Na^+/K^+-ATPase in the liver and kidneys of aged rats contributes to increased sensitivity to specific chemicals.

Gender

While the overall response to chemicals is generally similar between the sexes, some exhibit sex-based differences in toxicity. Adult females often display greater sensitivity than males, although exceptions exist.

Males generally metabolize chemicals faster than females. For example, the insecticide aldrin is metabolized more rapidly to the more toxic epoxide in male rats. Hexobarbital has a longer biological half-life and induces a longer sleep duration in female rats than in male ones. Glucuronidation of 1-naphthol and acetylation of sulfonamides are more efficient in male rats. Therefore, metabolically activated chemicals usually increase toxicity in males, while those detoxified by metabolism typically decrease toxicity in males. For instance, parathion, an organophosphate detoxified by metabolism, is twice as toxic in female rats compared to male ones; procaine is more extensively hydrolyzed in males, reducing its toxicity.

These metabolic sex differences are closely linked to sex hormones and typically manifest from sexual maturity through old age. Chloroform-induced nephrotoxicity in mice exhibits a marked sex difference, with males significantly more susceptible than females. Castration eliminates this difference in males, and androgen replacement restores it.

Sex differences in toxicity can also stem from variations in excretion. For example, the food additive butylated hydroxytoluene is primarily excreted in urine in male rats and in bile (feces) in females. The hepatocarcinogenic effect of the industrial chemical 2, 4-dinitrotoluene exhibits sex differences, with male rats being more susceptible. This is because glucuronide conjugates are more extensively excreted in bile in males, where they can be hydrolyzed, reduced, and reabsorbed, with the reduced metabolites contributing to liver cancer development.

Nutritional Condition and Lifestyle

Nutritional condition strongly influences the bioavailability of many chemicals. For example, iron deficiency enhances cadmium gastrointestinal absorption; individuals with low serum ferritin levels absorb cadmium twice as efficiently as those with normal levels. Dietary and lifestyle habits can alter xenobiotic metabolism, physiological or biochemical functions, and nutritional condition, thus affecting toxicity. Therefore, a balanced diet and adequate nutrition are crucial. In toxicological animal studies, nutritional deficiencies in experimental animals can lead to disease and compromise research results, highlighting the necessity of complete and sufficient nutrient provision.

Nutrient deficiencies or imbalances affect drug metabolism; the effects of protein deficiency on xenobiotic metabolism are well-documented. Animals fed a 5% protein diet exhibit lower microsomal protein levels and significantly reduced enzyme activity compared to those fed a 20% protein diet. Reduced plasma albumin levels following a low-protein diet increase the plasma levels of unbound chemicals, thus enhancing toxicity. Fatty acid deficiency lowers microsomal enzyme levels and activity, reducing the metabolism of ethylmorphine, hexobarbital, and aniline. This may be due to the essential role of lipids in cytochrome P450 function.

Deficiencies in vitamins and minerals also impair xenobiotic metabolism. Vitamins C, vitamins E, and vitamins B complex, either directly or indirectly, participate in cytochrome P450 system regulation; their deficiencies reduce biotransformation rates. Vitamin A deficiency affects endoplasmic reticulum structure, impairing mixed-function oxidase activity. Mineral deficiencies (calcium, copper, magnesium, zinc, etc.) reduce cytochrome P450-catalyzed oxidation-reduction reactions and biotransformation activity. Restoring mineral intake restores cytochrome P450 activity to physiological levels. Starvation reduces essential cofactors; for example, sulfates required for phase Ⅱ conjugation reactions may be depleted. Short-term food deprivation enhances the demethylation of dimethylnitrosamine, increasing hepatotoxicity. Overnight fasting increases the hepatotoxicity of acetaminophen and bromobenzene, possibly due to the depletion of 50% of normal glutathione levels, making insufficient glutathione available for detoxification. The detrimental effects of alcohol consumption and smoking are well-established; individuals with these habits may exhibit increased sensitivity to certain toxic effects upon exposure to other toxins. Furthermore, social, psychological, and mental factors also influence the toxic effects of xenobiotics to varying degrees.

Factors Influencing Exposure

Routes and Sites of Exposure

Toxins primarily enter the body through the digestive tract, lungs, skin, and via injection routes. Notably, when toxins directly access to the bloodstream through intravenous injection, their effects are most pronounced and elicit the fastest bodily response. In contrast, the toxicity effects vary across exposure routes, with skin exposure typically exhibiting the mildest effects, followed by oral, intradermal, muscle, subcutaneous, abdominal cavity, and inhalation exposure in ascending order of severity. Additionally, the route of exposure significantly impacts toxicity. For instance, toxins ingested orally undergo detoxification in the liver before entering systemic circulation, resulting in reduced toxicity compared to toxins that bypass the liver via inhalation and directly enter the bloodstream.

Organ and System Sensitivity

The route of exposure determines which organ or physiological system is most sensitive and exhibits the earliest dose-response effects. In the case of insecticides, at high doses, any exposure route can elicit characteristic cholinergic neurotoxicity symptoms across various organs. However, at lower doses, only specific organs respond. Skin exposure, for example, may initially manifest as local sweating and muscle twitching before systemic toxicity becomes apparent. Inhalation exposure can trigger bronchial constriction, while ingestion may cause gastrointestinal discomfort prior to or at lower doses than those required to induce systemic symptoms.

Furthermore, the route of exposure modulates the toxicity of chemicals. When ingested, toxins travel through the portal vein to the liver, where they undergo detoxification, resulting in reduced toxicity compared to their direct entry into the bloodstream via inhalation. This underscores the importance of considering exposure routes when assessing the potential health risks associated with toxic chemicals.

Duration and Frequency of Exposure

For numerous chemicals, the toxicological consequences diverge significantly between single and repeated exposures. For instance, the initial acute toxicity of benzene primarily manifests as an inhibitory effect on the central nervous system, whereas repeated exposure can harm the bone marrow and elevate the risk of leukemia. If a toxicant is rapidly absorbed during acute exposure, it may elicit prompt toxicity, but also delayed effects akin to or distinct from those seen in chronic exposure scenarios. Conversely, chronic exposure can result in both long-term, low-concentration toxicity and rapid toxicity following individual exposures. In describing the attributes of a chemical, understanding not only the nature of its effects but also the duration of exposure is crucial.

Another pivotal time-dependent factor is the frequency of exposure. When a chemical's half-life approximates the inter-exposure interval, even a single exposure can induce severe toxicity. Conversely, distributing the same dose over multiple exposures may render it non-toxic. If the chemical's clearance time significantly exceeds the inter-exposure interval, achieving toxic concentrations may require only a few administrations. Alternatively, if the half-life is much shorter than the interval, the chemical will fail to reach toxic concentrations regardless of the number of exposures. Importantly, even non-accumulative chemicals can damage tissues or cells, emphasizing the significance of whether these damages can be repaired during the inter-exposure period. Accumulative chemicals posing irreversible toxic effects or irreparable damage during the exposure interval may give rise to chronic toxicity. Thus, for any type of repeated exposure, the production of toxicity is influenced, and sometimes solely determined, by the frequency of exposure, regardless of its duration.

Carrier Substances or Vehicles

When chemicals enter the body, their solvents or carrier substances can significantly impact their toxic effects. Certain solvents can profoundly alter the absorption of chemicals following digestion, inhalation, or localized exposure.

Water, a ubiquitous chemical solvent, plays a pivotal role in skin permeability. Typically, the stratum corneum, the outermost layer of skin, contains approximately 7% water. Upon excessive exposure to water, the stratum corneum can absorb water, causing its weight to increase by 3–5 times and its permeability to rise by 2–3 times. Additionally, when the skin surface is covered with fabrics, face creams, ointments, or similar substances, the increased moisture in the epidermis can enhance the absorption of certain toxins.

Surfactants, though seemingly resistant to direct absorption, can modify the lipid pathways in the skin by fluidizing and defatting the proteins and fats within the stratum corneum, thereby altering its structure. Furthermore, some solvents have the ability to penetrate the lipids of biological membranes, modifying their lipophilic nature and barrier functions. The potency of these solvents in this regard is ranked as follows: ether/acetone > DMSO > ethanol > water. Notably, while high concentrations of ethanol and lipids do not inherently harm the skin, they can serve as solvents for lipophilic drugs present on the skin's surface.

Human beings and other organisms are often exposed to a myriad of chemicals simultaneously, each entering through various routes and exhibiting diverse modes of action and metabolic pathways. Exogenous chemicals can act as substrates, inhibitors, or inducers of enzymes, introducing a layer of complexity to their biological effects. Many compounds initially inhibit enzymes like microsomal monooxygenase, and only to make them become inducers.

The dynamics of chemical toxicity are intricate, with cases like Compound A, which is inherently toxic but undergoes detoxification within the body. In the presence of an inhibitor of its detoxification enzyme, Compound A's toxicity escalates. Conversely, exposure to an inducer of these detoxification enzymes diminishes Compound A's toxicity.

Compound B, which is non-toxic in its native form, undergoes metabolic activation to become more hazardous. When a metabolic inhibitor is present, this activation process is hindered, resulting in reduced toxicity of Compound B. However, exposure to an inducer of its metabolic activating enzyme intensifies the toxicity of Compound B.

In summary, the toxicity of chemicals can be modulated by the presence of enzyme inhibitors or inducers, leading to either detoxification or enhanced toxicity, depending on the specific chemical and its metabolic fate.

External Environment Factors

Temperature

The intricate body temperature regulation system of animals often shields them from direct metabolic alterations of exogenous chemicals due to external temperature fluctuations. Nevertheless, temperature shifts, acting as stressors, elicit hormonal interplay and disrupt internal metabolic processes. Consequently, variations in environmental temperature, whether upwards or downwards, significantly influence the toxicological responses of animals and humans. There are two distinct patterns observed: ① enhanced toxicity with increasing temperatures; ② toxicity augmentation at both elevated and reduced temperatures. For instance, caffeine toxicity in mice intensifies under both conditions, whereas D-amphetamine displays attenuated toxicity at lower temperatures but consistently elevates its toxicity with rising temperatures. Additionally, many toxins have the ability to directly perturb metabolic or thermoregulatory mechanisms, thereby modifying the body's toxicological responses in both hot and cold environments. As an example, rats subjected to cold stress exhibit accelerated metabolism of 2-naphthylamine into 2-amino-1-naphthol.

Barometric Pressure

Research has consistently shown that atmospheric pressure exerts a profound influence on the effects of certain chemicals and drugs. Specifically, when the partial pressure of oxygen is maintained at a level akin to that found at sea level, the toxicity of morphine to rats is mitigated. Similar outcomes have been reported in studies involving chlorpromazine, amphetamine, and meperidine (pethidine). Moreover, swift changes in barometric pressure can easily elicit varying degrees of stress, which in turn can modulate toxic reactions within the body.

Diurnal and Seasonal Rhythms

The sensitivity of biological systems to toxins undergoes dynamic changes based on the timing of exposure, whether it be within a single day, across different seasons of the year, or even over extended periods spanning years or decades. The diurnal fluctuations in toxic reactions are often influenced by internal factors within animals or tied to their feeding and sleeping patterns. Typically, rats that have been fed ad libitum display a lower LD_{50} value when subjected to gavage poisoning after an overnight fast. Similarly, in mice maintained under standard laboratory conditions, the duration of pentobarbital-induced sleep exhibits a diurnal pattern, with the longest sleep times occurring at 2 p. m. and the shortest at 2 a. m.

However, this pronounced diurnal difference diminishes significantly when mice are individually fed and exposed to continuous lighting throughout the day and night.

Certain enzymes involved in the metabolism of exogenous chemicals display circadian rhythms, which are primarily governed by the photoperiod rather than the intensity of light. For instance, the cytochrome P450 and microsomal monooxygenase systems in rats and mice exhibit circadian variations, with peak activities preceding the onset of darkness.

Furthermore, the pharmacodynamics and biotransformation rates of drugs in rats undergo seasonal or interannual variations. The induction of drug metabolism by phenobarbital, for example, follows a seasonal pattern. The basal metabolic rate of cycloheximide is elevated in winter and reduced in summer, whereas phenobarbital elicits an opposing seasonal cycle in cycloheximide oxidase. These seasonal variations in susceptibility may be linked to adaptive responses to cold or specific weather conditions prevalent in different geographical regions.

Interactive Toxicity of Chemical Mixtures

In reality, individuals rarely encounter a solitary chemical but are constantly exposed to a diverse array of chemicals from various sources such as workplaces, the natural environment, and residential settings. Consequently, humans are inevitably subjected to a complex mixture of substances. A mixture, in this context, comprises two or more chemical components that jointly influence human responses to these chemicals.

Types of Chemical Mixture Toxicity

When assessing the toxicological implications of chemical mixtures, it is commonly presumed that the individual chemical constituents contribute additively to the overall effect. This additive action signifies that the toxic impact of a mixture can be roughly estimated by summing up the exposure doses or biological effects of each constituent within the mixture. However, if the observed toxic effect of a mixture deviates from the predicted additive effect, based on the dose-response relationships of its individual components, this discrepancy is indicative of an interaction between the chemicals.

Basic Concepts of Interactive Toxicity

When two chemicals are administered simultaneously, their combined effects may be additive, greater than the sum of their individual effects. Understanding these interactions provides insights into toxicological mechanisms. The main types of interactions are as follows.

(1) Additive Effect: when the combined effect equals the sum of individual effects (2+3 =5). This is the most common interaction, exemplified by combined cholinesterase inhibition

from two organophosphate insecticides.

(2) Synergistic Effect: when the combined effect significantly exceeds the sum of individual effects (2+2=20). For instance, carbon tetrachloride and ethanol together produce liver injury far exceeding their summed individual effects.

(3) Potentiation: when a non-toxic substance enhances another chemical's toxicity (0+2 =10). For example, isopropanol, though not hepatotoxic alone, significantly increases carbon tetrachloride's hepatotoxicity.

(4) Antagonism: when chemicals interfere with each other's actions [4+6=8; 4+(−4)= 0]. Four major types exist. ① Functional Antagonism: chemicals produce opposite physiological effects. Example: vasopressors counteracting barbiturate-induced hypotension. ② Chemical Antagonism: direct chemical reaction produces less toxic products. Example: dimercaprol chelating heavy metals. ③ Dispositional Antagonism: altered absorption, distribution, biotransformation, or excretion reduces toxicant concentration at target sites. Example: activated charcoal preventing toxicant absorption. ④ Receptor Antagonism: competition at receptor sites reduces toxic effects. Example: naloxone antagonizing morphine at opioid receptors.

Mechanisms of Chemical Interaction

Interaction refers to the phenomenon in which one chemical substance has the capability to modify the toxicokinetics and/or toxicodynamics of another. Toxicokinetics pertains to the processes influencing the fate of a chemical within the body, including its absorption, distribution, metabolism (biotransformation), and elimination (excretion). These processes significantly shape the dose-response relationship, determining the extent and nature of a chemical's toxic effects.

Alterations at the toxicodynamic level can disrupt the competitive interactions between chemicals for specific targets, such as receptor binding sites, and interfere with signaling cascades, cell cycle control, and other vital biological processes. Additionally, some chemicals can hinder the intricate dynamics of tissue repair, leading to the unabated progression of toxic injury, culminating in organ dysfunction and, in severe cases, death.

Such mechanisms intricately influence the concentration of toxicants and their active forms within the body, as well as the responsiveness of tissues to these toxic insults. Understanding these mechanisms is fundamental to predicting the combined toxic effects of chemical mixtures, as it allows for a more comprehensive assessment of potential health risks associated with exposure to multiple chemicals simultaneously.

(Nie Jihua)

CHAPTER 7

General Toxicity

Introduction

The general toxicity of exogenous chemicals, as opposed to specific toxicities (usually referring to carcinogenicity, teratogenicity, mutagenicity, and reproductive toxicity), refers to the capability of these chemicals to induce a composite toxic effect on the organism under certain doses, exposure durations, and methods of exposure. Based on the duration of exposure to exogenous chemicals, general toxicity can be classified into acute, subacute, subchronic, and chronic toxicity. General toxicity research is crucial for exploring the damage caused by exogenous chemicals to the organism, providing clues for the study of toxic mechanisms and target organ toxicity. It is an integral part of the safety evaluation and hazard assessment of exogenous chemicals, and serves as a basis for establishing health standards and making health-related decisions.

Acute Toxic Studies

Concepts of Acute Toxicity

Acute toxicity tests are the primary toxicological evaluations conducted on exogenous chemicals. Acute toxicity refers to the toxic effects, including changes in general behavior, appearance, and mortality, caused in an organism following a single or multiple exposures within 24 hours, typically observed over a short period (usually 14 days). Acute exposure is defined as exposure lasting less than 24 hours, with routes mainly including oral, inhalant, and dermal exposure. Acute exposure is often achieved through a single administration. When the toxicity of an exogenous chemical is low, and no toxic effect is observed after administering the maximum poisoning dose to experimental animals, and the dose has not yet reached the specified limit dose, it is necessary to poison the animals multiple times within 24 hours.

The toxic effects induced by the test substance can vary significantly in timing and degree, depending on its chemical structure, physicochemical properties, dose, and the species and strain of the animals. Therefore, acute toxic effects should be observed over a sufficiently long period to comprehensively assess toxicity, up to a maximum of 14 days.

Objectives of Acute Toxicity Testing

Acute toxicity testing is a fundamental procedure in toxicology that aims to evaluate the immediate effects of potentially harmful substances on living organisms. The objectives of acute toxicity testing are multifaceted and crucial for understanding the safety profile of various chemicals. Firstly, researchers strive to determine a range of toxicity parameters to assess the magnitude of acute toxicity. This involves obtaining upper-limit toxicity parameters, such as the median lethal dose (LD_{50}) or median lethal concentration (LC_{50}), based on mortality data. These parameters are then used to perform acute toxicity grading, which helps categorize substances according to their level of toxicity. Secondly, acute toxicity tests allow for a preliminary assessment of the extent of harm caused by the exogenous chemical to the organism. By observing poisoning manifestations, the intensity of toxic action, and mortality rates in test animals, researchers can gain insights into the characteristics of the toxic effect, identify target organs, and establish dose-response relationships. Thirdly, the data obtained from acute toxicity testing provides a crucial foundation for designing more comprehensive toxicological studies. This information guides researchers in determining appropriate exposure doses and selecting relevant observation indicators for sub-chronic and chronic toxicity studies, as well as other specialized toxicological tests. Finally, acute toxicity testing helps determine whether the observed damage is reversible, which is essential for understanding the long-term implications of exposure to the substance in question. Through these comprehensive objectives, acute toxicity testing plays a vital role in safeguarding public health and informing regulatory decisions regarding chemical safety.

Parameters in Acute Toxicity Testing

Acute toxicity testing employs several key parameters to quantify the potential hazards of substances. The median lethal dose (LD_{50}) serves as the primary metric, representing the dose that is lethal to 50% of the test subjects. Other important parameters include the absolute lethal dose (LD_{100}), which is the lowest dose causing death in all test animals, and the minimum lethal dose (MLD or LD_{01}), which represents the dose that causes death in individual animals. Additionally, the maximum tolerated dose (MTD) or maximum tolerated concentration (MTC) denotes the highest exposure level that can be administered without causing animal death. These parameters are typically expressed in units of milligrams of substance per kilogram of body weight (mg/kg bw) for oral or dermal exposure, or in parts per million (ppm, μL/L) for inhalation studies. Collectively, these measures provide a comprehensive profile of a substance's acute toxicity.

Acute Toxicity Test Design

The design of acute toxicity tests is a critical process in toxicology that requires careful planning and execution. This process encompasses several key steps, each essential for obtaining reliable and meaningful results.

Initially, comprehensive substance information collection and understanding are essential. Researchers must thoroughly investigate the test substance's chemical structure, molecular weight, physical state, and characteristics under standard conditions. This includes assessing purity, impurity composition and content, solubility, and volatility. For novel substances, data from structurally, physically, and chemically similar compounds should be consulted to inform the selection of experimental animal strains and dosages. Additionally, identifying potential human exposure routes is crucial for determining appropriate administration methods.

The selection of experimental animals follows specific principles. Ideally, researchers choose animal strains whose metabolism and toxic responses closely mirror human reactions, while also considering factors such as ease of management, availability, and cost-effectiveness. Typically, both rodent and non-rodent species are employed, with mice and rats being the preferred rodent models. The use of commonly available strains is standard practice, often favoring opting for closed colony hybrids over purebred animals.

Gender and age considerations are crucial in animal selection. An equal number of male and female animals are usually chosen, with females being nulliparous and non-pregnant. Healthy adult animals are preferred, with body weight serving as an age indicator in rodents. The quantity and grouping of animals vary depending on the specific acute toxicity test method, typically involving 3–7 groups with at least 3 animals per group. Randomization in grouping is essential to balance non-treatment factors.

Quarantine and fasting procedures are implemented to ensure the health and preparedness of the animals. A quarantine period of 5–7 days is standard, followed by appropriate fasting periods before oral toxicity tests to minimize food interference with chemical toxicity.

The selection of test substance doses is fundamental to the success of acute toxicity testing. Researchers use the predicted median toxicity value, often based on LD_{50} data from similar substances, to design a range of doses. The goal is to select doses that will result in varying mortality rates, ideally including doses that cause approximately 50% mortality, as well as higher and lower mortality rates.

The routes of administration are chosen to simulate potential human exposure as closely as possible. Common routes include oral (often via gavage), inhalant, and dermal exposure. The specific method of administration is selected based on the substance's properties and intended use.

Observation of toxic effects is a critical component of the test design. The standard observation period is 14 days, though this may be extended based on the onset and severity of toxic reactions. Comprehensive observation includes detailed recording of poisoning symptoms, changes in body weight, mortality rates and timing, and pathological examinations. These observations provide crucial insights into the characteristics of the substance's acute toxic action and its target organs.

Pathological examinations, both gross and histological, are conducted on deceased animals and survivors at the end of the test period. Additional indicators, such as body temperature, electrocardiogram, electroencephalogram, or blood biochemical markers, may be included based on the specific toxic characteristics of the test substance.

Alternative Methods of Acute Toxicity Tests

The field of toxicology has undergone a significant transformation in its approach to acute toxicity testing, driven by the widespread adoption of the 3Rs principle (Replacement, Reduction, and Refinement) and growing international concern for animal welfare. This paradigm shift has led to the development and implementation of alternative methods aimed at optimizing testing procedures, minimizing animal usage, and potentially eliminating animal testing altogether.

At the forefront of this movement, the Organization for Economic Cooperation and Development (OECD) has issued several guidelines for alternative acute toxicity test methods. These include the Fixed Dose Procedure, the Acute Toxic Class Method, and the Up-and-Down Procedure. While the Fixed Dose Procedure and Acute Toxic Class Method are primarily utilized for toxicity classification, the Up-and-Down Procedure offers broader application by estimating the LD_{50} and its confidence interval.

The Fixed Dose Procedure represents a departure from classic acute toxicity tests by employing clear toxic signs as the evaluation endpoint rather than animal death. This method utilizes a series of predetermined doses (5, 50, 500, and 2000 mg/kg, with a provision for 5000 mg/kg in special circumstances) to assess the chemical's toxic response and classify its toxicity accordingly.

The Acute Toxic Class Method is a staged test procedure that uses death as an endpoint but requires fewer animals to reach acceptable conclusions. Based on bio-statistical principles and internationally validated by the OECD, this method preferentially employs rodents, typically rats. The procedure begins with testing three animals of a single sex at one of the set doses (5, 50, 300, or 2000 mg/kg). Subsequent steps are determined by the survival outcome of the animals, potentially leading to classification without further testing, testing at a higher or lower dose level, or testing additional animals at the same dose. This method allows for direct toxicity classification based on the approximate range of LD_{50} determined by the number of deaths at a certain dose.

The Up-and-Down Procedure typically uses death as an endpoint but can also accommodate other toxic endpoints, making it suitable for "all-or-none" responses. This method begins with a dose determined from preliminary data, observing the animal for 48 hours. Subsequent doses are increased or decreased based on the survival of the previous animal. The recommended dose sequence ranges from 1.75 to 5,000 mg/kg body weight, with the initial dose typically set below the estimated LD_{50}. If no LD_{50} data is available, dosing usually begins at 175 mg/kg. To facilitate the testing process and LD_{50} calculation, the United States Environmental Protection Agency (US EPA) has developed specialized software.

These alternative methods represent significant advancements in acute toxicity testing, offering more ethical and efficient approaches to toxicity assessment. By reducing animal usage and refining experimental procedures, these methods align with contemporary ethical standards while maintaining scientific rigor and reliability in toxicological evaluations.

Evaluation of Acute Toxicity

The primary objective of acute toxicity testing is to classify the acute toxicity of chemicals, allowing for the comparison of their acute toxic potential and the assessment of their acute toxic strength. The Globally Harmonized System of Classification and Labelling of Chemicals (GHS) categorizes the acute toxicity of chemical substances or mixtures into five categories based on the LD_{50} values for oral and dermal routes or the LC_{50} values for inhalant exposure (Table 7-1). Pharmaceuticals, food additives, cosmetics, and pesticide residues in food are not covered by the GHS. China's national food hygiene standard "Procedures and Methods for Toxicological Assessment of Food Safety" proposes a six-tier standard for acute toxicity classification (Table 7 - 2). The toxicity classification standard for pesticides categorizes pesticides into four levels (Table 7-3).

Table 7-1 **Acute Toxicity Hazard Categories**

Exposure Route	Category 1	Category 2	Category 3	Category 4	Category 5
Oral (mg/kg bw)	5	50	300	2, 000	5, 000
Dermal (mg/kg bw)	50	200	1, 000	2, 000	5, 000
Gases (ppm V)	100	500	2, 500	5, 000	5, 000
Vapours (mg/L)	0. 5	2. 0	10	20	5, 000
Gust & Mists(mg/L)	0. 05	0. 5	1. 0	5	5, 000

Table 7-2 **Acute Toxicity Classification for Food**

Category	Oral LD_{50} for Rats/(mg/kg)
Supertoxic	<1
Extremely toxic	1~50
Moderately toxic	>50~500
Slightly toxic	>500~5, 000
Practically nontoxic	>5, 000~15, 000
Nontoxic	>15, 000

Table 7-3 **Acute Toxicity Classification for Pesticide**

Category	Oral LD_{50} for Rats/(mg/kg)
Extremely toxic	<5
Highly toxic	5~50
Moderately toxic	>50~500
Slightly toxic	>500

Subacute, Subchronic, and Chronic Toxicity Studies

In the field of environmental and occupational health, human exposure to xenobiotics primarily occurs through long-term, low-dose, and repetitive contact. While acute toxicity data provide valuable initial insights, they are often insufficient for predicting the consequences of prolonged exposure. Consequently, investigations into subacute, subchronic, and chronic toxicity have become increasingly crucial in toxicological risk assessment.

Subacute toxicity studies, also known as repeated dose toxicity tests, are designed to evaluate the adverse effects of continuous exposure to a xenobiotic over a period of 14 to 30 days in experimental animals. These studies serve several critical purposes, including providing a preliminary determination of the No Observed Adverse Effect Level (NOAEL) and/or Lowest Observed Adverse Effect Level (LOAEL) for test substance under investigation, offering an initial assessment of the safety profile of the xenobiotic, and informing the selection of appropriate doses, observation indicators, and toxic endpoints for subsequent subchronic and chronic toxicity studies. Moreover, they help identify potential target organs and systems that may be affected by repeated exposure.

Subchronic toxicity studies extend exposure period to approximately one-tenth of the test animals' lifespan, typically 90 days for rodents, these studies provide a more comprehensive evaluation of the cumulative effects of xenobiotics over an extended period. These studies are of crucial in toxicology as they allow for the detection of delayed onset toxicity that may not be evident in shorter-term studies, thereby allowing for a more accurate determination of the NOAEL and LOAEL, which are crucial for risk assessment and regulatory decision-making. In many cases, subchronic toxicity studies can serve as a substitute for full-scale chronic toxicity tests, thereby reducing animal usage and resource expenditure.

Chronic toxicity studies represent the most extensive form of toxicity testing, typically lasting at least 12 months or a substantial portion of the test animals' lifespans. Despite their resource-intensive nature, chronic toxicity studies are indispensable as they provide the most comprehensive assessment of long-term exposure effects, including the potential for carcinogenicity. These studies allow for the evaluation of cumulative toxicity, the development of tolerance, and adaptive responses over an extended period, and enable the detection of subtle, slowly progressing adverse effects that may not be apparent in shorter-term studies. Importantly, chronic toxicity studies provide critical data for establishing safe exposure limits for humans, particularly for substances with potential lifetime exposure.

The progression from subacute to chronic toxicity testing allows toxicologists to build a comprehensive understanding of a xenobiotic's toxicity profile. This tiered approach enables the identification of potential hazards at earlier stages, informs the design of subsequent studies, and ultimately contributes to more accurate risk assessments. Furthermore, these studies collectively provide crucial data for regulatory agencies in establishing safety guidelines, determining acceptable daily intakes, and formulating public health policies aimed at mitigating the risks associated with chronic chemical exposure.

In summary, subacute, subchronic, and chronic toxicity studies form the cornerstone of modern toxicological risk assessment, bridging the gap between acute toxicity data and real-world exposure scenarios. They provide invaluable insights into the long-term health effects of xenobiotics and inform evidence-based decision-making in environmental and occupational health. By systematically evaluating the effects of prolonged exposure to xenobiotics, these studies enable toxicologists and regulatory bodies to better protect public health and safety in an increasingly complex chemical landscape.

Subacute and Subchronic, and Chronic Toxicity Tests Design

Subacute toxicity tests typically involve continuous exposure to a test substance for 14 to 30 days, while subchronic tests extend this period to approximately 90 days, or about one-tenth of the test animals' lifespan. Chronic toxicity tests, the most prolonged of the three, generally last for 12 months or more, sometimes spanning the entire lifetime of the test animals. All three types of studies share similarities in design, parameters selection, and results evaluation, aiming to determine the NOAEL and/or LOAEL of the test substance.

The selection of experimental animals is based on their sensitivity to the test substance and their similarity to humans in biotransformation and toxicological responses. Commonly used species include rodents, dogs, and occasionally non-human primates. For chronic toxicity tests, two mammalian species are typically involved, with rats as the preferred rodent species and dogs or monkeys as the non-rodent species. The number of animals per group is larger in chronic studies, with a minimum of 20 rodents of each sex per group and 4 to 6 non-rodents per group.

The route of exposure should mimic human exposure as closely as possible and remain consistent across all study durations. For chronic tests, oral exposure typically occurs once daily, 5 to 6 days per week, while inhalant exposure for industrial toxicants is administered for 4 to 6 hours per day, and for environmental toxicants, more than 8 hours per day.

To establish a clear dose-response relationship, these studies typically include at least three dose groups and one negative control group. The highest dose should induce apparent toxicity without excessive mortality, while the lowest dose should correspond to the NOAEL. In chronic studies, the medium dose should produce mild toxicity, such as changes in serum enzyme levels or slight weight reduction. Dose selection is often based on the substance's LD_{50}, MTD, or results from previous shorter-term studies, with an ideal dose interval of 2 to 4 times, not exceeding 10 times.

The duration of exposure varies significantly among the three test types. Subacute tests last 14 to 30 days, subchronic tests about 90 days, and chronic tests generally 12 months or more. The specific duration of chronic tests can vary based on the test requirements and animal species used, with industrial toxicants requiring at least 6 months of exposure and environmental toxicants and food substances requiring 1 to 2 years.

Throughout these studies, researchers observe a wide range of parameters to identify target organs and sensitive toxicological endpoints. General indices include changes in body weight, food consumption, behavior, and appearance. Blood tests and biochemical analyses are performed periodically to assess hematological and metabolic effects. At the study's conclusion, comprehensive pathological examinations are conducted, including organ weight measurements and histopathological analyses.

Specific indices related to the substance's known or suspected toxicity mechanisms may be included to provide deeper insights into its harmful effects. The rapid advancement of molecular biology and immunology has introduced new biomarkers of effect, enhancing our ability to detect subtle toxicological changes.

Recovery periods are incorporated into these studies to assess the reversibility of observed toxic effects and identify any delayed onset toxicity. For subacute studies, this is typically a 14-day period, extending to 28 days for subchronic studies. In chronic studies, the recovery period should be at least 28 days but not exceed one-third of the main test duration.

Observation of Toxic Effects

In subacute, subchronic, and chronic toxicity studies, the careful selection and observation of toxicological indices are crucial for identifying target organs and sensitive endpoints. These studies employ a comprehensive approach to detect and characterize potential adverse effects of test substances over extended exposure periods.

During subacute toxicity tests, researchers cast a wide net, employing a broad range of observation indices to ensure no significant effects are overlooked. As the study progresses to the subchronic and chronic phases, the focus narrows to emphasize the most significant and sensitive endpoints identified in earlier stages.

Throughout the exposure period, experimental animals undergo daily observations to monitor changes in general health and behavior. These observations include assessing body weight, food intake, coat condition, respiratory and circulatory function, and any abnormalities in movement or behavior. Body weight and food intake are typically recorded on a weekly basis.

Hematological and biochemical analyses form an integral part of these studies. Blood samples are collected at predetermined intervals, before, during, and after exposure, to evaluate parameters such as hemoglobin concentration, hematocrit, blood cell counts, and platelet levels. Biochemical tests assess markers of organ function and metabolic status, including glucose, urea nitrogen, liver enzymes (ALT, AST), creatinine, lipid profile, and protein levels.

Pathological examinations provide crucial insights into the morphological effects of the test substance. Upon study completion, all animals undergo gross necropsy, with particular attention paid to the appearance of the skull, thoracic, and abdominal organs. Key organs, including the adrenals, brain, reproductive organs, heart, kidneys, liver, spleen, thyroid, parathyroid, and thymus, are weighed to detect any substance-induced changes. Histopathological analysis is initially performed on tissues from control and high-dose groups, with examination extended to all dose groups if a dose-response relationship is observed.

In chronic toxicity studies, where test substance concentrations are typically low, meticulous attention to observational indices is essential for detecting subtle yet significant toxicological effects. Prior to initiating exposure, it is crucial to evaluate pre-designed indices to establish a baseline health status for the experimental animals, facilitating accurate comparisons with post-exposure results. Throughout the exposure period, researchers must conduct dynamic observations of various indices, comparing them concurrently with the control group to mitigate age-related confounding factors. This longitudinal monitoring approach enhances the study's ability to discern substance-induced changes from normal physiological variations. In the event of animal mortality during the study or tumor development following exposure cessation, immediate histopathological analyses should be performed to capture time-sensitive data that might otherwise be lost. Furthermore, the implementation of rigorous quality control measures for all indices testing is paramount to ensure consistent and reliable results across all animal cohorts throughout the study duration. By adhering to these practices, toxicologists can significantly enhance the sensitivity and reliability of chronic toxicity studies, enabling the detection of subtle toxicological effects that may manifest over extended exposure periods. This comprehensive approach to data collection and analysis is fundamental to accurately assessing the long-term safety profile of test substances and informing evidence-based regulatory decisions.

To further elucidate the specific toxic effects and mechanisms of action, additional specialized indices may be incorporated. These can include biomarkers of effect or indices that reflect toxicity to particular organ systems, such as the cardiovascular, endocrine, immune, or nervous systems. The selection of these specific indices is guided by existing toxicological data on the test substance and any noteworthy observations made during the study.

Recent advancements in molecular biology and immunology have expanded the repertoire of toxicologically relevant indices available to researchers. By judiciously selecting and measuring these advanced markers, toxicologists can gain deeper insights into the mechanisms of toxicity and conduct more comprehensive safety evaluations.

This multi-faceted approach to observing and measuring toxic effects in subacute, subchronic, and chronic studies enables toxicologists to construct a detailed profile of a substance's potential adverse effects, providing crucial data for risk assessment and regulatory decision-making. The data generated from these progressively longer-term toxicity tests are invaluable for establishing safety guidelines and informing regulatory decisions, contributing significantly to our understanding of xenobiotic effects and our ability to protect public health in an increasingly complex chemical landscape.

Evaluation of Subacute, Subchronic, and Chronic Toxicity

The primary goals of subacute, subchronic, and chronic toxicity tests are to establish dose-response relationships and identify target organs of toxicity, aiming to determine corresponding subacute/subchronic/chronic NOAEL and/or LOAEL. Therefore, evaluating the results necessitates a comprehensive analysis and study of the experimental data, employing statistical methods, and integrating theoretical knowledge from toxicology and related disciplines to arrive at reliable and scientific conclusions.

Given the numerous observation indices in chronic toxicity tests, attention should be paid to the inter-group comparisons of relevant indices, especially between the various dose groups and the normal control group. If inter-group differences are statistically significant, further analysis is required to determine whether there is a dose-response relationship or not, which is a prerequisite for establishing a causal relationship between the test substance and adverse effects. Moreover, comparisons of related series of indices are important. For instance, changes in serum enzymes reflecting liver function should be considered in conjunction with changes in hepatic histopathological findings to scientifically and reasonably conclude whether the test substance causes liver damage. The specific aspects of result evaluation include toxic effects manifestation, dose-response relationship, target organs, and reversibility of damage. Each parameter should be separately evaluated for its statistical, biological, and toxicological significance.

Additionally, for certain special tests and experimental species, variations among animals and within the same animal should be considered, which might lead to apparent differences in indices. For example, increased variability among individuals in aged rodent populations due to a higher probability of spontaneous diseases can mask smaller group differences, not truly reflecting the actual effect. Many experimental factors, such as the route of administration of the test substance, blood sampling methods, and randomness in blood sampling, can affect variability and must be taken into account. For example, continuous intravenous infusion can increase variability among certain experimental animals (like white blood cell count, hematocrit, serum protein content), making it difficult to interpret minor differences in results. Proper management of the experimental process is crucial for obtaining accurate indices, and the implementation of Good Laboratory Practice (GLP) provides a basic assurance for controlling experimental quality.

In summary, in the process of evaluating results from subacute, subchronic, and chronic toxicity tests, a comprehensive and integrated analysis of all observations and test results during the experimental period is essential. This should be combined with the physicochemical properties of the test substance and structure-activity relationship analysis of similar chemicals. The evaluation should utilize statistical, biological, toxicological, and other relevant scientific theories and methods. Additionally, incorporating available human data and epidemiological study findings are crucial to draw scientific, reasonable conclusions, providing a toxicological experimental basis for the risk management of harmful chemicals.

Local Toxicity Studies

Local toxicity studies are conducted to assess the damage caused by chemical exposure to specific body parts like the skin and eyes. Local toxic reactions often precede systemic toxicity, making the study of local toxic effects crucial for early disengagement from exposure, timely treatment, and the prevention of systemic toxic effects.

Acute Eye Irritation/Corrosion Tests and Alternative Methods

The assessment of acute eye irritation and corrosion is a critical component of toxicological evaluation, essential for determining the ocular safety profile of various compounds. Eye irritation refers to reversible inflammatory changes in the anterior ocular surface, while corneal corrosion indicates irreversible tissue damage following exposure to a test substance. Historically, the Draize eye test has been the standard method for this assessment, utilizing rabbits to evaluate ocular responses to test substances. This in vivo assay involves applying the substance to one eye and observing changes in the conjunctiva, cornea, and iris over a specified period. However, concerns about result subjectivity and animal welfare have led to the development of alternative methods.

These alternatives include ex vivo organ tests, such as the Bovine Corneal Opacity and Permeability (BCOP) test and the Isolated Chicken Eye (ICE) test, which use isolated ocular tissues to assess irritation potential by measuring changes in corneal opacity, swelling, and permeability. Cell toxicity-based assays, like the Neutral Red Uptake (NRU) test, evaluate eye irritation potential by measuring cellular viability in various cell lines. Chorio-Allantoic Membrane (CAM) tests, including the Hen's Egg Test on the Chorio-Allantoic Membrane (HET-CAM), utilize chicken embryo membranes as a model for the human conjunctiva, assessing irritation by monitoring vascular changes.

More recently, reconstructed human corneal tissue models, such as EpiOcular and SkinEthic HCE, have been developed to provide a more physiologically relevant context for evaluating eye irritation potential. These alternative methods reflect the toxicological community's commitment to the 3R's principle (Replacement, Reduction, and Refinement) in animal research. While no single alternative method fully replicates the complexity of the in vivo ocular response, the integration of multiple approaches within a tiered testing strategy offers a promising path forward.

Dermal Irritation/Corrosion Test and Alternative Methods

Dermal irritation and corrosion tests are crucial components of toxicological assessment, evaluating the potential for chemicals to induce reversible inflammatory changes or irreversible tissue damage upon skin contact. These tests encompass both single and multiple exposures, as well as assessments on intact and compromised skin barriers. The primary endpoints of these evaluations are the manifestation of dermal irritation, characterized by localized and reversible inflammatory responses, and dermal corrosion, which involves irreversible tissue damage following chemical exposure.

Certain circumstances preclude the necessity for dermal irritation testing. These include substances with extreme pH values ($\leqslant 2$ or $\geqslant 11.5$), chemicals with known severe dermal toxicity (dermal $LD_{50} < 200$ mg/kg bw), and compounds that have demonstrated no signs of skin irritation in acute dermal toxicity studies at doses up to 2, 000 mg/kg bw. These exclusion criteria serve to minimize unnecessary animal testing and focus resources on chemicals with uncertain dermal effects.

The Draize skin test has long been the standard method for evaluating dermal irritation potential. This in vivo assay typically employs albino rabbits, with test substances applied to a shaved area of dorsal skin for a specified duration, usually 4 hours. Observations of erythema and edema are conducted at predetermined intervals following substance removal, with the evaluation period extending up to 14 days to capture the full progression of reversible or irreversible irritation.

In response to ethical concerns and regulatory changes, such as the European Union's ban on animal testing for cosmetic ingredients and finished products, alternative methods for assessing skin irritation have been developed and validated. These in vitro approaches aim to reduce animal use while maintaining or improving predictive accuracy.

Monolayer skin cell culture models, utilizing keratinocytes, melanocytes, or fibroblasts, offer a simplified system for initial screening of skin irritants. While these models lack the structural complexity of intact skin, they provide a platform for high-throughput evaluation and eliminate species-specific differences. However, their simplicity limits direct extrapolation to human responses.

Epidermal tissue culture models, such as Reconstructed Human Epidermis (RHE) and EpiDerm (EPI), represent a more advanced alternative. These three-dimensional cultures, grown at an air-liquid interface, simulate the structure and function of human epidermis.

These models have been validated for use in skin irritation testing and offer improved physiological relevance compared to monolayer cultures.

Organotypic artificial skin models represent the cutting edge of in vitro dermal toxicity testing. These complex systems incorporate both epidermal and dermal components, closely mimicking the structure and function of normal human skin. The development and refinement of these models continue to be an active area of research, with the potential to provide the most comprehensive in vitro representation of human skin responses to chemical exposures.

Skin Sensitization Tests and Alternative Methods

Skin sensitization is a complex immune-mediated toxic response to chemical exposure, manifesting as allergic contact dermatitis in humans. This phenomenon is characterized by a range of dermal reactions, including pruritus, erythema, edema, papules, vesicles, and bullae. In non-human species, the presentation may be limited to erythema and edema. The primary objective of skin sensitization testing is to predict the potential of exogenous substances to elicit such reactions in humans through the use of animal models.

The mechanism of skin sensitization involves a two-phase process: induction and elicitation. During the induction phase, initial contact with a sensitizing agent may produce minimal or no apparent dermal response. However, upon subsequent exposure, a delayed hypersensitivity reaction can occur, often extending beyond the original site of contact. This process is mediated by the hapten hypothesis, wherein chemicals penetrate the skin and form covalent bonds with carrier proteins, creating complete antigens. These antigens interact with Langerhans cells in the epidermis or macrophages, initiating antibody formation and establishing immune memory.

The elicitation phase occurs upon re-exposure to the sensitizing agent, even at lower concentrations, resulting in a Type IV hypersensitivity reaction. This delayed-type hypersensitivity response, mediated by T-cells, typically reaches its peak 24–48 hours post-secondary antigen contact.

Skin sensitization assays are broadly categorized into two types: those utilizing Freund's Complete Adjuvant (FCA) and those without adjuvants. Adjuvant-based methods enhance the sensitivity of the animal model to allergens, facilitating the detection of weak sensitizers and improving the predictive power for human responses. Traditional methodologies include the Buehler Test (BT) and the Guinea Pig Maximization Test (GPMT), with the latter involving intradermal injection of the allergen combined with FCA.

These assays typically employ guinea pigs as the model organism and are structured into induction and elicitation phases. The induction phase involves repeated dermal exposure to the test substance at low to moderate concentrations, either via topical application or subcutaneous injection, over a period of approximately two weeks. Following a 10–14 day interval, the elicitation phase is initiated, wherein a previously unexposed skin area is treated with a lower concentration of the test substance. Dermal reactions are then observed and scored at 24, 48, and 72 hours post-challenge, with the severity of edema and erythema compared to the induction phase to determine the substance's skin sensitization potential.

In addition to local dermal reactions, other endpoints such as ear swelling and lymph node cell proliferation (as in the Local Lymph Node Assay) are utilized to assess the potential for delayed hypersensitivity reactions.

Current research in the field of skin sensitization testing is focused on developing in vitro alternatives to traditional animal-based methods. These efforts are centered on three main areas of investigation. The first area involves elucidating the chemical sensitization processes based on immunological recognition by key immune cells, particularly dendritic cells and T-cells, which are integral to both the induction and elicitation phases of contact hypersensitivity. Researchers are working to develop assays that can accurately model these cellular interactions and responses in vitro. The second area of focus is on establishing sophisticated skin models that accurately simulate the penetration of chemicals through the epidermal granular layer and dermis. These models aim to replicate the complex structure and barrier function of human skin, allowing for more physiologically relevant assessments of chemical penetration and potential sensitization. The third area involves developing and refining keratinocyte culture models to better represent the initial interactions between potential sensitizers and the skin. These models seek to capture the early stages of the sensitization process, including the activation of keratinocytes and the release of pro-inflammatory mediators. By advancing these three areas of research, scientists aim to create a comprehensive suite of in vitro tools that can reliably predict skin sensitization potential without the need for animal testing.

(Chen Tao)

CHAPTER 8

Chemical Mutagenesis

Introduction

Mutations are permanent, transmissible alterations in DNA sequences that result in changes to the amount or structure of genetic material in the cell. Both small-scale (i. e. one or few base-pair changes of a single gene) and large-scale (i. e. chromosomal rearrangements affecting multiple genes) DNA alterations can lead to mutations. Mutations may arise spontaneously due to errors during DNA replication and cell division, or they may be induced by exposure to mutagens, which are physical, chemical or biological agents that can induce mutations, such as ultraviolet light, alkylating agents and aflatoxin. The capacity of an agent to induce mutation is called mutagenicity.

It is important to distinguish mutagenicity from the broader concept of genotoxicity. Genetic toxicology studies genetic damage to hereditary material resulting in genetic alterations. While mutagenicity specifically refers to the induction of transmissible genetic changes, genotoxicity encompasses a wider range of endpoints including DNA damage, unscheduled DNA synthesis (UDS), and sister chromatid exchanges (SCEs). Genotoxic effects may be repaired or may ultimately lead to mutations. Thus, all mutagens are genotoxic, but not all genotoxic substances are mutagenic. Standardized assay outcomes that detect mutations in populations of cells and/or organisms have been applied to systematic hazard classifications of chemicals under the United Nations Globally Harmonized System of Classification and Labelling of Chemicals. Under GHS, the chemical hazards associated with germ cell mutagenicity are assigned to one of two hazard categories: ① substances known to induce heritable mutations (subcategory 1A) or regarded as if they induce heritable mutations (subcategory 1B) in the germ cells of humans; ② substances which cause concern that they may induce heritable mutations in the germ cells of humans.

It is worth mentioning that in the last decades, there has been an increased emphasis on the role of epigenetic changes that control gene expression through DNA methylation and histone modifications in the production of altered phenotypes. Although these epigenetic changes can be transmitted between generations, these are not mutations by definition as they do not involve changes in DNA sequence, and have not been observed to lead to amended point-of-departure values for risk assessment.

Types of Mutation

Mutations encompass a wide spectrum of alterations in DNA sequence, ranging from subtle changes within a single gene to large-scale chromosomal abnormalities. These genetic modifications can be broadly categorized into two main types: gene mutations and chromosomal abnormalities. Gene mutations are typically confined to a single gene and involve small-scale DNA sequence changes, such as base substitutions, insertions, or deletions. In contrast, chromosomal abnormalities involve larger-scale changes affecting the structure or number of chromosomes.

Gene Mutations

Gene mutations represent permanent alterations in the DNA sequence of a specific gene. These changes can occur through various mechanisms, primarily base-pair substitutions and frameshift mutations. Base-pair substitutions involve the replacement of one nucleotide with another, while frameshift mutations result from the insertion or deletion of nucleotides, altering the reading frame of the genetic code.

Base-Pair Substitutions

Base-pair substitutions are characterized by the replacement of one nucleotide with another in the DNA sequence. These substitutions can be further classified into two subtypes: transitions and transversions. Transitions involve the exchange of a purine for another purine (A↔G) or a pyrimidine for another pyrimidine (C↔T). And transversions involve the replacement of a purine with a pyrimidine or vice versa (e. g. A↔C, A↔T, G↔C, G↔T).

Frameshift Mutations

Frameshift mutations occur when nucleotides are inserted or deleted in numbers that are not multiples of three, thereby altering the reading frame of the genetic code. This shift in the reading frame can result in a completely different amino acid sequence downstream of the mutation site, often leading to the production of non-functional proteins. Additionally, frameshift mutations can introduce premature stop codons, resulting in truncated protein products.

Chromosomal Abnormalities

Chromosomal abnormalities encompass large-scale changes in chromosome structure or number. These alterations can have profound effects on gene expression and cellular function, often leading to severe phenotypic consequences.

Structural Chromosome Aberrations

Structural chromosomal aberrations involve changes in the organization of genetic material within chromosomes. These alterations can result from incorrect repair of DNA double-strand breaks or errors during chromosomal recombination. Figure 8 – 1 illustrates various types of chromosomal alterations, which represent major changes in the genetic material. The main types of structural aberrations include deletions, duplications, inversions, and translocations. Deletions involve the loss of chromosomal segments, while duplications result in the repetition of genetic material. Inversions occur when a chromosomal segment is reversed in orientation, and translocations involve the exchange of genetic material between non-homologous chromosomes. Among these, deletions and translocations are particularly significant in mutagenicity testing due to their relative ease of detection through microscopic analysis.

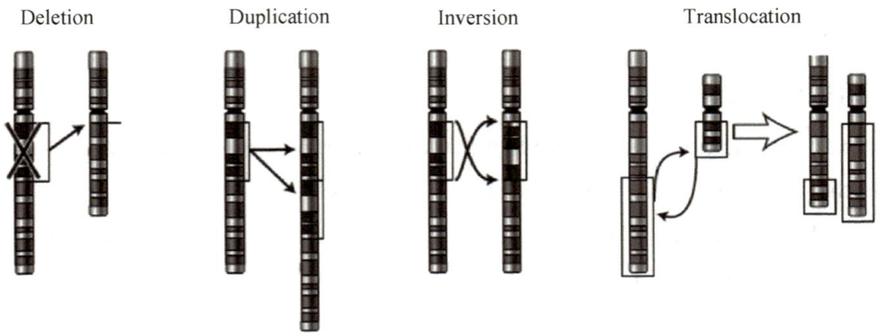

Figure 8-1 **Major types of chromosomal alterations**

Numerical Chromosome Changes

Numerical chromosomal changes refer to alterations in the number of chromosomes within a cell. These changes can be classified into two main categories: aneuploidy and polyploidy. Aneuploidy involves the gain or loss of one or a few individual chromosomes, resulting in an abnormal chromosome number that is not an exact multiple of the haploid set. Cells with aneuploidy can be further classified as monosomic (lacking one chromosome) or trisomic (possessing an extra chromosome). Polyploidy, involves the presence of one or more additional complete sets of chromosomes. Both aneuploidy and polyploidy can have significant impacts on cellular function and organism development, often leading to severe phenotypic consequences or embryonic lethality.

Health Impact of Mutations

Mutations can significantly impact human health, with their effects varying based on the location and type of target cells affected. These genetic alterations can occur in both somatic and germ cells, each with distinct consequences.

Somatic Mutations

Somatic mutations arise in the genomes of normal dividing and transformed cells due to endogenous and exogenous factors. Their association with cancer is well-established, evidenced by the correlation between chemical mutagenicity and carcinogenicity in biological systems with metabolic activation capabilities. Cancer cytogenetics has revealed various chromosomal modifications, including deletions, translocations, inversions, and amplifications, which are implicated in leukemia, lymphoma, and solid tumors. Mutations in noncoding gene promoter regions have also been identified across multiple cancer types. Large-scale copy-number alterations and chromosomal rearrangements can induce varying fitness changes depending on the tumor type, with some recurrent aneuploidies likely subject to positive selection.

Molecular studies of oncogenes and tumor suppressor genes have elucidated the central role of mutations in cancer development. Mutational alterations of proto-oncogenes can lead to overexpression of growth-stimulating activity, while inactivation of tumor-suppressor genes removes inhibitory influences on cellular proliferation. Many cancers involve both oncogene activation and tumor-suppressor genes inactivation. Beyond cancer, somatic mutations contribute to various genetic alterations and human diseases, including aging, atherosclerosis, and congenital anomalies.

Germ Mutations

Germ cell mutations can have profound consequences on subsequent generations. Lethal dominant mutations result in nonviable offspring, while viable dominant mutations can be transmitted to future generations. Recessive mutations are of particular concern as they can be carried by unaffected heterozygous individuals and accumulate in the gene pool. Germ cell mutations also contribute to complex disorders with genetic components, such as heart disease, hypertension, and diabetes. Many congenital abnormalities arise from de novo mutations in parental germ cells.

It is important to note that mutations can be harmful, beneficial, or neutral, depending on their context and location. While mutations drive evolutionary processes, they are undirected and often have negative effects on individuals, including fertility disorders, embryonic and perinatal death, malformations, hereditary diseases, and cancers. Occasionally, mutations can confer evolutionary advantages. Mutations in nonessential DNA or those with negligible effects on gene function may have no impact on the organism.

Mechanism of Mutagenesis

Preservation of genome integrity is central to cellular survival and successful propagation of hereditary material, yet ubiquitously present ultraviolet radiation, ionizing radiation, and chemical agents will pose threats to genomic stability.

DNA Damage

DNA damage, resulting from environmental factors and normal metabolic processes within the cell, occurs at a rate of 1, 000 to 1, 000, 000 molecular lesions per cell each day. Although this represents only 0. 000165% of the approximately 6 billion bases in the human genome (or 3 billion base pairs), if these damages are not repaired, they can lead to mutations in critical genes, such as tumor suppressor genes. These mutations can hinder a cell's ability to function properly and significantly increase the risk of tumor formation and diseases like cancer.

The vast majority of DNA damage affects the primary structure of the double helix; that is, the bases themselves are chemically modified. These modifications can, in turn, disrupt the molecules' regular helical structure by introducing non-native chemical bonds or bulky adducts that do not fit in the standard double helix. Unlike proteins and RNA, DNA usually lacks tertiary structure, and therefore damage or disturbance does not occur at that level. DNA is, however, supercoiled and wind around "packaging" proteins called histones (in eukaryotes), and both superstructures are vulnerable to the effects of DNA damage.

DNA as Target

DNA damage can occur through various mechanisms, both from normal cellular processes and environmental exposure to genotoxic agents. The primary types of DNA damage include oxidative damage, alkylation of bases, hydrolytic base loss, bulky adduct formation, DNA crosslinking, and DNA strand breaks (single and double-stranded).

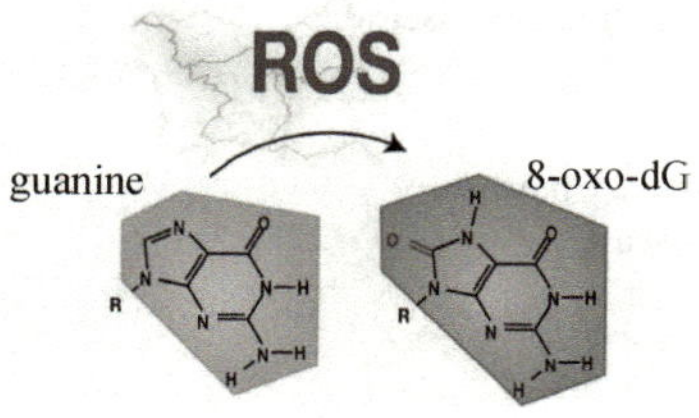

Figure 8-2 Reactive oxygen species and DNA damage

Under conditions of oxidative stress, 8-oxo-dG is the result of reactive oxygen species (ROS) modifying guanine.

(1) Oxidative Damage: Oxidative damage, particularly caused by reactive oxygen species (ROS), is a significant source of cellular stress and DNA damage. Hydroxyl radicals (·OH), among the most reactive and electrophilic ROS, can be generated by ultraviolet and ionizing radiation or enzymatic reactions. These radicals can induce the formation of 8-oxo-7, 8-dihydroguanine (8-oxo-dG) from guanine residues, which is one of the most prevalent DNA lesions, as shown in Figure 8-2. Guanine is especially susceptible to oxidation due to its low ionization potential compared to other DNA bases.

The 8-oxo-dG lesion is widely recognized as a biomarker of oxidative stress, with estimates suggesting that up to 100,000 such lesions can occur daily in DNA per cell. Elevated levels of 8-oxo-dG are frequently associated with carcinogenesis and various disease states, making it a valuable indicator of oxidative damage in tissues, as shown in Figure 8-3.

During DNA replication, 8-oxo-dG can lead to mispairing, with adenine often incorporated opposite the lesion. In subsequent repair processes, the 8-oxo-dG is excised, and thymine is incorporated in its place. This sequence of events typically results in a G to T transversion mutation, highlighting the mutagenic potential of oxidative DNA damage.

(2) Alkylation of Bases: Alkylating agents, ubiquitous in the environment and produced endogenously as byproducts of cellular metabolism, introduce lesions into DNA or RNA bases. These modifications can be cytotoxic, mutagenic, or neutral to the cell, depending on the specific site of alkylation and the alkyl group involved.

(3) Hydrolytic Base Loss: Apurinic/apyrimidinic (AP) sites, also known as abasic sites, are locations in DNA lacking either a purine or a pyrimidine base. These sites can arise spontaneously or due to DNA damage, as shown in Figure 8-4. Under physiological conditions, it is estimated that approximately 10,000 apurinic sites and 500 apyrimidinic sites may be generated daily in a single cell.

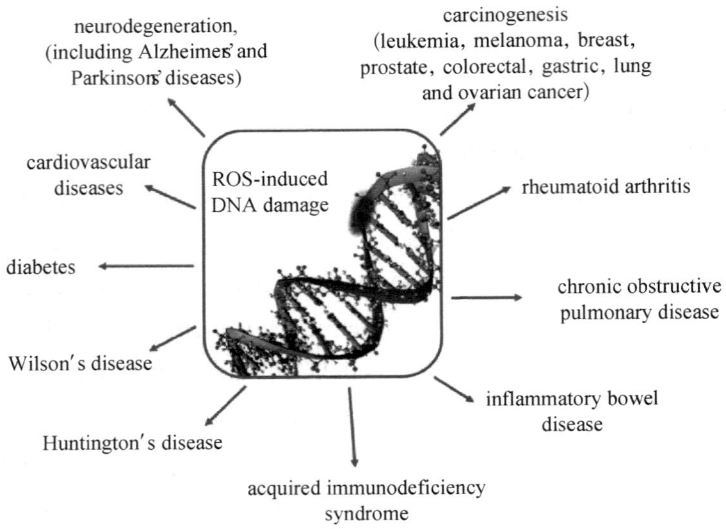

Figure 8-3 **Oxidative stress and human health**

DNA damage caused by oxidative stress has been associated with many human disease states.

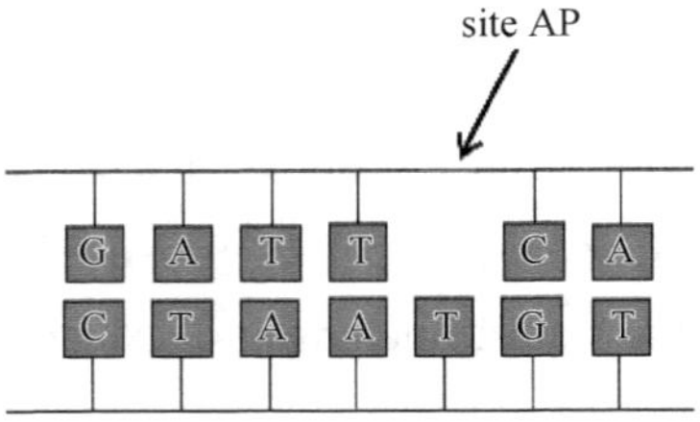

Figure 8-4 **Abasic sites**

Apurinic and Apyrimidimic (AP) sites occur due to unstable hydrolysis

(4) Bulky Adduct Formation: Certain biologically reactive chemicals form covalent linkages with DNA and proteins, creating large, bulky adducts that protrude from the main molecule. These adducts can significantly distort the DNA structure and interfere with normal cellular processes.

(5) DNA Crosslinking: DNA crosslinking occurs when exogenous or endogenous agents react with two nucleotides, forming a covalent linkage. This can happen within the same strand (intrastrand) or between opposite strands of double-stranded DNA (interstrand), as shown in Figure 8-5. These crosslinks interfere with DNA replication and transcription, potentially triggering cell death.

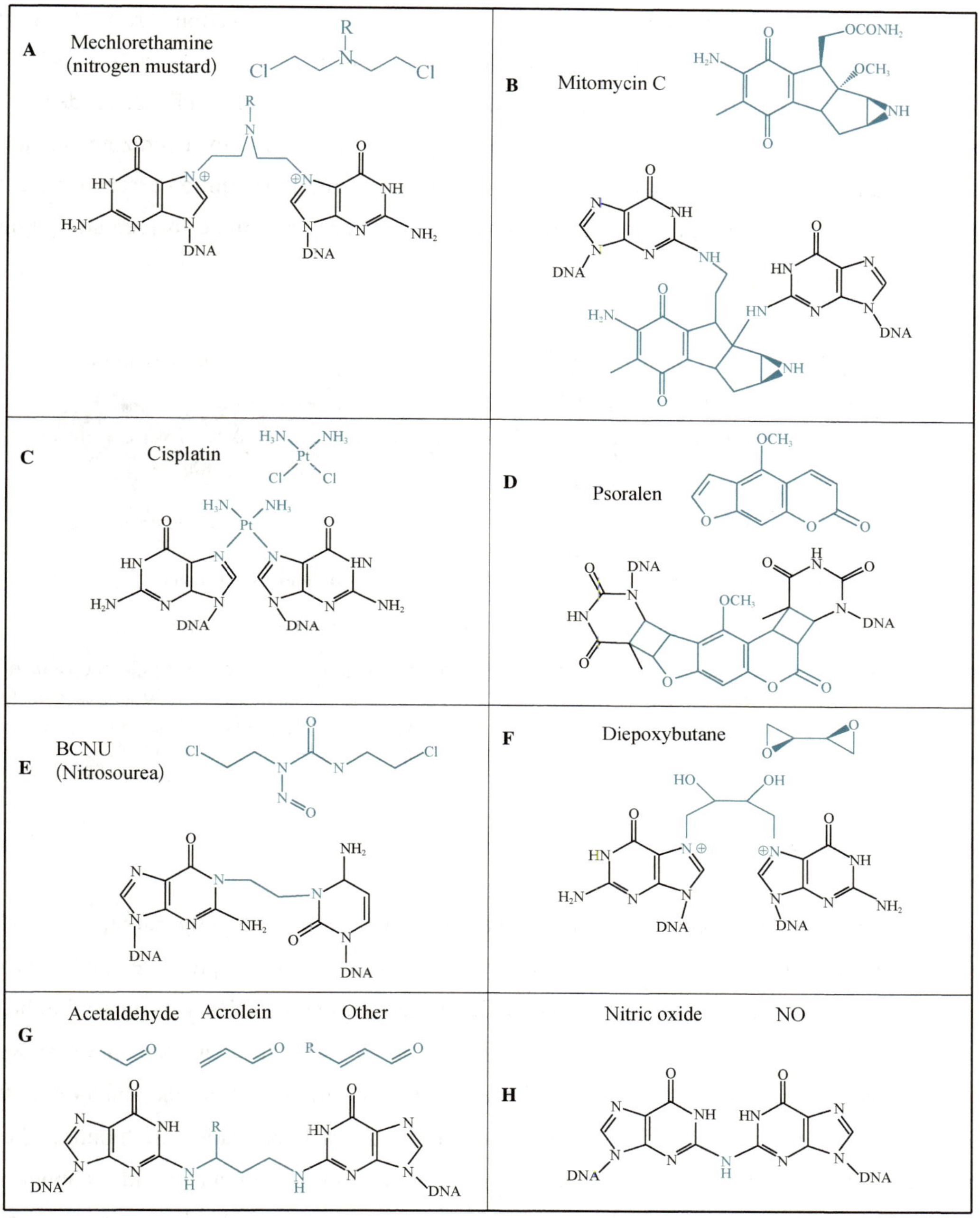

Figure 8-5 Intrastrand and interstrand DNA crosslinks

Ultraviolet (UV) light can induce molecular crosslinks between adjacent pyrimidine residues, commonly thymine dimers, as shown in Figure 8-6. Two prevalent UV products are cyclobutane pyrimidine dimers (CPDs) and 6-4 photoproducts. These premutagenic lesions alter DNA structure and base pairing. While cells can correct many of these lesions through photolyase reactivation or nucleotide excision repair, uncorrected lesions can inhibit polymerases, cause transcription or replication errors, or lead to replication arrest. Notably, pyrimidine dimers are a primary cause of melanomas in humans.

(6) DNA Strand Breaks: Ionizing radiation, such as that from radioactive decay or cosmic rays, can cause breaks in DNA strands (Figure 8-6). Low-level ionizing radiation may induce irreparable DNA damage, leading to replication and transcription errors associated with neoplasia, or may trigger viral interactions. These effects contribute to premature aging and cancer development.

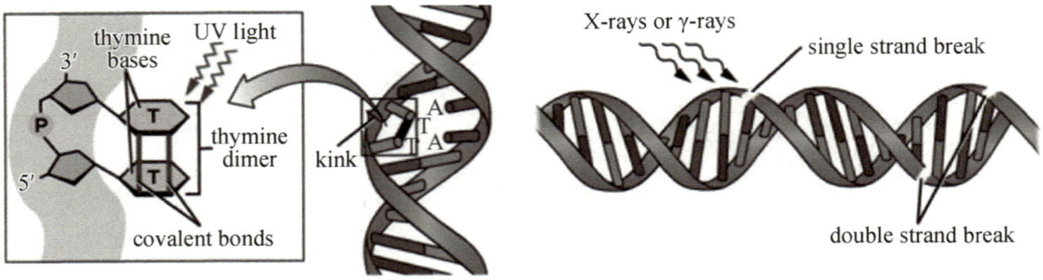

(a) Non-ionizing radiation (b) Ionizing radiation

Figure 8-6 Double-stranded DNA breaks and thymine dimer formation

(b) Ionizing radiation, such as X-rays and γ-rays contain enough energy to cause single and double-stranded breaks in the DNA backbone. (a) Energy from non-ionizing radiation such as UV light is directly absorbed by the DNA causing thymine residues that are adjacent within a single DNA strand to become cross-linked.

DNA not as Target

DNA damage can occur through mechanisms that do not directly target the DNA molecule itself. These indirect pathways involve alterations in cellular processes and enzyme systems that are crucial for maintaining genomic integrity. One significant avenue of indirect DNA damage is through disruption of cell division processes. Mutagens can interfere with various stages of mitosis and meiosis, particularly affecting the formation and function of the mitotic spindle apparatus. By disrupting the synthesis and polymerization of tubulin, these agents can lead to abnormal chromosome segregation, resulting in aneuploidy (abnormal chromosome number) and polyploidy (multiple sets of chromosomes). These chromosomal aberrations can have profound effects on cellular function and viability, potentially contributing to carcinogenesis and developmental abnormalities.

Another critical mechanism of indirect DNA damage involves the impairment of enzyme systems responsible for DNA synthesis and repair. The fidelity of DNA replication is maintained by a complex network of enzymes and regulatory proteins, all of which are encoded by specific genes. Mutagens can interfere with the function of these enzyme systems, compromising the accuracy of DNA replication and the efficiency of DNA repair processes. This interference can indirectly lead to the accumulation of DNA damage, including base mismatches, insertions, deletions, and more complex chromosomal rearrangements. The disruption of DNA repair pathways is particularly concerning, as it can result in the persistence of DNA lesions that would normally be corrected, thereby increasing the likelihood of mutation fixation and genomic instability.

DNA Repair and Tolerance Pathway

Cellular DNA is constantly subjected to various forms of damage, which, if left unrepaired, could lead to mutations, genomic instability, and ultimately cell death or transformation. To counteract these threats, cells have evolved an intricate network of DNA repair pathways that work in concert to maintain genomic integrity. These pathways include direct repair (DR), base excision repair (BER), nucleotide excision repair (NER), mismatch repair (MMR), and DNA double-strand break (DSB) repair. In cases where the sustained damage is too extensive for repair, cells may undergo apoptosis as a protective mechanism against becoming mutant.

Direct Repair (DR)

Direct repair system can act directly on damaged nucleotides, converting each one back to its original structure. There are two distinct DR mechanisms in the majority of organisms: photoreactivation of UV-induced pyrimidine dimers by photolyases, and the removal of the alkyl groups from DNA and RNA by methyltransferases and dioxygenases.

Photoreactivation

This process directly reverses the formation of UV-induced pyrimidine dimers. The enzyme DNA photolyase harnesses light energy to break the covalent bonds linking adjacent pyrimidines, effectively mending the damaged bases. While photolyases are present in various species, including fungi, plants, and some vertebrates, they are notably absent in humans.

Methylguanine-DNA Methyltransferase Repair

This mechanism, carried out by O^6-methylguanine-DNA methyltransferase (MGMT), directly repairs O^6-methylguanine. MGMT protects cells against the toxic effects of simple alkylating agents by transferring the methyl group from O^6-methylguanine to one of its own cysteine residues, thus restoring the original guanine structure.

Base Excision Repair (BER)

BER is a critical DNA repair mechanism that maintains genomic integrity by addressing oxidative and alkylative damage to DNA bases or the sugar-phosphate backbone. This pathway involves a series of coordinated enzymatic steps that efficiently recognize, remove, and replace damaged bases. The process begins with DNA glycosylases identifying and excising the damaged base, creating an AP site. An AP endonuclease then cleaves the DNA backbone at this site, followed by termini clean-up to prepare for repair synthesis. DNA polymerases, typically polymerase β, fill the resulting gap, and finally, DNA ligase seals the nick to complete the repair. This streamlined process involves various specialized enzymes, including glycosylases, endonucleases, phosphatases, polymerases, and ligases, working in concert to restore the DNA to its original state. BER's importance extends beyond basic DNA maintenance, playing roles in aging, neurodegenerative diseases, and cancer development. Understanding BER provides insights into cellular health and offers potential targets for therapeutic interventions in various pathological conditions.

Nucleotide Excision Repair (NER)

NER is a vital DNA repair mechanism that addresses bulky DNA lesions, including UV-induced pyrimidine dimers and chemical adducts from carcinogens or chemotherapeutic drugs. This complex process involves over 30 proteins working in a coordinated sequence. NER begins with damage recognition, followed by local unwinding of the DNA duplex around the lesion. The damaged strand then undergoes dual incision, excising a segment containing the lesion. DNA polymerases fill the resulting gap, and DNA ligase seals the nick, completing the repair. This versatile system is crucial for maintaining genomic integrity, protecting cells against diverse DNA damaging agents. NER's importance is underscored by disorders like xeroderma pigmentosum, which result from NER defects and lead to increased UV sensitivity and cancer risk. The pathway's efficiency is essential for preventing mutations that could cause cellular dysfunction or carcinogenesis, thus playing a key role in overall genomic stability and cellular health.

Mismatch Repair (MMR)

DNA mismatch repair systems operate to repair mismatched bases formed during DNA replication, genetic recombination, and as a result of DNA damage induced by chemical and physical agents. The principal steps are damage recognition by a specific protein that binds to the mismatch, stabilizing of the binding by the addition of one or more proteins, cutting of the DNA at a distance from the mismatch, excision past the mismatch, resynthesis, and ligation.

DNA Double-Strand Break (DSB) Repair

Breaks in both DNA strands are a particularly dangerous threat to genome stability. Unrepaired double-strand breaks trigger one or more DNA damage response systems to either check cell-cycle progression or induce apoptosis. In response to the threat of double-stranded breaks (DSBs), cells have evolved at least two independent pathways for repairing DSBs, by homologous recombination (HR) or by nonhomologous DNA end joining (NHEJ).

Homologous Recombination (HR)

HR comprises a series of interrelated pathways that function in the repair of DNA DSBs and interstrand crosslinks (ICLs). HR utilizes a sister chromatid or homologous chromosome as a template for DNA resynthesis and rejoining to accurately resynthesize DNA spanning a DSB. Followings are the basic steps of HR. The initial step is the production of a 3' ended single-stranded tail by exonucleases or helicase activity. Through a process of strand invasion, whereby the single-stranded tail invades an undamaged homologous DNA molecule, together with DNA synthesis, a so-called Holliday junction DNA complex is formed. By cleavage of this junction, two DNA molecules are produced (with or without a structural crossover), neither of which now contain a strand break.

Non-homologous End Joining (NHEJ)

NHEJ is the primary mechanism of DSB repair in vertebrate cells.

In contrast to homologous recombination, NHEJ simply restores integrity in the DNA by joining the two ends without necessarily preserving the original sequence. The NHEJ process is rather complex and requires a tightly coordinated interplay between the key enzymes to timely initiate each subset of the entire process. Many of these interactions have not been fully investigated and are still poorly understood. The NHEJ process may be divided into three steps: ① the capture of both ends of the broken DNA molecule, ② the formation of a molecular bridge that brings the two DNA ends back together, and ③ the subsequent religation of the broken DNA molecule.

Translesion Synthesis (TLS)

TLS is a vital DNA damage tolerance mechanism that allows cells to maintain genomic replication and survival in the face of persistent DNA lesions. This process becomes crucial when cells encounter DNA damage that cannot be promptly repaired, particularly during DNA replication. TLS enables cells to bypass these lesions, preventing replication fork stalling and potential cell death.

The mechanism is mediated by a set of 11 highly specialized DNA polymerases, each with specific affinities for certain types of lesions and varying across species. These TLS polymerases possess unique characteristics that distinguish them from high-fidelity replicative polymerases, including large active sites to accommodate bulky DNA lesions, fewer contacts with the DNA template for increased flexibility, low processivity, and a lack of 3'-5' exonuclease activity.

The TLS process involves a temporary polymerase switch at the site of DNA damage, where the replicative polymerase is briefly replaced by one or more TLS polymerases to facilitate lesion bypass. Once the damaged site is traversed, the replicative polymerase resumes its function, restoring normal DNA synthesis.

Mutagenicity Testing

Mutagenicity testing is a critical component of toxicological assessment, designed to evaluate the potential of chemical substances and physical agents to induce genetic alterations. This process plays a pivotal role in the hazard assessment of chemicals for regulatory purposes, serving as a cornerstone in safeguarding public health and environmental integrity. The significance of mutagenicity testing is further underscored by its close association with carcinogenesis, as many carcinogens exhibit mutagenic properties. Consequently, these tests are routinely employed as primary screens in the assessment of a compound's carcinogenic potential.

The field of mutagenicity testing has evolved to encompass a diverse array of methodologies, with over two hundred "test systems" documented in scientific literature. These systems span a broad biological spectrum, ranging from bacteriophages to complex mammalian models. Despite this extensive repertoire, practical considerations and standardization requirements have led to the regular use of fewer than 20 test systems in routine toxicological assessments. Some of these specialized assays are exclusively available in advanced laboratories equipped with specific expertise and resources.

Strategy for Mutagenicity Testing

A comprehensive mutagenicity assessment requires consideration of multiple genetic endpoints, including gene mutations, changes in chromosome structure (such as breaks, deletions, and rearrangements), and alterations in chromosomal number (polyploidy or aneuploidy). Given that no single test can detect all genotoxic endpoints, it is standard practice to employ a battery approach, utilizing a specific series of complementary assays.

An effective test battery must incorporate: ① assays capable of detecting each genetic endpoint, ② tests in both prokaryotic and eukaryotic systems, ③ a combination of in vitro and in vivo methodologies, and ④ evaluation of effects in both somatic and germ cells. Regulatory bodies such as International Council for Harmonization of Technical Requirements for Pharmaceuticals for Human Use, Organization for Economic Co-operation and Development (OECD), Food and Drug Administration (FDA), and Environmental Protection Agency (EPA) have developed similar recommendations for the standard battery of mutagenicity tests. The battery includes testing for gene mutations in bacteria, testing for gene mutations in mammalian cells in vitro using a system that can also detect structural chromosome aberrations, and an in vivo test for chromosome aberrations.

While efforts have been made to harmonize testing strategies, there is no universal consensus on the optimal combination of tests for all purposes. Additional assays may be employed based on specific requirements or to address unique endpoints. These supplementary tests may offer an extensive database on chemical mutagenesis (i. e. Drosophila sex-linked recessive lethal test), a unique genetic endpoint (i. e. aneuploidy, mitotic recombination), applicability to diverse organisms and tissues (i. e. DNA damage assays such as the comet assay), or special importance in the assessment of genetic risk (i. e. germ cell assays). The most widely accepted systems are summarized below under three major categories, namely, gene mutations, chromosomal abnormalities, and DNA damage, as shown in Table 8-1.

Table 8-1 **General Mutagenesis Assays**

Classification	Assays
Assays for gene mutations	Bacterial Reverse Mutation Assay (Ames Test) Mammalian Cell Mutation Test tk mutations in mouse lymphoma or human cells hprt or xprt mutations in Chinese hamster or human cells Drosophila sex-linked recessive lethal test Saccharomyces cerevisiae gene mutation assay
Assays for chromosomal abnormalities	Cytogenetic analysis in cultured mammalian cell Cytogenetic analysis in rodent bone marrow Cytogenetic analysis in mammalian germ-cell Micronucleus test Dominant lethal test
Assays for DNA damage	Unscheduled DNA synthesis test Sister chromatid exchange assay Single cell gel electrophoresis (Comet assay) Assays for chemical adducts in DNA Mitotic recombination in Saccharomyces cerevisiae

Gene Mutation Test

Bacterial Reverse Mutation Assay (Ames Test)

The Ames test stands as a cornerstone in the field of genetic toxicology. Developed in the 1970s by Professor Bruce Ames at the University of California, Berkeley, this assay has become a widely accepted and indispensable tool for detecting chemicals capable of inducing mutations in DNA. The Ames test's popularity stems from its remarkable efficiency, combining cost-effectiveness, simplicity, and rapid results, making it an invaluable preliminary screen in mutagenicity testing.

At the heart of the Ames test are several engineered strains of Salmonella typhimurium, each bearing specific mutations in genes involved in histidine biosynthesis. These strains are auxotrophic for histidine, meaning they are unable to synthesize this essential amino acid and thus cannot grow in histidine-deficient media. The principle of the assay relies on the potential of mutagenic compounds to reverse these pre-existing mutations, thereby restoring the bacteria's ability to synthesize histidine and form colonies on histidine-deficient medium. Figure 8-7 illustrates the key components and process of the Ames test, providing a visual representation of this elegant and informative assay.

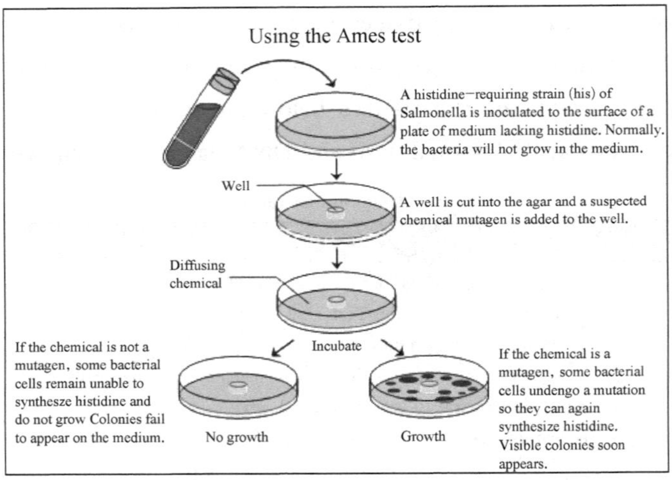

Figure 8-7 **The Ames test**

The test typically employs different Salmonella strains designed to detect various types of mutations. Some strains are sensitive to base-pair substitutions (missense mutations), while others are engineered to detect frameshift mutations. This diversity ensures a broad spectrum of mutagenic events can be identified.

A critical feature of the Ames test is its incorporation of mammalian metabolic activation systems, typically in the form of rat liver microsomes (S9 fraction). This addition is crucial for detecting pro-mutagens-compounds that require metabolic activation to exert their mutagenic effects. The S9 mixture simulates the biotransformation processes that occur in the mammalian liver, allowing the test to identify mutagenic potential that might otherwise be missed in a purely bacterial system.

The assay procedure involves exposing the bacterial strains to the test compound, with and without metabolic activation, on agar plates lacking histidine. If the test compound is mutagenic, it will induce reverse mutations in some bacterial cells, enabling them to grow and form visible colonies. The number of revertant colonies is quantified and compared to negative (solvent) and positive controls to assess the mutagenic potential of the test substance.

Interpretation of Ames test results involves both statistical analysis and biological relevance assessment. A dose-dependent increase in revertant colonies, typically two-fold or greater compared to the negative control, is generally considered a positive result. However, the evaluation must also consider factors such as reproducibility, dose-response relationships, and the specific characteristics of the bacterial strains used.

While the Ames test is highly sensitive and correlates well with rodent carcinogenicity for many classes of chemicals, it is important to note its limitations. False positives can occur, particularly with certain classes of compounds, and some carcinogens that act through non-mutagenic mechanisms may not be detected. Therefore, the Ames test is typically used as part of a battery of tests in comprehensive mutagenicity and carcinogenicity assessments.

Mammalian Cell Mutation Test

Mammalian cell mutation tests complement microbial assays in genetic toxicology studies by leveraging the genetic complexity of eukaryotic cells. These tests employ cultured mammalian cells to detect forward mutations at specific gene loci, primarily hprt (coding for hypoxanthine guanine phosphoribosyl transferase) and tk (coding for thymidine kinase). The principle involves exposing cells to the test substance, then sub-culturing them in selective media where only mutant cells can survive and form colonies. Mutations at the hprt locus confer resistance to toxic purine analogues like 8-azaguanine, while tk mutations provide resistance to pyrimidine analogues such as trifluorothymidine.

The key advantage of these assays lies in their closer resemblance to human cellular metabolism and DNA repair mechanisms, potentially offering more relevant insights for human risk assessment. They can detect a broader spectrum of genetic alterations, including point mutations and small deletions. However, like all in vitro systems, they have limitations, including the potential for false positives and the inability to fully replicate in vivo conditions. Despite these constraints, mammalian cell mutation tests serve as an essential bridge between bacterial tests and in vivo studies, contributing significantly to the comprehensive genotoxicity assessment and safety evaluation of chemicals and pharmaceuticals.

Drosophila Sex-linked Recessive Lethal Test (SLRL)

The SLRL test is a sophisticated in vivo assay that utilizes Drosophila melanogaster to detect mutations in the germ line, encompassing both point mutations and small deletions. This forward mutation assay offers a comprehensive screening of approximately 800 loci on the X-chromosome, leveraging the unique genetic characteristics of Drosophila. The test's principle is predicated on the hemizygous expression of X-linked mutations in male offspring, where lethal mutations are inferred from the absence of one class of male progeny typically produced by heterozygous females. The SLRL test presents several advantages: it employs an intact eukaryotic organism with interrelated organ systems and activation mechanisms, is relatively straightforward to perform, and avoids the use of mammalian test subjects. However, it is important to acknowledge its limitations, primarily the significant differences between insect and mammalian hormonal and immune systems, which may impact the extrapolation of results to human risk assessment. Despite these constraints, the Drosophila SLRL test remains a valuable tool in genetic toxicology, offering insights into mutagenic potential within a complex biological system while balancing ethical considerations in toxicological research.

Chromosomal Abnormalities Assays

Chromosomal abnormalities assays, particularly the chromosome aberration test (i. e. cytogenetic assays, CA), represent a cornerstone in genotoxicity assessment, providing crucial insights into the ability of test compounds to induce structural and numerical chromosomal alterations. This classical method employs microscopic analysis to directly visualize changes in chromosome structure and number, offering a comprehensive evaluation of genomic integrity. The assay can be conducted using cells exposed in vitro or harvested from in vivo sources, such as bone marrow from animals or peripheral blood lymphocytes from humans. Typically, metaphase chromosomes are examined after Giemsa staining, allowing for the detection of aberrations in chromosome size, form, and number. Advanced techniques, such as fluorescent in situ hybridization (FISH) with chromosome-specific painting probes, enhance the assay's sensitivity, enabling the vivid visualization of complex rearrangements and translocations. The CA test's primary advantage lies in its broad cellular target, providing a holistic view of genotoxic effects across the entire genome. This comprehensive approach makes the chromosome aberration test an indispensable tool in genetic toxicology, offering valuable data for risk assessment and mechanism understanding of genotoxic agents, despite the labor-intensive nature of microscopic analysis and the expertise required for accurate interpretation of chromosomal aberrations.

Micronucleus Test

The micronucleus test is a powerful and widely adopted method in genetic toxicology for detecting chromosomal damage and disruptions to the mitotic apparatus induced by chemical agents. This assay is based on the identification of micronuclei, which is small, extranuclear bodies composed of acentric chromosome fragments or whole chromosomes that fail to incorporate into daughter nuclei during cell division. These micronuclei form when chromosomal fragments or whole chromosomes lag behind during anaphase and are subsequently excluded from the main nuclei after telophase.

The versatility of the micronucleus test is evident in its application to both in vitro and in vivo systems, allowing for the detection of clastogens (agents that induce chromosomal breakage) and aneugens (agents that affect chromosome segregation). Figure 8-8, which illustrates a micronucleus in a human lymphocyte, provides a visual representation of this key indicator of genetic damage.

One of the most frequently employed variants is the Mammalian Erythrocyte Micronucleus Test, typically conducted in vivo using mice. This assay capitalizes on the unique developmental process of erythrocytes in bone marrow. As erythroblasts mature into polychromatic erythrocytes, they extrude their main nucleus. However, any micronuclei formed during this process remain in the cytoplasm of the resultant anucleated cell, facilitating their visualization and quantification.

The procedure involves treating animals with the test compound, followed by the extraction of bone marrow cells. These cells are then prepared as smears and stained appropriately. The frequency of micronucleated polychromatic erythrocytes (PCEs) is visually scored under a microscope. An increase in this frequency in treated animals, compared to controls, serves as a clear indication of induced chromosomal damage.

The micronucleus test offers several advantages in genotoxicity assessment. Its relative simplicity in execution, coupled with its sensitivity in detecting both structural and numerical chromosomal aberrations, makes it an invaluable tool in screening for potential genotoxic agents. Moreover, the assay's applicability to various cell types and its adaptability to both in vitro and in vivo systems enhance its utility in comprehensive genotoxicity evaluations.

In recent years, advances in automated scoring systems and the integration of flow cytometry have further enhanced the efficiency and objectivity of micronucleus detection. These technological improvements have not only increased the throughput of the assay but also improved its sensitivity and reproducibility.

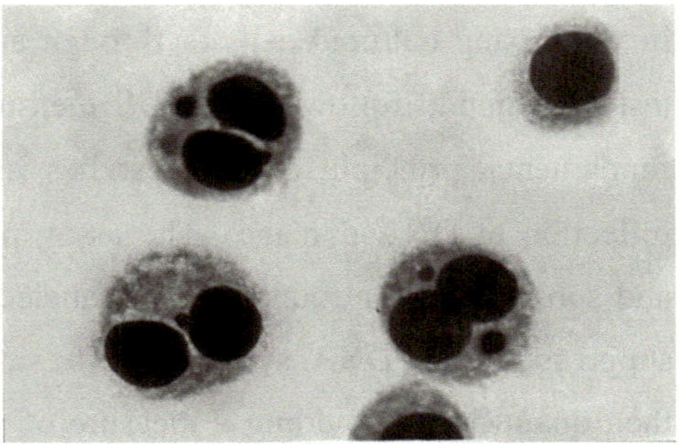

Figure 8-8 **Micronucleus in a human lymphocyte**

Dominant Lethal Test (DLT) in Rodent

The DLT in rodents is a sophisticated in vivo assay designed to evaluate the genotoxic potential of compounds on male germ cells. Typically conducted in mice or rats, this test provides critical insights into the ability of chemicals to induce chromosomal damage or mutations in spermatogenic cells that can lead to embryonic lethality. The assay's principle revolves around exposing male rodents to the test substance, followed by mating them with untreated females. The subsequent analysis focuses on the early stages of embryonic development in these mated females, specifically examining implantation sites and early embryonic losses. Key endpoints include the fertility index (ratio of pregnant to mated females), the proportion of females with dead implantations, and the ratio of dead implantations to total implantations. These parameters serve as indicators of dominant lethal mutations, which are typically the result of chromosomal aberrations or genetic damage in the male gametes that prove fatal to the developing zygote. The DLT's strength lies in its ability to detect germ cell mutagens in a physiologically relevant context, accounting for in vivo metabolic processes and DNA repair mechanisms. However, interpretation of results requires careful consideration of potential confounding factors such as toxicity-induced mating behavior changes. Despite its complexity and resource-intensive nature, the Dominant Lethal Test remains a valuable tool in comprehensive genotoxicity assessments, particularly for compounds with suspected reproductive or developmental toxicity.

DNA Damage Assays

Unscheduled DNA Synthesis (UDS) Assay

The UDS assay is a sophisticated method for detecting and quantifying DNA damage induced by chemical agents. This assay capitalizes on the cellular response to DNA damage, which involves the initiation of enzymatic repair mechanisms resulting in the synthesis of short DNA segments outside the normal replication cycle. The UDS assay can be conducted either in vitro using cultured cells or through an in vivo approach where animals are exposed to the test compound, followed by UDS measurement in cells extracted from specific tissues. The fundamental principle of this test lies in its ability to measure repair synthesis as a direct reflection of DNA damage. The assay protocol involves exposing cells to the test substance and subsequently introducing radiolabeled thymidine (typically tritiated) under conditions that suppress normal DNA synthesis. The incorporation of this labeled nucleotide into DNA is then quantified, providing a measure of repair synthesis activity. The amount of incorporated radioactivity correlates with the extent of DNA repair and, by extension, the degree of primary DNA damage induced by the test compound. This method offers unique insights into the genotoxic potential of chemicals by directly assessing the cellular repair response, making it a valuable complement to other genotoxicity assays. However, interpretation of UDS results requires careful consideration of factors such as cytotoxicity and the specific DNA repair pathways involved. Despite these challenges, the UDS assay remains an important tool in comprehensive genotoxicity evaluations, particularly for compounds suspected of inducing DNA damage that may not be detected by other standard assays.

Sister Chromatid Exchange (SCE) Assay

The SCE assay is a highly sensitive and widely used method in genetic toxicology for detecting DNA damage and potential genotoxic agents. SCEs represent the reciprocal exchange of DNA segments between sister chromatids during replication, serving as indicators of DNA damage and repair processes. While the molecular mechanisms of SCE formation are not fully understood, their susceptibility to chemical induction and correlation with genotoxic and oncogenic potential make them valuable markers in toxicological assessments. The assay involves treating cells with a test compound and incorporating 5-bromodeoxyuridine (BrdU) into newly synthesized DNA for two cell cycles, resulting in differential staining patterns between sister chromatids. This creates the characteristic "harlequin chromosomes" pattern, as illustrated in Figure 8-9.

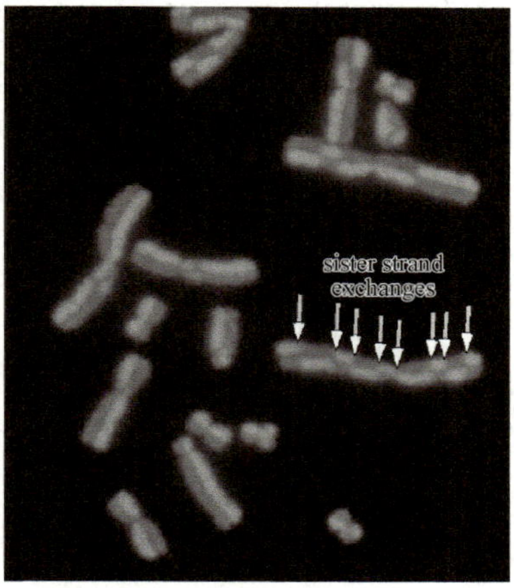

Figure 8-9 Visualization of sister chromatid exchange

The SCE assay's high sensitivity to a wide range of genotoxic agents, particularly DNA-alkylating compounds, makes it an invaluable tool in comprehensive genotoxicity testing strategies. However, it's important to note that SCEs don't always directly correlate with mutagenicity or carcinogenicity, necessitating interpretation alongside other genotoxicity tests. Recent advancements in automated scoring systems and molecular techniques have further enhanced the assay's utility and efficiency, providing more detailed insights into SCE formation mechanisms and their relationship to specific types of DNA damage. These improvements have increased the assay's throughput and deepened our understanding of genotoxic processes, cementing the SCE assay's role as a crucial component in the evaluation of compounds' genotoxic potential.

Single Cell Gel Electrophoresis (SCGE)

The SCGE assay, commonly known as the Comet assay, is a powerful technique in genetic toxicology for detecting DNA damage and repair at the individual cell level. This method combines DNA gel electrophoresis with fluorescence microscopy to visualize the migration of DNA strands from agarose-embedded cells. In the presence of DNA breaks, the relaxed DNA migrates towards the anode during electrophoresis, forming a comet-like shape, while undamaged DNA remains immobile. Figure 8-10 illustrates this phenomenon, showing cells with varying degrees of DNA damage. The assay offers several advantages, including single-cell analysis, high sensitivity, and applicability to various eukaryotic cell types both in vitro and in vivo. It requires only a small number of cells, making it suitable for situations with limited sample availability. However, it's important to note that samples containing predominantly necrotic or apoptotic cells may yield inaccurate results due to extensive DNA fragmentation. Despite this limitation, the Comet assay remains a valuable tool in environmental and human biomonitoring studies, offering unique insights into DNA damage across diverse biological contexts.

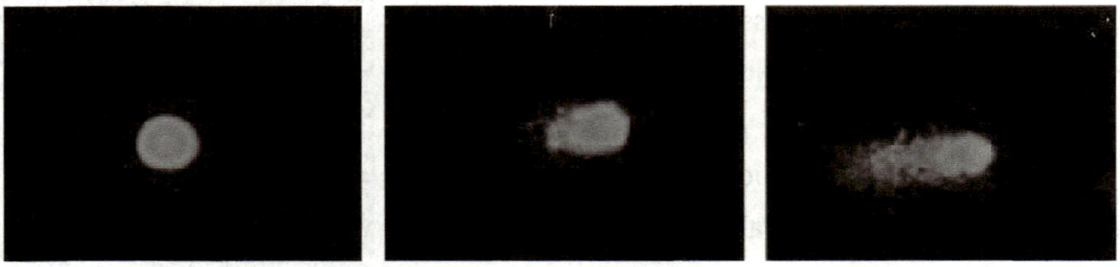

Figure 8-10 **Comet assay image**

Advances in Mutagenesis Test

Advances in mutagenesis test have significantly transformed genetic toxicology over the past two decades, ushering in a new era of molecular precision and efficiency. This evolution has been driven by innovations in molecular biology, biotechnology, and other related fields, enhancing our ability to detect and characterize genetic alterations with unprecedented accuracy.

The detection of chromosomal alterations has been refined through advanced Fluorescence in situ hybridization (FISH) techniques, including multi-color FISH and spectral karyotyping. These methods have improved the resolution and specificity of chromosomal analysis, enabling the identification of complex rearrangements and small deletions previously difficult to detect.

Next-generation sequencing (NGS) technologies, including third- and fourth-generation platforms like Oxford Nanopore and PacBio, have revolutionized mutation analysis at the DNA sequence level. These high-throughput methods offer increased sensitivity in detecting rare mutations, improved distinction between natural and induced mutations, and enhanced detection of large structural variants through long-read sequencing capabilities.

In silico approaches have become more sophisticated, incorporating machine learning algorithms and quantitative structure-activity relationship (QSAR) models integrated with toxicogenomics data. These computational methods have improved the accuracy of genotoxicity predictions based on chemical properties, contributing to enhanced testing strategies that reduce animal use.

Transgenic animal models for mutagenicity assays have been further refined, offering improved sensitivity and tissue-specific mutation detection. New models, such as the Pig-a assay and CRISPR/Cas9-mediated transgenic rodents, have expanded the toolkit for in vivo mutagenesis testing.

The integration of omics technologies, including transcriptomics, proteomics, and metabolomics, has provided a holistic view of cellular responses to genotoxic agents. Single-cell RNA sequencing has enabled the examination of cell-specific responses within heterogeneous populations, leading to the identification of novel biomarkers and molecular signatures associated with different types of genetic damage.

Advanced cell culture models, such as 3D cultures and organ-on-a-chip systems, have improved the recapitulation of in vivo tissue architecture and cell-cell interactions in vitro. These sophisticated models offer better predictivity of human responses to potential mutagens.

Epigenetic considerations have gained prominence, with new methodologies developed to assess DNA methylation and histone modifications. These approaches provide insights into non-mutational mechanisms of genotoxicity.

Artificial intelligence and machine learning have enhanced data analysis capabilities, improving pattern recognition, predictive modeling, and the identification of novel biomarkers of genotoxicity.

As the field continues to evolve, the integration of these diverse technologies into cohesive testing strategies remains a key challenge. Future directions in mutagenesis test will likely involve a system biology approach, combining multiple lines of evidence to provide comprehensive assessments of genotoxic potential. This integrative approach will need to address standardization of protocols, development of adverse outcome pathways specific to different mechanisms of genotoxicity, and refinement of in silico models to improve predictive accuracy.

(Zhang Jie)

CHAPTER 9

Chemical Carcinogenesis

Introduction

Historical Background

The relation between cancer and chemical exposure has been recognized for centuries. In 1761, John Hill observed a high incidence of nasal cancer among users of tobacco snuff, marking one of the earliest documented links between a specific chemical exposure and cancer. In 1775, Percivall Pott documented that chimney sweeps exposed to soot had an increased risk of scrotal cancer, marking one of the first occupationally linked cancers. About twenty years later, Samuel Thomas von Sömmerring noted a frequent occurrence of lip cancer among pipe smokers. In 1895, Rehn discovered the occurrence of bladder tumors among workers in aniline dye factories.

The 20th century witnessed a surge in the identification of chemical carcinogens. Researchers uncovered cancers induced by a diverse array of chemicals under various exposure conditions. Notable examples include the link between asbestos and mesothelioma, vinyl chloride and angiosarcoma of the liver, and benzene and leukemia.

Given the gravity of carcinogenesis and the rapid emergence of novel chemicals, numerous governmental agencies, academic institutions, and industrial laboratories have undertaken extensive research and test on laboratory animals. These efforts aim to elucidate the mechanisms of action of potential carcinogens, determine dose-response relationships, and assess the relevance of human exposure to cancer risk. Additionally, in vitro assays, such as the Ames test, have been developed to screen for mutagenic potential, often an indicator of carcinogenicity.

These scientific endeavors have not only enhanced our understanding of chemical carcinogenesis but also provided valuable leads for epidemiological studies. The integration of animal studies, mechanism research, and human epidemiology has been crucial in identifying carcinogens, establishing regulatory guidelines, and implementing preventive measures to protect public health.

Moreover, recent advancements in molecular biology, toxicogenomics, and systems biology have revolutionized our approach to studying chemical carcinogenesis. These technologies allow for a more comprehensive understanding of the genetic and epigenetic alterations induced by chemical carcinogens, paving the way for personalized risk assessment and targeted prevention strategies.

Fundamental Concepts

Carcinogenesis is the complex process through which cancer develops. Chemical carcinogenesis is the study of the mechanisms through which chemical carcinogens induce cancer and also involves the development/utilization of experimental systems to assess whether a substance is a potential human carcinogen. An important aspect of toxicology is the identification of potential human carcinogens.

Cancer is not a single disease but rather comprises a large group of diseases, all of which can be characterized by the uncontrolled growth and proliferation of an abnormal cell to produce a population of cells that have acquired the ability to multiply and invade surrounding and distant tissues. It is this invasive characteristic that imparts its lethality on the host.

Cancer is a type of neoplasm. There are two basic types of neoplasms, termed benign and malignant. The general characteristics of these tumors are defined in Table 9-1. The term "tumor" is often used interchangeably with "neoplastic lesion" and refers to a grossly observable abnormal growth. Only through histopathological examination can the precise type, grade, and stage of a neoplasm be determined. Cancer is the general name for a malignant neoplasm. In terms of cancer nomenclature, most adult cancers are carcinomas that are derived from epithelial cells (colon, lung, breast, skin etc.). Sarcomas are derived from mesenchymal tissues, while leukemias and lymphomas are derived from blood-forming cells and lymphoid tissue, respectively. Melanoma is derived from melanocytes, and cancers like retinoblastoma, glioblastoma, and neuroblastoma are derived from the stem cells of the retina, glia, and neurons, respectively.

Table 9-1 **Some General Characteristics of Benign and Malignant Neoplasms**

Benign	Malignant
Generally slow growing	May vary from slow to rapid growth
Few mitotic figures	Numerous mitotic figures
Well-differentiated, resembling parent tissue	Often poorly differentiated, with disorganized architecture and loss of parent tissue structure
Sharply demarcated mass, does not invade surrounding tissues	Locally invasive, infiltrating into surrounding normal tissues
No metastases	Metastases

In general, a carcinogen is an agent, either chemical or physical, that induces neoplasia. A more precise definition is as follows: A carcinogen is an agent that, when administered to previously untreated animals, results in a statistically significant increase in neoplasm incidence, covering one or more histogenetic types, compared to appropriately untreated animals. It has been proposed that the majority, approximately 90%, of human cancers are attributed to environmental factors, with a significant proportion being associated with chemical carcinogens.

Several organic compounds have been identified as potential carcinogens, including polycyclic aromatic hydrocarbons (PAHs), dialkylnitrosamines, nitrite, and aflatoxin B_1. In addition, numerous inorganic elements and their compounds, such as those of cadmium, chromium, nickel, lead, beryllium, and arsenic, have been shown to be carcinogenic. Some cancers may result from abnormal internal production of specific hormones, highlighting the intricate relationship between hormonal balance and carcinogenesis. Disruptions in the homeostatic mechanisms of an organism, such as excessive hormone production, can lead to neoplastic transformation.

Among the most prevalent environmental mixtures exhibiting carcinogenic properties are tobacco smoke, combustion products, engine exhaust, and air pollution. Interactions between the chemicals within these mixtures may be additive, synergistic, or inhibitory. Dietary factors, including excessive caloric intake, excessive alcohol intake, and a variety of chemical contaminants of the diet, including aflatoxin B_1, are carcinogenic.

Mechanism of Chemical Carcinogenesis

Chemical carcinogenesis, as shown in Figure 9-1, is a multistage and multistep process. Carcinogenic chemicals act by initiating certain genetic alterations in a cell, promoting the formation of a neoplasm, converting the neoplasm to a cancer.

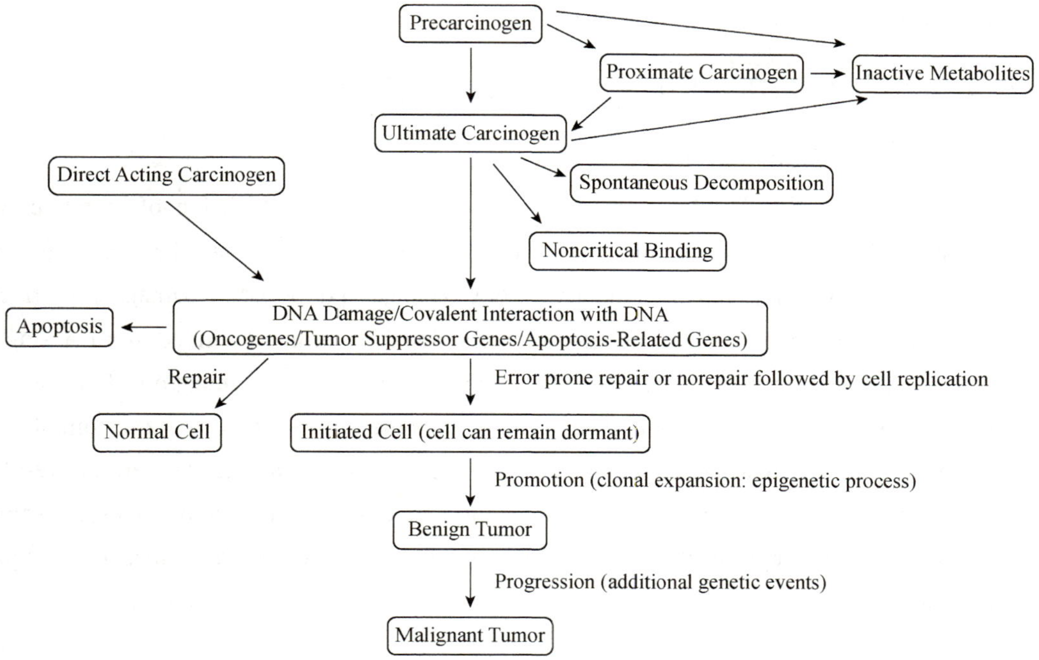

Figure 9-1 Schematic diagram depicting fate of a genotoxic carcinogen and its relation with carcinogenesis

Metabolism of Chemical Carcinogens in Relation to Carcinogenesis

Most carcinogenic chemicals are initially inactive. However, they undergo bioactivation in the body to yield metabolites. From concept of metabolic activation, the important terms procarcinogens, parent, proximate and ultimate carcinogen were developed. Procarcinogens refer to chemical carcinogens that necessitate metabolism to exert their carcinogenic effects. A parent carcinogen is a compound that must be metabolized to manifest carcinogenic activity. A proximate carcinogen is an intermediate metabolite requiring further metabolism, eventually leading to the formation of the ultimate carcinogen. The ultimate carcinogen is the actual metabolite that covalently binds to macromolecules. A number of metabolic reactions are involved in the "activation" of chemicals to their ultimate carcinogenic forms.

Interaction with Macromolecules

A critical step in the induction of cancer by chemicals is the covalent interaction of the reactive metabolites of chemicals with macromolecules. Some of them, such as proteins, may not play a critical role in carcinogenesis. However, when DNA is the target, the reaction may lead to point mutation, frame-shift mutation and other alterations. These changes may not persist, they may be reversed by an error-free DNA repair or disappear when the cell dies. However, these DNA alterations can persist if they are not repaired by cellular mechanisms, contributing to the development of cancer.

Genotoxic Mechanism of Carcinogenesis

Mutation and Carcinogenesis

Molecular analyses of human tumors have confirmed the accumulation of mutations in critical genes during the development of cancer. These mutations can be the result of imperfect DNA replication/repair, oxidative DNA damage and/or DNA damage caused by environmental carcinogens. Most cancers are monoclonal in origin (derived from a single cell) and do not arise from a single critical mutation but from the accumulation of sequential critical mutations in relevant target genes within a single cell (Figure 9-2). Initially a mutation occurs in a critical gene, which provides a growth advantage to the cell and results in the expansion of the mutant clone. Each additional critical mutation provides a further selective growth advantage resulting in clonal expansion of cells with mutations in multiple critical genes.

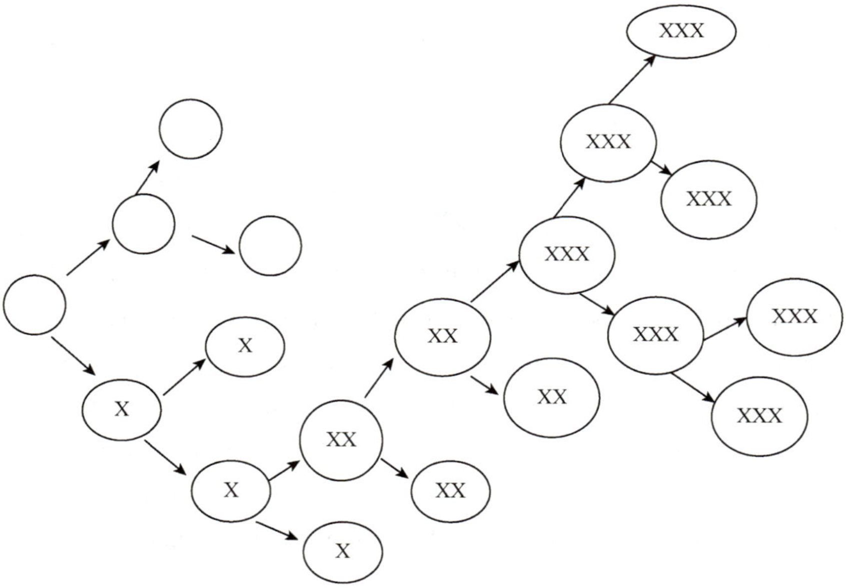

Figure 9-2 Monoclonal origin of cancer

X designates the occurrence of a mutation in a critical gene.

Oncogenes and Tumor Suppressor genes

There are two categories of genes targeted by oncogenic mutations: proto-oncogenes and tumor suppressor genes. The classification depends on whether mutations amplify or diminish the gene product's function in cells. Proto-oncogenes code for proteins that stimulate cell division. When mutated, they transform into carcinogenic oncogenes, producing overactive abnormal protein products, leading to uncontrolled cell proliferation. Conversely, tumor suppressor genes code for proteins inhibiting cell division. When a mutation occurs in a tumor suppressor gene, the inhibitory proteins may not function properly, and inappropriate growth of cells remains unchecked.

Oncogenes: Mutations Causing Gain of Function

An oncogene is mutated or abnormally expressed a gene encoding a protein capable of transforming cells or inducing cancer. Most oncogenes derive from normal genes, namely proto-oncogenes. Mutations in proto-oncogenes activate cancer-promoting activities, either by increasing gene expression levels or enhancing biochemical activity. Quantitative or qualitative changes in gene products contribute to gain of function, positively influencing cell proliferation. The most defined oncogenes include the following categories: Growth factor (e. g. *sis*, *ks/hst*, *TGF*α), Growth factor receptor (e. g. *erbB*, *kit*), Intracellular tyrosine kinases (e. g. *src*, *abl*), Signal transduction molecule (e. g. *ras*, *gsp*, *gip*), Serine/threonine kinases (e. g. *raf*, *mos*) and Transcription factor (e. g. *myc*, *fos*, *jun*).

Tumor Suppressor genes: Mutations Causing Loss of Function

Tumor suppressor genes, also known as anti-oncogenes, encode proteins that generally function as negative regulators of cell proliferation or positive regulators of apoptosis. Inactivation of these genes, caused by allelic loss, point mutation, or chromosome deletion, leads to uncontrolled cell proliferation. Generally, if one allele of a tumor suppressor gene is inactivated, the cell is normal. However, when both alleles are inactivated, the ability to control cell proliferation is lost. The p53 gene, a critical tumor suppressor, is frequently mutated in human cancers, highlighting its crucial role in cell cycle control and DNA damage repair. Rb, another important tumor suppressor, controls the transition from G1 to S phase of the cell cycle. Mutations in these genes can lead to uncontrolled cell proliferation and tumor development.

Nongenotoxic Mechanism of Carcinogenesis

Some chemicals induce tumors in experimental animals following chronic exposure without directly interacting with DNA. These chemicals are classified as nongenotoxic carcinogens. They do not exhibit genotoxicity, meaning they do not directly damage DNA, but they can still induce tumors in rodent models. The organs and tissues affected by these carcinogens are often those with a high incidence of spontaneous tumors in the animal model. Long-term exposure to relatively high levels of these chemicals is typically required for tumor formation. These carcinogens may operate through various mechanisms, such as sustained cytotoxicity, receptor-mediated effects, hormonal perturbation, induction of oxidative stress, and modulation of methylation status.

Dysregulation of Cell Cycle and Carcinogenesis

Precise regulation of the cell cycle is essential for maintaining DNA integrity and ensuring that cell proliferation occurs only under specific conditions. Dysregulation of the cell cycle is a hallmark of cancer, leading to uncontrolled tumor growth due to unchecked cell division. This dysregulation can result from defects in cell cycle, checkpoints, DNA repair, or apoptosis. The p53 gene plays a crucial role in regulating the cell cycle by acting as a checkpoint regulator, linking systems that detect DNA damage to genes inducing cell death or cell cycle inhibition. Mutations in this gene are frequent in cancers, disrupting its regulatory functions and contributing to cell cycle dysregulation.

The Role of Telomeres in Cellular Immortalization and Development of Cancer

Normal human cells have a finite lifespan in tissue culture. As cells divide, the ends of chromosomes, called telomeres, progressively shorten. Telomere length acts as a molecular clock that governs the lifespan of replicating cells. Telomerase, an enzyme that adds repetitive telomeric sequences to maintain telomere length, is typically inactive in somatic cells. However, in germ cells and some cancer cells, telomerase activity is maintained, allowing these cells to preserve telomere length and achieve immortality. Telomerase activation is a crucial step in the development of many cancers, enabling their indefinite proliferation.

Epigenetic Gene Silencing

Epigenetic gene silencing, a process involving aberrant methylation of promoter DNA and transcriptional repression, is another important mechanism for loss of gene function in cancer. This silencing can occur during the early stages of human tumor progression and can disrupt or over-activate key developmental pathways and cell signaling properties. DNA methylation is a critical epigenetic modification that plays a significant role in carcinogenesis. Chemical carcinogens can modify DNA methylation, methyltransferase activity, and chromosomal structure, leading to hypomethylation and/or hypermethylation of the genome. Hypermethylation of tumor suppressor genes can lead to their silencing, while hypomethylation may contribute to the overexpression of proto-oncogenes or global genomic instability, potentially increasing mutation rates.

Sustained Cytotoxicity and Regenerative Hyperplasia

Cytotoxicity followed by regenerative hyperplasia is a well-documented mode of action for many non-DNA-reactive chemical carcinogens. These chemicals cause cell death without directly damaging DNA, but they induce persistent regenerative growth as a compensatory response. This regenerative growth increases the chance of acquiring spontaneous DNA mutations, leading to the accumulation and proliferation of mutated cells. These preneoplastic focal lesions can eventually lead to tumor formation.

Apoptosis Inhibition

Homeostasis, the balance between proliferation and programmed cell death, usually in the form of apoptosis, is tightly regulated to ensure the integrity of organs and tissues. Mutations in DNA that lead to cancer disrupt these processes, altering the program that regulates proliferation and apoptosis. Non-mutagenic carcinogens typically increase the frequency of spontaneous mutations and inhibit apoptosis, expanding the population of transformed cells and promoting cancer development.

Cellular Communication and Carcinogenesis

Gap junctional intercellular communication appears to play an important role in the regulation of cell growth and cell death, in part through the ability to exchange small molecules (<1 kDa) between cells. If cell communication is blocked between tumor and normal cells, the exchange of growth inhibitory signals from normal cells to initiated cells is prevented, thus allowing the potential for unregulated growth and clonal expansion of initiated cell populations.

Multi-stage Processes of Carcinogenesis

The pathogenesis of neoplasia is believed to consist of at least three operationally defined stages: initiation, promotion, and progression. It is in the first and last stages of neoplastic development, initiation and progression, that structural changes in the genome (DNA) can be observed. The structural changes are most likely to be responsible for the induction of these stages, especially the stage of initiation. The intermediate stage of promotion does not appear to involve direct structural changes in the genome of the cell but instead depends on an altered expression of genes.

Initiation

Initiation, the first stage of carcinogenesis, is defined as a stable, heritable change. This rapid and irreversible process results from the interaction of a carcinogen, known as an initiator, with cellular components, particularly DNA. Initiation requires one or more rounds of cell division to "fix" the genetic alterations, which may include point mutations, deletions, or chromosomal translocations.

The efficiency of initiation can be modulated by factors such as xenobiotic metabolism and DNA repair mechanisms. The dose-response relationship and relative potency of initiators have been demonstrated in various experimental systems. However, these parameters may be influenced by alterations in xenobiotic metabolism and trophic hormones.

A key characteristic of initiation is its irreversibility, the genotype and/or phenotype of the initiated cell is established at the time of initiation. However, not all initiated cells survive, many undergo apoptosis, highlighting the body's natural defense against potentially cancerous cells. The spontaneous or fortuitous initiation of cells in various tissues is a common occurrence, suggesting that the development of neoplasia can sometimes be a function solely of the action of agents at the stages of promotion or progression.

Promotion

The promotion stage involves the selective clonal expansion of initiated cells, resulting in the formation of preneoplastic lesions. Unlike initiation, promotion is generally reversible and does not involve direct DNA alterations. Instead, tumor promoters act by changing gene expression patterns, leading to increased cell proliferation and/or inhibition of apoptosis.

Promoting agents or their metabolites likely do not directly interact with DNA. Tumor promoters generally show organ-specific effects, for example, a liver tumor promoter like phenobarbital will not function as a tumor promoter in the skin or other tissues.

Promotion is highly susceptible to modulation by physiological factors, including age, diet, and hormones. Many modulating factors are themselves promoting agents. The dose-response relationships of promoting agents exhibit sigmoid-like curves with an observable threshold and a maximal effect. This threshold effect may be considered a consequence of the reversible nature of their effects at the cellular level, while the maximal effect is due to a saturation of ligand binding and the promotion of all initiated cells.

Progression

The progression stage of carcinogenesis involves the conversion of the preneoplastic lesions to neoplasms. During this stage, additional genotoxic events occur resulting in additional DNA damage including chromosomal damage such as aberrations and translocations. In the neoplastic state, cells accumulate mutations and epigenetic changes that disrupt normal growth control mechanisms, enabling them to outgrow the surrounding normal cells. The tumor microenvironment is an important component of this process and the presence of "normal" cells and stroma within the lesion is critical for the neoplastic cells to survive and propagate. During progression, the initially clonal nature of the neoplastic lesion is typically lost, giving rise to a polyclonal cell population within the lesion. Agents that impact on the progression stage are predominantly genotoxic, although additional mutagenic events may arise through sustained stimulation of cell proliferation. These events result in the transfer from preneoplastic, clonally derived cell populations into neoplastic cell populations.

By definition, the progression stage is an irreversible stage in that neoplasm formation, whether benign or malignant, occurs. With the formation of neoplasia, an autonomous growth and/or lack of growth control is achieved. Spontaneous progression can occur through spontaneous karyotypic changes in mitotically active initiated cells during promotion. The accumulation of nonrandom chromosomal aberrations and karyotypic instability are hallmarks of progression. As such, chemicals that function during the progression stage are frequently clastogenic and are capable of causing chromosomal abnormalities.

Complete carcinogens have the ability to function at all three stages of carcinogenesis, initiation, promotion, and progression, and therefore exhibit genotoxic properties.

Table 9 – 2 summarizes the key morphological and biological characteristics of each stage, providing a comparative overview of their reversibility, cellular changes, dose-response relationships, and other important aspects.

Table 9–2 **Characteristics of Initiation, Promotion, and Progression in Carcinogenesis**

Characteristic	Initiation	Promotion	Progression
Reversibility	Irreversible in viable cells	Operationally reversible at gene expression and cellular levels	Irreversible
Morphological changes	No discermible morphological changes	Clonal expansion of altered cells	Discermible alterations in cellular structure; benign or malignant neoplasms
Genetic changes	Stable, heritable changes (mutations)	Generally no direct DNA alterations; changes in gene expression	Further genetic/epigenetic changes; karyotypic instability
Dose-response relationships	No readily measurable threshold	Exhibits measurable threshold and maximal effect	Complex, depends on specific alterations
Environmental sensitivity	Efficiency sensitive to xenobiotic factors	Highly sensitive to environmental factors (diet, hormones, age)	Sensitive in early phases, may decrease with progression
Cell division requirement	Requires cell division for "fixation"	Involves increased cell proliferation	Continued proliferation with decreased growth control
Agent specificity	Initiators cause direct DNA damage	Promoters often show tissue specificity	" Progressor " agents enhance karyotypic instability
Spontaneous occurrence	Spontaneous initiation is common	Can occur spontaneously (e. g. by endogenous promoters)	Spontaneous progression possible, enhanced by increased cell replication

Carcinogen Classification

International Agency for Research on Cancer(IARC) Carcinogen Classification

IARC is a department of the World Health Organization(WHO). The IARC produces a series of monographs that describe the methodology for the evaluation of specific chemicals and the rationale for their final classification. The IARC approach assigns the chemical or mixture to one of five groupings based upon strength of evidence for the agent's possible, probable or definite carcinogenicity to humans. The classification reflects the strength of the evidence available from animals, epidemiology and other relevant data. The classification may change for a chemical when new information becomes available.

Group 1–Carcinogenic to Humans Agents in this category are deemed definitely carcinogenic to humans. This classification is assigned when there is sufficient evidence of carcinogenicity in humans, showing a causal relationship between exposure and cancer. Examples include aflatoxin, benzene, arsenic, and tobacco smoke.

Group 2A–Probably Carcinogenic to Humans Agents in this group are considered probably carcinogenic to humans. This classification is applied when there is limited evidence of carcinogenicity in humans but sufficient evidence from experimental animals. Examples include acrylamide and benzo[a]pyrene.

Group 2B–Possibly Carcinogenic to Humans Agents classified in this group are possibly carcinogenic to humans. This designation is used when there is limited evidence in humans and less than convincing evidence in experimental animals. Examples include carbon tetrachloride and styrene.

Group 3–Not Classifiable as to its carcinogenicity to humans The agent falls into this category when evidence for carcinogenicity in humans and experimental animals is inadequate or limited. Examples include caffeine and fluorescent lighting.

Group 4–Probably Not Carcinogenic to Humans This category is used when there is evidence suggesting lack of carcinogenicity in humans and in experimental animals. Few agents have been classified in this group.

Classes of Agents Associated with Carcinogenesis

Chemical agents influencing the development of cancer fall into two main categories based on their mutagenicity in vitro.

Genotoxic Carcinogenic Agents

Genotoxic agents, also known as DNA-damaging agents, directly or indirectly cause alterations in the genetic material. These agents can be categorized based on their mechanisms of action. Direct-acting carcinogens are intrinsically reactive compounds that covalently interact with DNA without requiring metabolic activation. Examples include N-methyl-N-nitrosourea and methyl methanesulfonate. In contrast, indirect-acting carcinogens require metabolic activation by cellular enzymes to form the ultimate carcinogenic species. Benzo[a]pyrene and aflatoxin B_1 are notable examples of this category.

Radiation and oxidative stress can also induce DNA damage through various mechanisms. Ionizing radiation, for instance, can directly ionize DNA to produce strand breaks or indirectly generate reactive oxygen species that damage DNA bases. Similarly, certain chemicals and cellular processes, including respiration and lipid peroxidation, can produce reactive oxygen species leading to DNA damage. Inorganic agents such as arsenic, chromium, and nickel are also considered DNA-damaging agents, although their mechanisms of action are often complex and may involve multiple pathways.

Nongenotoxic Carcinogenic Agents

Nongenotoxic agents contribute to carcinogenesis without directly altering DNA sequences. These agents operate through various mechanisms that disrupt normal cellular processes. Hormones, such as conjugated estrogens and diethylstilbestrol, can promote carcinogenesis by altering gene expression patterns and cell proliferation rates. Immunosuppressive xenobiotics, including azathioprine and cyclosporin A, may contribute to cancer development by compromising the immune system's ability to detect and eliminate abnormal cells.

Solid-state agents, which include materials like plastic implants and asbestos fibers, can induce carcinogenesis through chronic irritation and inflammation. Tumor promoters, such as peroxisome proliferators, TCDD, and phenobarbital, have been identified in rodent models and act by enhancing the growth and survival of initiated cells. In humans, various environmental and lifestyle factors are thought to act through promotional mechanisms. These include dietary factors (such as caloric intake, fat consumption, and protein intake), excess alcohol consumption, and late age at first pregnancy. It's worth noting that some agents, like tobacco smoke and ultraviolet radiation, exhibit both initiating and tumor-promoting activities, underscoring the complex nature of carcinogenesis.

Identification of Carcinogen

Short-term Tests for Mutagenicity (Rapid Screening Tests for Carcinogen Identification)

Numerous rapid screening tests for mutagenicity have been developed to aid in identifying potential carcinogens, based on the close relationship between mutagenesis and carcinogenesis. These tests utilize various systems, including microbes, insects, mammalian cells, and whole animals. They can be classified into three groups: ① gene mutation assays, ② chromosome aberration tests, ③ primary DNA damage assays.

While useful in carcinogen identification, these tests create challenges for risk estimation. Most are in vitro screens for mutagenicity, based on the assumption that all carcinogens are mutagenic. However, not all compounds that test positive for carcinogenicity in a two-year bioassay are mutagenic, either directly or after metabolic activation.

Mammalian Cell Transformation

Most cell transformation assays use fibroblast cultures derived from embryonic tissue. The cells from mouse fibroblast cultures underwent changes in morphologies and growth patterns when treated with carcinogens. The direct relationship of these changes to carcinogenesis was demonstrated by the development of tumors in a host animal transplanted with transformed cells.

In a typical assay situation, cells will multiply in culture until a monolayer is formed. At this point, they cease dividing unless transformed. Chemicals that are transforming agents will, however, cause growth to occur in thicker layers above the monolayer. These clumps of transformed cells are known as foci. The doses are selected from the results of a preliminary experiment and range from a high dose that reduces colony formation (but not more than 50%) to a low dose that has no measurable effect on colony formation. After exposure for 1–3 days to the test chemical, the cells are washed and incubation is continued for up to 4 weeks. At that time, the monolayers are fixed, stained and scored for transformed foci.

Long Term (the Two-Year) Bioassays

Long-term bioassays are considered the gold standard for carcinogenicity testing, typically conducted over a significant portion of the test animals' lifespan. These studies are designed to evaluate the potential carcinogenic effects of substances through prolonged exposure in rodent models. The experimental design typically involves testing in two rodent species, with rats and mice being preferred due to their relatively short lifespans. This dual-species approach helps to account for potential species-specific responses and provides a more comprehensive assessment of carcinogenic potential.

The studies begin with young adult animals, usually starting at weaning, and continue for an extended period. For mice, the dosing is carried out for 1.5 to 2.0 years, with an observation period of 18–24 months. Rats, having a slightly longer lifespan, are dosed for 2.0 years or more, with an observation period of 24–30 months. This prolonged exposure and observation allow for the detection of late-onset tumors and provide insight into the cumulative effects of the test substance over time.

To ensure statistical robustness, each dose group includes 50 animals of each sex. The study typically employs three dose levels, with the highest dose designed to produce minimal toxicity without significantly altering lifespan. Lower doses are often set at fractions of the highest dose, such as one-half and one-quarter. A concurrent control group is also included to provide a baseline for comparison. This multi-dose approach allows for the assessment of dose-response relationships, which is crucial in determining the carcinogenic potential of the test substance.

Throughout the study, animals are closely monitored for various parameters including food consumption, body weight changes, and clinical signs of toxicity. At the conclusion of the study, or upon death or sacrifice in extremis, a comprehensive necropsy is performed on all animals. Tissues are examined microscopically to identify and characterize any neoplastic lesions, providing detailed information on the nature and distribution of tumors.

The evaluation of carcinogenic potential is based on a comprehensive analysis of several key parameters. A statistically significant increase in the incidence of tumors in treated groups compared to controls, particularly if dose-related, is a primary indicator of carcinogenicity. This is often accompanied by an increase in the number of tumors per animal or the development of tumor types not observed in the control group. The timing of tumor occurrence is also considered, with earlier appearance in treated animals being a significant factor. Additionally, increased tumor multiplicity, the presence of metastatic tumors (especially if benign tumors show metastatic potential), and the development of rare tumors uncommon in the test species or strain are all important considerations.

However, it's crucial to note that the interpretation of these studies goes beyond mere statistical significance. The biological relevance of the findings is carefully considered, and these factors are taken into account, such as the type and location of tumors, the historical incidence of spontaneous tumors in the test species, and the potential relevance to human cancer risk. A weight-of-evidence approach is typically employed, integrating the results of the bioassay with data from genotoxicity studies, mechanism investigations, and any available epidemiological evidence.

These long-term bioassays provide invaluable data for risk assessment and regulatory decision-making regarding potential carcinogens. While they have limitations, such as the high cost and long duration, they remain a cornerstone of carcinogenicity testing, complementing other lines of evidence in the complex process of identifying and characterizing potential human carcinogens.

Epidemiology Investigation

Epidemiological studies play a crucial role in identifying potential carcinogens in human populations. These observational studies examine the distribution and determinants of cancer, providing valuable insights that complement laboratory-based research. Epidemiological approaches to carcinogen identification include several types of studies, each with its strengths and limitations.

Case reports and case series can provide initial indications of potential carcinogenic exposures. While these cannot establish causality, they often serve as the basis for more rigorous investigations. Ecological studies examine correlations between exposure and cancer rates at the population level, but are limited by the ecological fallacy and inability to control for confounding factors.

Case-control studies compare individuals with cancer (cases) to those without (controls), examining their histories of exposure to potential carcinogens. These studies are efficient for rare cancers but may be subject to recall bias. Cohort studies, however, follow groups of exposed and unexposed individuals over time to compare cancer incidence. While these provide stronger evidence for causality, they require large sample sizes and long follow-up periods, especially for rare cancers or those with long latency periods.

Cross-sectional studies can provide a snapshot of exposure and disease status in a population at a single point in time. Although limited in their ability to establish temporality, they can be useful for generating hypotheses and examining the prevalence of exposures and outcomes.

Epidemiological studies face several challenges in establishing causal relationships between specific chemical exposures and cancer. These include long latency periods between exposure and cancer development, difficulties in accurately measuring past exposures, and the presence of numerous confounding factors. Additionally, ethical considerations prevent deliberate human exposure to potential carcinogens, necessitating reliance on observational data.

Despite these limitations, epidemiological studies have been instrumental in identifying many human carcinogens, including tobacco smoke, asbestos, and certain occupational exposures. They provide critical evidence for risk assessment and regulatory decision-making, complementing data from animal studies and mechanism investigations. The integration of epidemiological findings with data from experimental studies and emerging molecular and genetic techniques continues to advance our understanding of environmental carcinogenesis and inform cancer prevention strategies.

(Cao Yi)

CHAPTER 10

Developmental Toxicity and Teratogenesis

Introduction

Developmental toxicology constitutes a contemporary branch discipline within toxicology that emerged on the foundation of teratology. Developmental toxicology is an emergent science, which involves the study of abnormal developmental outcomes induced by exposure to detrimental factors, along with their pharmacokinetics, mechanism, pathogenesis, and consequences. Teratology is the science that studies the causes and mechanisms of abnormal fetal development and congenital malformations. As a descriptive science, it precedes the advent of written language. Malformations denote defects in the anatomical morphology and structure of developing organisms. They can be classified into severe malformations and minor malformations. The former exerts pronounced effects on appearance, physiological functions, or lifespan, while the latter have only marginal or no effects. The earliest evidence of teratology can be traced back to a marble sculpture depicting conjoined twins in southern Turkey around 6, 500 BC, while Egyptian frescoes depicting human conditions such as cleft palate and achondroplasia date back as early as 5, 000 years ago. The Babylonians, Greeks, and Romans held the belief that abnormal babies reflected celestial events and were thus regarded as omens of the future. Hippocrates and Aristotle maintained that abnormal development might arise from physiological causes, such as uterine trauma or stress. However, Aristotle also generally opined that the impression and emotion of the mother would influence the development of the child. Another belief, namely the hybridization theory, proposed that hybridization between humans and animals was the cause of congenital malformations.

With the flourishing of biological sciences during the 16th—17th centuries, birth defects were also perceived by some as divine retribution upon the parents and society of malformed babies. The emergence of the germplasm theory expounded by Weissmann in the 1880s and the rediscovery of Mendel's laws in 1900 led genetics to be recognized as the basis of certain birth defects. Modern experimental teratology originated in the early 19th century when Saint-Hilaire generated malformed chicken embryos by subjecting eggs to various environmental conditions, encompassing physical trauma (shocks, inversions, stabbings) and toxic exposures. In the early 20th century, it was discerned that diverse environmental conditions (temperature, microbial toxins, drugs) would interfere with the development of birds, reptiles, fish, and amphibians. In contrast, mammalian embryos were considered resilient against the induction of malformations and were safeguarded by the maternal system from adverse environmental conditions. The first report of induced birth defects in mammal species was published in the 1930s as a consequence of experimental maternal nutritional deficiency. Hale induced malformations in the offspring of sows through feeding a diet lacking vitamin A, including anophthalmia and cleft palate. Commencing from 1940, Josef-Warkany and colleagues initiated a series of experiments, in which they demonstrated that maternal dietary insufficiency and other environmental factors could impact the intrauterine development of rats, leading to adverse pregnancy outcomes, such as miscarriage, stillbirth, stillbirth at term, intrauterine growth retardation, abnormal development, neonatal and infant death, rendering it impossible to produce descendants with normal appearance and function. Subsequent studies showed that chemical and physical reagents, like nitrogen mustard, trypan blue, hormones, antimetabolites, alkylating agents, hypoxia, and X-rays can cause malformations in mammals.

Gregg was the first to report an epidemic of human malformations caused by environmental factors, by linking the epidemic of Australian rubella virus infections to an increased incidence of eye, heart, and ear defects, as well as mental retardation. Defects of the heart and eyes are mainly associated with the first or second month of pregnancy when the mother is infected, while hearing and language defects and mental retardation are most commonly associated with infection in the third month of pregnancy. Later, the risk of congenital malformations associated with rubella infection within 4 weeks before pregnancy was estimated at 61%; at 26% for the 5th to 8th weeks; and at 8% for the 9th to 12th weeks. It is estimated that about 20, 000 children in the United States alone suffered from the effects of prenatal rubella infection. Maternal rubella is now rare in developed countries thanks to vaccination programs, but rubella epidemics continue to occur in developing countries.

Principles of Developmental Toxicology

Principles of Teratology

The Principles of Teratology, first proposed by Jim Wilson in his seminal work *Environment and Birth Defects* (1973), have stood the test of time and continue to form the cornerstone of our understanding of developmental toxicology. These principles elucidate the complex interplay between genetic and environmental factors in the etiology of birth defects. Wilson's six fundamental laws encompass the following concepts, ① teratogenic susceptibility is determined by the interaction between the embryo's genotype and adverse environmental factors, ② this susceptibility varies with the developmental stage at which the embryo encounters these adverse factors, ③ teratogenic agents operate through specific pathogenic mechanisms, ④ the nature of the teratogen influences its interaction with the developing organism, ⑤ abnormal development manifests in four primary ways: death, malformation, growth retardation, and functional defects, ⑥ the severity of developmental defects is dose-dependent, increasing with higher exposures.

Building upon these principles, we can identify four key specificities of teratogenic effects. ① Stage specificity refers to the existence of brief, sensitive periods during which teratogenic effects are most pronounced. ② Substance specificity describes how different chemicals may induce distinct types of malformations at defined developmental stages. ③ Species specificity acknowledges that teratogenic effects may be reproducible in some species but not in others, highlighting the importance of careful extrapolation in teratology research. ④ Dose specificity recognizes that certain malformations occur only within a narrow dose range, underscoring the complex relationship between exposure and effect in developmental toxicology.

These principles and specificities collectively provide a robust framework for understanding and predicting teratogenic effects, guiding both research and clinical practice in the field of developmental toxicology.

The Critical Period of Susceptibility and Endpoint

The critical period of susceptibility to developmental toxicity refers to a specific stage in an organism's development during which it is particularly vulnerable to the toxic effects of certain chemicals. The critical period of susceptibility in an organ occurs just prior to and during its initial formation. The susceptibility critical period may be extended because of organ functional defects.

The endpoint of developmental toxicity is a specific indicator of developmental abnormalities in an organism exposed to certain chemicals. Developmental toxins can act at different developmental stages, resulting in a range of effects. Although embryogenesis is complex, involving cell migration, proliferation, differentiation, and organ formation, the process of development can be divided into three major stages: pre-implantation, implantation to organ formation, and fetal to neonatal stage. Different stages of exposure have different outcomes(Table 10-1).

Table 10-1 **The Outcomes Associated with Exposure During Different Periods**

Stage of Exposure	Primary Outcome
Pre-implantation	Embryonic lethality
Implantation to time of organogenesis	Morphological defects
Fetal to neonatal stage	Functional disorders, growth retardation, carcinogenesis

[Table 10-1 is derived from Table 10-1 in Chapter 10 of the second edition of *Texbook of Toxicology: Basic and Case Studies*]

(1) Pre-implantation period (1-2 weeks in human): This period spans from fertilization to the completion of implantation. The pre-implantation period is characterized by rapid cell division, resulting in an increase in cell numbers with minimal differentiation, and the damage is typically inflicted on relatively undifferentiated cells. The undifferentiated pre-implantation embryo has a good potential for recovery and growth. In general, specific teratogenic effects rarely occur at this time, usually having no or only minor effects on growth, or death (due to irreparable damage or implantation failure). However, fetal malformations can also occur due to exposure to toxins during the pre-implantation period. It has been demonstrated that immediate exposure to chemicals such as ethylene oxide, ethyl methanesulfonate, ethylnitrosourea, and triethylene triamine within a short timeframe (e. g. 6 hours) following fertilization can lead to malformed fetuses. Pregnant mice treated with ethylnitrosourea on days 2. 5, 3. 5, and 4. 5 of pregnancy developed neural tube defects and cleft palate. Because rapid mitosis occurs during the pre-implantation period, chemicals that affect DNA synthesis or integrity, or affect microtubule assembly, will produce special toxicity if they reach the embryo.

(2) Organ formation period (3-8 weeks in human): After implantation, the pregnant body enters the organ formation period, until the hard palate has closed. This period involves rapid changes in organogenesis, which includes processes of cell proliferation, cell migration, intercellular interaction, and morphological remodeling of tissue formation. During the organ formation period, the various tissues and structures being formed are at their most susceptible. The peak incidence of each malformation corresponds to the developmental timing of the tissue structure. A toxin may affect one or some developmental processes, so the pattern of

tissue structure susceptibility will vary with different toxins. The length of pregnancy varies among different species, and the timing of the sensitive period also varies. During this period, the most prominent manifestation of the developmental toxicity of exogenous chemicals is structural malformations, but there can also be embryonic death and growth retardation. The type and incidence of malformations are determined by the chemical and its exposure dose and time.

(3) Fetal to neonatal stage (9–38 weeks in human): After organ formation concludes, the fetal period begins, marked by tissue differentiation, growth, and physiological maturation. During this period, the organs continue to develop, acquiring the necessary functions for life before birth, which includes fine structural morphogenesis and biochemical maturation (such as the induction of tissue-specific enzymes and structural proteins). Fetal exposure is most commonly associated with effects on growth and functional maturation. Adverse outcomes may impact the function of the central nervous system and reproductive organs, including behavioral, cognitive, and motor deficits, and reduced fertility. These effects are not always evident before birth and may require careful observation and tests in the offspring following birth. Structural changes can occur during the fetal period, but these are usually deformations or abnormalities rather than malformations. Some effects may take years to become apparent, while others may even cause the onset of aging and organ failure in later life(Table 10–2).

Table 10–2 **Summary of In Vivo Regulatory Protocol Guidelines for Evaluation of Developmental Toxicity**

Maldevelopment	Target System	Observe Effects
Spermatid	Whole body of pregnancy	Low birth weight, neonatal deaths
Oocyte	Whole body of pregnancy	Cell death; congenital malformations
After birth	Cardiovascular system metabolism	Interference with active transport; altered maternal-fetal circulation; altered nutrient biosynthesis; altered biotransformation of exogenous chemicals
Embryo	Whole body of pregnancy	In utero growth retardation; congenital malformations; mortality
Fetus	Whole body of pregnancy Reproductive system and kidneys Bones	Growth retardation; mortality; transplacental carcinogenesis Urogenital malformations Skeletal malformations
Infants	CNS Reproductive system Respiratory organs Muscle tissue Whole body	Neurobehavioral abnormalities; withdrawal symptoms; altered mental capacity Altered fertility Respiratory depression Hypotonia Neonatal death

[Table 10–2 is derived from Table 10–1 in Chapter 10 of the seventh edition of *Textbook of Fundamentals of Toxicology*]

The Concept of Dose-Response Relationship and Threshold

In developmental toxicology studies, the main observed effects of prenatal exposure at birth include mortality, malformation, and growth retardation. The relationship between these effects is complex and varies depending on the type of agent, exposure time, and dose. For some agents, these endpoints can represent a continuum of increasing toxicity, where growth retardation may occur at low doses, malformations at higher doses, and death at the highest doses.

Because of the high regenerative growth potential of mammalian embryos, the presence of cell homeostasis mechanisms, and maternal metabolic defense, developmental toxicity in mammals is generally considered a threshold phenomenon. The threshold hypothesis suggests that there is a maternal dose below which no adverse effects occur. Although many mechanisms are unclear, it is evident that the repair mechanisms of embryos and cells, as well as dose-dependent kinetics, support the existence of a threshold. Conversely, a non-threshold relationship suggests that any dose, including exposure to a single molecule of a toxic substance, has the potential to cause developmental toxicity. There is a wide range of individual differences in the population, and the overall threshold is determined by the threshold of the most sensitive individuals in the population. The common types of dose-response relationships are as follows:

(1) Normal fetal growth, structural abnormalities, and embryonic death can coexist. Low doses initially cause growth retardation, embryonic resorption, and malformations. As the dose increases, embryonic death becomes the dominant outcome, leading to the death of the entire litter of embryos. Chemicals with high teratogenicity shift the teratogenic response to the left on a dose-response curve, but they still overlap with the embryonic death curve.

(2) Teratogenicity can occur at doses well below the embryonic lethal dose, resulting in either whole litter malformations or individual malformations. Malformed fetuses often exhibit growth retardation, and the growth retardation curve parallels the teratogenic curve. When the dose increases to exceed the dose causing whole litter malformations, embryonic death occurs, usually accompanied by significant maternal toxicity.

(3) Only fetal growth retardation and embryonic death occur, without the occurrence of malformations. Growth retardation often appears first, and the curve is relatively flat. Embryonic death occurs only at higher doses, and the curve is steeper, almost showing an "all or none" response. Chemicals exhibiting this type of response spectrum are considered to have embryotoxicity but no teratogenicity.

DOHaD Hypothesis

DOHaD is an acronym that stands for the concept of "the developmental origins of health and disease ". The purpose of introducing the DOHaD concept is to improve early diagnosis and intervention rates for high-risk populations and to provide scientific evidence for policy development aimed at preventing such diseases. Numerous epidemiological studies have demonstrated a correlation between the intrauterine growth and development of fetuses and the occurrence of certain adult diseases. Based on these research findings, the Fetal Origins of Adult Disease (FOAD) hypothesis was proposed by Barker in 1998, which is famously known as the Barker hypothesis. The concept of FOAD gradually evolved into the DOHaD theory. The following are the relevant hypotheses of the DOHaD theory:

(1) Developmental Plasticity: The plasticity of development refers to the phenomenon in which a genotype can produce many different physiological and morphological states in different environmental conditions during fetal development; this phenomenon is known as developmental plasticity. It is generally believed that rapid fetal growth begins in the 9th week of pregnancy, which is sensitive to changes in the external environment and has the ability to adapt to environmental changes: this ability is called "plasticity", and this period becomes the "plasticity period".

(2) Adaptive response: Due to the fetal plasticity during development, the body can make an adaptive response when facing environmental disturbances. The body's adaptive responses to the environment include immediate adaptive responses (IARs) and predictive adaptive responses (PARs). When fetal development is inadequate within the uterus, the most prominent adverse pregnancy outcomes include fetal growth restriction and slowed fetal growth. Phenotype alterations resulting from inappropriate adverse pregnancy outcomes primarily occur during the plasticity period and can be categorized as appropriate or inappropriate PARs. Inappropriate PARs occur when the predicted phenotype induced by the environment does not align with the actual environment, suggesting that mature organs cannot adapt to conditions outside the plasticity period, which can lead to the development of corresponding diseases in adulthood.

(3) Economizing genotype hypothesis: In 1962, Neel introduced the economizing gene hypothesis to explain the rise in obesity and diabetes, which marked the earliest application of the "economizing genotype" theory. After repeated famine selection, those individuals with a survival advantage (i. e. the most "frugal" in using energy) were retained by natural selection. The genes that regulate insulin secretion in these preserved individuals' genomes (thrifty genes) have the ability to secrete insulin in large quantities after a full meal. In the recent period of human evolution, due to the basic guarantee of food supply, the thrifty

genotype that has shown evolutionary advantages has no obvious effect on survival, but it is still preserved, and the result is that post-meal hyperinsulinemia leads to secondary insulin resistance, followed by cell failure and diabetes.

Maternal Toxicity and Developmental Toxicity

The Impact of Maternal Factors on Developmental Toxicity

Maternal toxicity refers to the harmful effects of chemical toxins on the mother during pregnancy, manifested by reduced weight gain, impaired function, clinical symptoms, and even death. Developmental toxicity refers to any adverse effects induced prior to attainment of adult life. It includes effects induced or manifested in the embryonic or fetal period and those induced or manifested postnatally. Although all developmental toxicity ultimately arises from cellular damage within the pregnant body, the occurrence of damage may be a direct effect on the embryo (fetus), an indirect effect brought about by toxicity to the mother and placenta, or a combination of direct and indirect effects.

A number of studies have directly linked specific forms of maternal toxicity to developmental toxicity, including instances in which developmental toxicity has been exacerbated by subject-induced maternal effects, as well as instances in which deleterious maternal effects have directly caused developmental toxicity. However, it is challenging to differentiate between the indirect effects of maternal toxicity and the direct toxicity to the embryo (fetus) and to determine the relative contributions of each factor.

Maternal factors affecting development mainly include the mother's genetic background, age, parity, body shape, nutrition, disease, stress, and other health parameters, as well as exposures, and can also affect development through placental toxicity.

(1) Genetics: The genetic structure of the pregnant mother plays a role in determining the developmental outcome. For example, the incidence of cleft lip and palate depends on the mother's genotype rather than the embryo's, and the incidence is higher in whites than in blacks. Two related mouse strains, A/J and CL/Fr, exhibit spontaneous CL(P) rates of 8%-10% and 18%-26%, respectively. The incidence of CL(P) in offspring is determined by the mother's genotype rather than the embryo's.

(2) Disease: Uncontrolled maternal diabetes and certain infectious fevers can adversely affect the fetus due to disease-related maternal changes or direct placental infection. For instance, cytomegalovirus infection is linked to fetal death, microcephaly, mental retardation, blindness, and deafness. High heat is a strong teratogen in experimental animals, and there is a lot of evidence linking febrile illness in mothers during the first three months of

pregnancy with birth defects, especially malformations of the central nervous system.

(3) Nutrition: Various dietary deficiencies, from protein-calorie malnutrition to deficiencies of vitamins, trace elements, and enzyme cofactors, are known to adversely affect pregnancy. The Medical Research Council (MRC) discovered that daily supplementation with 4 mg of folic acid during pregnancy reduced the recurrence rate of neural tube defects (NTDs) by more than 70% in pregnancies that were at risk of having NTD infants.

(4) Stress: Different forms of maternal toxicity can elicit a common physiological stress response. Test rats or mice exposed to noise during pregnancy have been found to exhibit developmental toxicity. Survey research has revealed a positive correlation between maternal stress and adverse pregnancy outcomes, including low birth weight and congenital malformations.

(5) Placental toxicity: The placenta is involved in attachment, nutrition, gas exchange, and waste removal. It also produces hormones necessary for maintaining pregnancy and can metabolize and store exogenous chemicals. Toxicity to the placenta can compromise these functions and lead to adverse effects on the pregnant body. Cadmium (Cd) exposure in the late stages of pregnancy has been shown to cause fetal necrosis, reduce blood flow, and inhibit nutrient transfer across the placenta.

The Relationship Between Maternal Toxicity and Developmental Toxicity

In animal developmental toxicity tests, the relationship between maternal toxicity and developmental toxicity is often observed in the following types.

(1) Developmental toxicity can occur without maternal toxicity, indicating that developmental toxicity has a specific mechanism and is independent of maternal toxicity, such as thalidomide. These chemicals are often overlooked and can be the most dangerous.

(2) Developmental toxicity and maternal toxicity can coexist, especially when developmental toxicity is only observed as maternal toxicity is present. The developmental effects may be indirect and often do not have a specific teratogenic mechanism. Many human developmental toxins that people knows, such as alcohol and cocaine, primarily exert their harmful effects on the embryo (fetus) through maternal toxicity, and their developmental toxicity may be partly due to the secondary effects of maternal physiological disorders. For example, alcoholics are often malnourished, and alcohol affects the transplacental transport of nutrients, which can enhance the direct effects on the fetus.

(3) Certain chemicals may have maternal toxicity but not teratogenic effects. These substances often raise concerns during pregnancy and are therefore avoided.

(4) Certain chemicals may not exhibit maternal toxicity or developmental toxicity at

certain doses.

Cases of Human Developmental Toxicants

Currently, more than 40 substances that can cause human developmental abnormalities have been identified through epidemiological investigations, including radiation, infection, maternal trauma and metabolic disorders, drugs, and environmental chemicals. Below are some typical human developmental toxicants and teratogens(Table 10-3).

Table 10-3 Known Human Developmental Toxicants or Teratogens

Radiation	Drugs/Environmental Chemicals
Heal	Androgen chemicals
Radioiodine	Angiotensin-converting enzyme inhibitors: Captopril, Itopril
Atomic radiation dust	Antibiotic: tetracycline
Infection	Antitumor drugs: aminopterate, methotrexate, cyclophosphamide
Rubella virus	Chelating agent: penicillamine
Cytomegalovirus	Chlorobenzene
Herpes simplex virus	Cocaine
Toxoplasmosis	Coumarin anticoagulants
syphilis	Iodide
Maternal trauma and metabolic disorders	lithium
Alcoholism	Ethylene oxide
Amniocentesis, early chorionic sampling	Fluconazole, high dose
Cretinism, endemic diseases	Metals: Mercury (organic), lead
Diabetes	Misoprostol
Folate deficiency	Isotretinoin
Hyperthermia	Thalidomide
Phenylketonuria	Toluene abuse
Rheumatism and congenital heart block	Vitamin A (large dose)
Sjogren's syndrome	

[Table 10-3 is derived from Table A12-6 of *The Concise Course in Modern Toxicology, but has been amended*]

Several typical human developmental toxicants and teratogens are described as below.

(1) Thalidomide: Thalidomide, as a sedative/hypnotic drug, was first marketed in 1957 in the then Federal Republic of Germany under the trade name of "Reaction Stop", and was used to alleviate sleep disturbances and symptoms of nausea and vomiting in the early stages of pregnancy because of its sedative, hypnotic and antiemetic effects. According to incomplete statistics, during the period of 1960—1962, thalidomide consumption by pregnant women in over 20 countries led to approximately 12, 000 cases worldwide of severe congenital malformations, including limb reduction defects (phocomelia), anophthalmia, cleft palate, stunted skeletal growth, and gastrointestinal atresia. In addition to teratogenicity, adverse effects of thalidomide include peripheral neuritis, venous and arterial thrombosis, hypotension, severe skin reactions, centropenia, and bradycardia.

Thalidomide is the most potent human teratogen, with teratogenic effects in humans and rabbits at 0.5 to 1.0 mg/kg, but no teratogenic effects were observed in rats and mice, even at doses up to 4,000 mg/kg. Thalidomide was withdrawn from the market in November 1961 because of its association with birth defects. Case reports ended in mid-1962 as exposures were terminated. An estimated 5,850 malformed babies were said to have been born worldwide, making it the most serious clinical drug event causing fetal malformations in human history.

(2) Diethylstilbestrol (DES): Diethylstilbestrol can cross the placenta and enter the fetus, resulting in a condition known as DES syndrome, characterized by malformations and cancers of the reproductive organs in offspring. Male offspring may experience hypospadias, epididymal and testicular abnormalities, sperm abnormalities, and an increased risk of prostate and testicular cancer. Female offspring may experience fallopian tube malformations, cervical and vaginal clear cell carcinoma.

(3) Methylmercury: Methylmercury is very easy to enter the fetus through the placenta. A large amount of accumulation in the body of children, which occurred in Japan in the 1950s due to long-term consumption of fish and shellfish contaminated by methylmercury caused chronic methylmercury poisoning. The disease first occurred in Minamata Bay, Kyushu, Japan, so also known as Minamata disease. The most common manifestations of Minamata disease are peripheral sensory disorders, central visual field reduction, high-frequency domain hearing impairment and motor disorders, collectively known as Hunter-Russel syndrome.

(4) Lead: Lead is a common industrial poison and environmental pollutant that can cause toxic effects on multiple organs and systems in the body, including the heart, bones, small intestine, kidneys, reproductive system and nervous system. The nervous system is extremely vulnerable to the toxicity of lead, especially the central nervous system of children, because of the imperfect development of the blood-brain barrier in fetuses and infants, lead is easier to enter the central nervous system. A large number of epidemiological studies have shown that lead can cause significant reductions in intelligence quotient (IQ), attention deficit hyperactivity disorder, and significantly reduced reading and learning ability in children. Studies have shown that for every 10 mg/mL increase in blood lead concentration between 50 and 350 mg/mL, IQ decreases by 2 to 4 points. There was a significant negative correlation between maternal blood lead level and neonatal neurobehavioral development in the second trimester.

(5) Retinoic acid: Retinoic acid is a natural or synthetic compound with a vitamin A structure or similar function. Research has shown that vitamin A can cause various embryonic malformations in animals, and vitamin A derivatives, 13-cis-retinoic acid, and retinoic acid can all cause human embryonic malformations, mainly including central nervous system,

craniofacial, and urogenital system malformations, and low IQ.

Mechanisms of Developmental Toxicity

Development is characterized by a series of coordinated changes, including alterations in size, biochemistry, physiology, shape, and function. These changes are controlled by a cascade of gene expression regulators, some of which are inherited from the mother and present in the ovum prior to fertilization. Environmental chemicals can disrupt normal development through various mechanisms, such as interacting with endogenous receptors, modifying DNA or proteins, triggering lipid peroxidation, inhibiting enzymes, altering cell membranes, and other processes.

Cell-cell Interactions

Cell-cell interactions are primarily achieved through cellular communication, including direct intercellular communication such as gap junction communication and membrane surface molecule contact communication, as well as receptor-mediated cell signal transduction systems. Research has found that different stages of embryonic development involve various types of cellular communication, and disruption of this communication can affect normal cellular biological processes, leading to malformations or other developmental toxicities.

For instance, the metabolic activation products of thalidomide cause downregulation of adhesive receptors in embryonic cells, impeding interactions between cells and between cells and the matrix during development, disrupting cell communication and resulting in limb bud abnormalities. Embryonic cell apoptosis and malformations caused by teratogens like retinoic acid also involve impacts on cell signal transduction systems.

DNA Damage

DNA stores the genetic information essential for the survival and reproduction of organisms, thus maintaining the integrity of DNA molecules is crucial for cells. DNA damage refers to permanent changes in the nucleotide sequence of DNA occurring during replication, leading to changes in genetic traits. External environmental factors and internal factors within the organism frequently cause damage or changes to DNA molecules. Unlike RNA and proteins, which can be synthesized in large quantities within cells, a prokaryotic cell typically contains only one copy of DNA, and a diploid eukaryotic cell has just one pair of the same DNA. If DNA damage or genetic information changes cannot be corrected, it may affect normal cell development and potentially impact offspring if it occurs in reproductive cells.

Phosphoramide mustard (PM) and acrolein (AC) appear to be teratogenic metabolites of cyclophosphamide (CP). AC preferentially binds to proteins and shows high binding into the yolk sac, while PM preferentially binds to DNA. Both CP and PM have been shown to cause DNA single-strand breaks and DNA-DNA and DNA-protein cross-links. PM and AC have different targets in the embryo, and DNA damage induced by CP is caused by PM.

Interference with Gene Expression

Interference with the expression of certain genes in the early embryo can exhibit teratogenic effects, and teratogens can alter positional information and prevent embryogenesis. Genes controlling positional information often encode transcription factors, the regulation of which will stimulate tissue differentiation and morphogenesis. Teratogens, can directly affect cell differentiation, proliferation, or apoptosis. Hydrophilic signaling molecules, such as growth factors, and hydrophobic molecules, such as vitamin A analogs, can modulate these processes, and activated signaling pathways often induce uncoordinated loss of tissue-specific gene expression. In addition to altering other signaling pathways, teratogens may cause some signaling pathways to interact inappropriately and exhibit synergistic or antagonistic effects with other teratogens.

Gametogenesis and fertilization are susceptible to toxic damage. It is now known that the maternal and paternal parental genomes do not contribute equally to the zygotic syncytial genome. The process of imprinting occurs during gametogenesis, and differential expression of alleles depends on whether they are of maternal or paternal origin. Imprinting requires a process of cytosine methylation and chromatin conformation changes, a process that is likely to be affected by the toxicants that are targeted in this way. The effect of toxicity on imprinting undoubtedly plays a role in paternally mediated developmental toxicity.

Inhibition of Cell Cycle Progression and Cell Death

During embryonic development, cell proliferation, differentiation, and death are all necessary, and there is a delicate balance between them. Inhibition or excess of each process can affect normal development. Research has found that cell death plays an important role in normal embryonic development, especially in morphogenesis. Cell death is necessary for the shaping process from the hand plate to the fingers. Cell proliferation is obviously necessary for development. In embryos, there is a delicate balance between cell proliferation, cell differentiation, and cell death. DNA damage induced by CP may cause cell cycle confusion and cell death in specific cell groups. If DNA damage is repaired, the cell cycle can return to normal, but if the damage is severe or the cell cycle is inhibited for too long, it may trigger apoptosis.

Secondary Effects of Maternal Physiological Dysregulation

The teratogenic effects of diflunisal in rabbits may be attributed to maternal anemia, which leads to hypoxia. The anticonvulsant drug phenytoin can affect maternal folate metabolism in animal experiments, and these changes may play a role in the teratogenicity of the drug. Reduced uterine blood flow may be a mechanism of hydroxyurea teratogenesis, which increases cardiac contractility, changes heart rate, reduces stroke volume, thereby greatly reduces uterine blood flow, and increases vascular resistance in pregnant rabbits.

Hormones play an important role in maintaining homeostasis and regulating the developmental process. Endocrine disruptors in the environment can affect endogenous hormone levels, change the homeostasis of the maternal environment, and cause developmental toxicity. Many teratogens have a common mechanism of developmental toxicity, which is secondary maternal zinc (Zn) deficiency caused by the induction of maternal metallothionein (MT). This induction can increase liver MT concentrations significantly, causing a large amount of maternal Zn to accumulate in the liver, which in turn causes a significant reduction in plasma Zn concentration, leading to maternal Zn deficiency.

Developmental Toxicity of Endocrine Disrupting Chemicals

"Endocrine disruptors" have been broadly defined as "exogenous substances that interfere with the production, secretion, transport, metabolism, binding, action, or elimination of natural hormones that maintain homeostasis and the developmental process". Because hormones play a key role in guiding differentiation in many tissues, developing organisms are particularly sensitive to fluctuations in the timing and intensity of exposure to chemicals with hormonal (or anti-hormonal) activity. Many types of chemicals, such as pesticides, herbicides, fungicides, plasticizers, surfactants, organometals, halogenated polycyclic aromatic compounds, and plant estrogens, induce developmental toxicity through at least four modes of action involving the endocrine system: acting as ligands for steroid hormone receptors; modifying steroid hormone metabolizing enzymes; interfering with the release of hypothalamic-pituitary trophic hormones; acting through as yet unclear modes of action resembling hormonal action.

Placental Toxicity

At least 46 substances known to be toxic to the yolk sac or chorionic (hair) membrane placenta include cadmium (Cd), arsenic, mercury, cigarette smoke, ethanol, cocaine, endotoxin, and sodium salicylate. For example, Cd causes developmental toxicity during late pregnancy through placental toxicity (causing necrosis and reduced blood flow) and inhibition of nutrient transport.

It was found that injection of Cd into rats in late gestation caused fetal death, but almost no cadmium entered the fetus; instead, fetal death occurred within 10 hours accompanied by a reduction in uteroplacental blood flow. If Cd was injected directly into the fetus, there was only a slight increase in fetal death, even though the fetal Cd load was almost 10-fold higher than after maternal administration. In addition, Cd induces MT in the placenta, which has a high affinity for Zn and interferes with Zn transfer across the placenta by binding Zn in the placenta. Cd, which is physicochemically and chemically similar to the essential element Zn, competitively inhibits transmembrane translocation of Zn uptake across the placenta microvesicles in humans, as well as competitively inhibiting other Zn-dependent processes in the placenta. Co-administration of Zn ameliorates the developmental toxicity of Cd.

Safety Assessment and Testing

Lessons from developmental toxic chemicals show that animal experiments and epidemiological surveillance of populations are necessary for providing adequate public health protection.

Guidelines for the Management of in Vivo Testing

In 1966, the US Food and Drug Administration formulated guidelines for reproductive research in safety assessment (Phases Ⅰ, Ⅱ, and Ⅲ). The general goal of the studies defined by these guidelines is to determine NOAEL, the maximum dose that does not cause a significant increase in harmful effects in offspring. The NOAEL is then used in the hazard assessment process to assess the likelihood of human impact under a given exposure scenario.

The actual test plan is determined by the following aspects: the intended use of the drug, especially reproductive system drugs, the type of chemical and the expected clinical administration route, and any available existing toxicity, pharmacodynamic, pharmacokinetic, and structural or activity similarities with other chemicals. Certain drugs may be used only once in a lifetime (such as diagnostic drugs and surgical drugs), and can adopt a shortened exposure time and higher dose regimen. For the vast majority of drugs, three-phase trials are sufficient(Table 10-4).

Table 10-4 **Relationship Between Exposure at Various Developmental Stages and Pregnancy Outcomes**

Study	Exposure	Endpoints Covered	Comments
Phase Ⅰ: Fertility and general reproductive toxicity test	Males: 10 weeks prior to mating Females: 2 weeks prior to mating	Gamete development, fertility, pre-and post-implantation viability, parturition, lactation	Assesses reproductive capabilities of male and female following exposure over one complete spermatogenic cycle or several estrous cycles
Phase Ⅱ: Teratogenicity test	Implantation (or mating) through end of organogenesis (or term)	Viability, weight, and morphology (external, visceral, and skeletal) of conceptuses just prior to birth	Shorter exposure to prevents maternal metabolic adaptation and to provide high exposure to the embryo during gastrulation and organogenesis. Earlier dosing option for bioaccumulative agents or those impacting maternal nutrition, Later dosing option covering male reproductive tract development and fetal growth and maturation
Phase Ⅲ: Perinatal toxicity test	Last trimester of pregnancy through lactation	Postnatal survival, growth and external morphology	Intended to observe effects on development of major organ functional competence during the perinatal period, and thus may be relatively more sensitive to adverse effects at this time

[Table 10-4 is derived from Table 10-3 in Chapter 10 of the seventh edition of *Textbook of Fundamentals of Toxicology* which is published by the People's Health Publishing House, but has been amended]

Phase Ⅰ: Fertility and Early Embryonic Development Toxicity Test (Fertility and General Reproductive Toxicity Test)

Rats are the preferred experimental animals. The number of animals per group should be sufficient for meaningful interpretation of the data, with a recommended 16-20 animals per sex per group. Generally, three dose groups, one solvent control group, and one positive control group are set up.

Exposure time for male animals starts 2 weeks before mating and continues until before implantation. In recent years, there has been a significant change in the exposure time for male animals before mating. In 1981, the OECD stipulated that rats should be exposed for at least 10 weeks and mice for 8 weeks. Mating male rats with female rats after 8-10 weeks of continuous exposure is not a sensitive method for detecting the effects on sperm production. Sperm survival rate and morphological examination can provide more sensitive endpoints for reproductive toxicity studies. Moreover, exogenous chemicals that affect sperm production almost always affect the post-meiotic stage (3-5 weeks before sperm maturation). Careful histopathological examination of male gonadal tissues and organs can provide valuable supplementary information on male fertility and sperm production. Therefore, the International Conference on Harmonization (ICH) guidelines shorten the exposure time for male animals to 4 weeks before mating and combine it with histopathological examination.

Female animals generally terminate pregnancy at 13–15 days, and males are euthanized after confirming successful mating and pregnancy. During the exposure period, it is important to observe the water intake, food intake, weight changes, and mating period vaginal smear examination of male and female parents. Histopathological examination of the testes, epididymis, ovaries, and uterus of all animals is required, as well as examination of the number, motility, and morphology of sperm in the epididymis or testes, the number of corpora lutea, implantation sites, resorbed fetuses, dead fetuses, and live fetuses. The results of the test are mainly based on the toxicity and NOAEL of the F_0 generation, the toxicity and NOAEL of the F_1 generation, and the number of affected litters in each group for comprehensive evaluation.

Phase Ⅱ: Embryo-fetal Toxicity Test (Teratogenicity Test)

Two species are generally selected, one rodent and one non-rodent. Healthy, sexually mature, and unmated female rats or rabbits are preferred, with a male-to-female animal ratio of 2 : 1 or 1 : 1 for mating. At least 15 pregnant rats and 12 pregnant rabbits per group are required.

At least three dose groups, one negative control group, and one positive control group should be set up for the test. Positive control substances can include cyclophosphamide, aspirin, or vitamin A. Control group animals should receive the same treatment as the dose groups, except for the test substance. A preliminary test can be conducted to determine the dose of the test substance that causes embryo or fetal death. Under conditions that allow for the physicochemical and biological properties of the test substance, the high-dose group should cause significant toxic reactions in the mother, such as slight weight loss, but not cause more than 10% maternal death; the low dose should not cause any observable toxic reactions in the animals; and intermediate doses can be set between the low and high doses using a geometric series. If the toxicity of the test substance is low, a dose of 1000 mg/kg body weight with no significant embryotoxic or teratogenic effects can be used for a limit test, without the need for other dose groups. If the high-dose preliminary test has some toxic effects on the mother but no adverse effects on the embryo, a limit test can also be used.

The dosing period is from day 6 to 15 of pregnancy for rats and from day 6 to 18 for rabbits. During the test, the weight of the pregnant rats is measured every 2–3 days. On the one hand, the dose of the test substance can be adjusted according to the weight gain, and on the other hand, the pregnancy and embryonic development of the pregnant animals can be observed. Pregnant animals are euthanized 1–2 days before natural delivery, generally on 19–20 days after pregnancy for rats, 18–19 days for mice, and 29 days for rabbits. The uterus is removed by laparotomy, weighed, and examined for resorbed fetuses, early dead fetuses, late dead fetuses, and live-born pups. After the live-born pups are removed, their sex, weight, body length, external malformations, visceral malformations, skeletal malformations, and development (ossification) are examined.

Phase Ⅲ: Prenatal and Postnatal Development Toxicity Test (Perinatal Toxicity Test)

Rats are the preferred experimental animals. The number of animals per group should be sufficient for meaningful interpretation of the results, with a recommended 16–20 pregnant animals per group. Three dose groups, one solvent control group, and one positive control group (if necessary) are set up.

Administration period is from implantation to the end of lactation. Rats are dosed from day 15 of pregnancy until day 28 postpartum, at which point lactation is ceased, and the dams and a portion of the offspring are sacrificed. Eight pups per litter (striving for a balanced sex ratio) are raised to sexual maturity and mated to evaluate the fertility of the F_1 generation, which is then sacrificed after the birth of the F_2 generation. Primary observations include maternal water consumption, food intake, body weight changes, symptoms of poisoning, mortality rates, pregnancy and parturition timings, litter size, and conception rates; for the F_1 generation, sex ratio, phenotypic abnormalities, survival rates at birth and during nursing, growth indices, physiological development, pre-weaning neurological behaviors, post-weaning behaviors, mating behaviors, and conception rates are noted. Post-weaning F_1 major organs, testes, epididymides, ovaries, and uteri weights, and visceral abnormalities are examined. Study results are primarily evaluated based on maternal toxicity and NOAEL, embryotoxicity, teratogenicity, offspring neurobehavioral effects, and NOAEL.

Subsequently, as an outcome of ICH for pharmaceutical registration technical requirements, a new rationalized testing protocol was established and accepted internationally. Moreover, improved testing guidelines in other areas have been recommended, such as developmental immunotoxicity, carcinogenicity, specific neurotoxicity studies, endocrine disruptor studies, pharmacokinetics, and direct neonatal drug application studies. These protocols are used as supplementary or further studies when standard experiments indicate a necessity.

Data Consistency

Concerning the similarity in the response to developmental toxicants between laboratory animals and humans, there have been several comprehensive reviews. Generally, these studies support the hypothesis that laboratory results can predict potential human effects. The strongest consistency is observed when positive data are available from more than one test species. However, even in such cases, cross-species extrapolation of specific types of developmental toxicity effects is inappropriate.

In quantitative terms, a few comparisons have shown that humans tend to be more sensitive to developmental toxicants than the most sensitive test species. Although there is a high consistency in reports of positive agents across species, retrospective steps are usually necessary to develop animal models that reflect human outcomes. Frankos reviewed data on 38 compounds, proven or suspected to be active in humans; apart from tobramycin causing otic defects, all tested animals were positive in at least one species, with 76% being positive in more than one species.

Epidemiology

Reproductive epidemiology is the science of studying the statistical associations between specific exposures in fathers, mothers, and during pregnancy, and reproductive outcomes. Generally, the rarer the birth defects, the less frequent the population exposure, the smaller the sample size, and the shorter the study duration, and the greater the biological plausibility, the easier it is to establish a link between specific exposures and adverse reproductive outcomes. Some rare exposures, such as rubella or thalidomide, have strong developmental toxicities and lead to rare adverse pregnancy outcomes that can often be identified without formal epidemiological studies. In most other cases, case-control or cohort studies are required to find correlations. Both types of studies require definite reproductive outcomes and exposures, and a significant toxic effect and large sample sizes to draw relatively reliable conclusions. Therefore, developmental epidemiologists often face challenges. For example, in the United States, the exposure rate to valproate is less than 1%, and its risk of causing spinal bifida is only twice that of controls, thus observing a statistically significant increase in malformation rates due to valproate requires at least one million observed births. Another challenge epidemiologists face is the high rate of pregnancy failures in the population. Statistically, about 31% of pregnancy failures occur around the time of implantation, and another 15% are clinically evident miscarriages. Therefore, in the general population, many pregnancy failures due to specific exposures are overlooked. Moreover, with the prevalence of prenatal testing, some may choose to selectively abort fetuses with abnormalities. Therefore, the incidence of birth defects may not accurately reflect the rate of developmental anomalies in pregnant bodies; prevalence rates are more appropriate, as they use the number of live births rather than total pregnancies as the denominator.

The primary objectives of using epidemiological studies to investigate abnormal reproductive outcomes are threefold: ① to identify the causes of birth defects, usually by analyzing case reports or clusters of similar phenomena; ② to monitor trends in birth defects worldwide through extensive surveillance of national registries; ③ to raise public awareness and protect public health.

Risk Assessment Elements

Extrapolation of animal data on developmental toxicity follows two basic directions: one is voluntary exposure to drugs, usually at high doses (biologically effective), and the other is environmental formulations, which are usually involuntary and at lower levels. For drugs, a pregnancy rating system is used (FDA, US, 1979). In this system, letters A, B, C, D, and X are used to categorize the evidence of chemical risks to human embryos (Table 10-5). For example, a drug is categorized as class A if adequate and well-controlled studies in pregnant humans have not demonstrated a risk; a drug is categorized as class X (contraindicated during pregnancy) if studies or post-marketing reports in animals or humans show that the fetal risk clearly outweighs any possible benefit to the patient. The default category is C (risks cannot be ruled out), assigned when there is a lack of human studies and animal studies either lack fetal risk or show positive risks, but benefits may justify potential risks. Categories B and D represent areas where risks are relatively smaller or larger, respectively. Manson (1994) reviewed the Physicians' Desk Reference from 1992 and found that of 1,033 drugs, 7% were categorized as X, 66% as C, and only 0.7% as A. The FDA's categorization process has been criticized for being too reliant on risk/benefit comparisons, especially considering that the magnitude of risks is often unknown or the benefits are not in question.

Table 10-5 Animal Eexperiment Results

Population Study Results	Animal Experiment Results		
	+	−	No Information Available
+	X or D	X or D	X or D
−	B	A	A or B
No information available	C1	B	C2

A, B, C2: May be used during pregnancy only if clearly needed.

C1: May be used during pregnancy if the potential benefits are considered to outweigh the potential risks to the fetus.

D: Should notify the patient of the potential risk to the fetus if used during pregnancy.

X: Contraindicated for use during pregnancy or in women who may become pregnant.

[Table 10-5 is derived from Table 10-5 in Chapter 10 of the seventh edition of *Textbook of Fundamentals of Toxicology*]

For environmental factors, in the assessment of developmental toxicity—a non-cancer endpoint—the goal of hazard assessment is typically to articulate the doses, routes, frequency, and duration of exposure that induce the lowest observable effect levels in the most appropriate experimental animal models (United States. Environmental Protection Agency, 1991). This level of exposure, termed the "critical effect ", is then extrapolated to derive a relative human safety exposure level through the application of safety factors or uncertainty factors.

Alternative Tests

A variety of alternative testing systems have been established to refine, reduce, or replace standard mammalian prenatal toxicity assessments. These tests can be incorporated into whole-animal studies to provide valuable information and decrease the number of animals used, either as part of a screening battery or for further analysis.

In recent years, validation studies have been conducted on three types of in vitro embryotoxicity tests: the rat embryonic limb bud micromass test, the mouse embryonic stem cell test, and the rat whole embryo culture test. For example, the micromass culture involves cultivating limb bud cells from rat embryos over five days to assess their differentiation and cellular proliferation. Some alternative tests are listed as below.

(1) Rat Whole Embryo Culture (RWEC): Rat embryos are extracted from the uteri on gestational days 9–10, and the test substance is added to the culture medium. The embryos are then cultured in a gas-perfused rotating incubator. Observations include heart beating, yolk sac diameter, somites, neural tube closure, and overall length. Embryo survival is recorded, and organ morphological differentiation is evaluated using the Brown's morphological scoring system. This test can ascertain developmental toxicity, explore dose-response relationships, and understand the mechanisms of action of chemicals.

(2) Embryonic Micromass Cell Culture (ECCC): This test involves co-culturing high-density primary embryonic cells with test substances to assess their impact on cell proliferation and differentiation. This can help in evaluating the teratogenicity of chemicals based on reductions in cell and colony numbers.

(3) Mouse Embryonic Stem Cell Test (MESCT): Mouse embryonic stem cells derived from the inner cell mass of the blastocyst can differentiate into various cell types under specific conditions, making them useful tools for studying developmental toxicity. A well-established embryonic stem cell line for these studies is the mouse embryonic stem cell line D3, which can differentiate into various types of cells including cardiomyocytes, endothelial cells, pancreatic islets, and neurons. The advantages include: ① using established cell lines as research subjects, eliminating the need to euthanize pregnant animals; ② embryonic stem cells have the potential to differentiate into multiple cell types, providing a strong representation of early embryonic development.

(4) Fish Embryo Test (FET): Newly fertilized zebrafish embryos are exposed to test chemicals and monitored via developmental markers for lethality. The test can determine acute toxicity based on specified observations recorded during the exposure period.

(5) Fruit Fly Test (FFT): The test observes the growth of larvae from the moment fly

eggs are laid until the adults emerge from the eggs. Structural defects in adult flies, such as wing abnormalities, are assessed in this test.

Developmental toxicology is the science that studies the pharmacokinetics, mechanisms, epidemiology, and outcomes of factors leading to abnormal development. Developmental toxicity refers to any morphological or functional changes caused by chemical or physical factors that disrupt normal growth, homeostasis, development, differentiation, and behavior. The critical period of susceptibility in an organ occurs just prior to and during its initial formation.

The principle based on the developmental stages of the pregnant body is a major consideration due to critical periods of fetal and organ development. The primary outcomes for the fetus depend on the gestational stage affected. The teratogenic sensitivity period refers to a specific stage in an organism's development when it is most sensitive to the toxicity of a chemical substance, making it susceptible to damage.

Developmental toxicity endpoints are specific indicators of abnormal development exhibited by an organism after exposure to certain chemicals. Developmental toxicants can act at different stages of development, producing varying effects. The process of development can be divided into three major stages: pre-implantation, from implantation to organogenesis, and from fetus to neonate.

Developmental toxic effects observed at birth, caused by exposure prior to birth, primarily include embryonic lethality, malformations, and growth retardation. The relationships among these effects are complex and vary with the type of exogenous factor, time, and dose of exposure. For some agents, these endpoints may represent a continuum of increasing toxicity, with low to high doses successively causing growth retardation, malformations, and lethality. Malformations and deaths do not necessarily occur simultaneously.

While all developmental toxicity ultimately depends on cellular-level damage in the pregnant body, the damage may occur as a direct effect on the embryo-fetus, an indirect effect due to toxicity to the mother and placenta, or a combination of direct and indirect effects. Maternal factors influencing development include genetics, diseases, nutrition, stress, and toxicity of the placenta.

Mechanisms of teratogenic action may include chromosomal breakage, mitotic alterations, changes in nucleic acid structure or function, insufficient precursor or substrate supply, lack of energy supply, changes in membrane characteristics, osmotic imbalances, and enzyme inhibition. These cellular damages can rapidly trigger unique pathogenic responses in the embryo.

Both experimental animal testing and epidemiological studies in humans are necessary for providing appropriate public health protection. The FDA established guidelines for safety evaluation of reproductive studies in 1966, and a modernized, rationalized testing protocol was established in 1994 by ICH.

Actual testing protocols are determined by various aspects including the expected use of the drug, type of substance, expected clinical route of administration, and available information on toxicity, pharmacodynamics, pharmacokinetics, and similarities with other chemicals. For the vast majority of drugs, a three-phase trial is sufficient. For developmental toxicity of environmental factors, the goal of risk assessment is to determine NOAEL in the most appropriate experimental animal model and derive a relatively safe human exposure level using safety factors or uncertainty factors.

(Chen Tao)

CHAPTER 11

Regulatory Toxicology

Introduction

Regulatory toxicology is a crucial subset of regulatory science, focusing on the intricate relationship between scientific and regulatory decision-making. This chapter, explores the dynamic interplay between science and policy, which gives rise to many of the central challenges in regulatory toxicology.

As a pivotal component of regulatory science, regulatory toxicology plays a critical role in evaluating and applying scientific findings to formulate effective regulations for safeguarding human health and environmental safety. The field navigates the inherent tension between rigorous scientific evaluation and practical policy considerations, striving to strike a delicate balance between these often-competing demands.

This chapter will provide a comprehensive analysis of regulatory toxicology, emphasizing its role in addressing the complex interplay between toxicological science and regulation. By understanding the nuances of this relationship, regulatory toxicologists can more effectively navigate challenges, contributing to the development of sound regulations that promote human health and environmental safety.

The Science/Policy Interface in Regulatory Toxicology

Science and regulatory policy serve distinct purposes, each characterized by unique objectives and methodologies. Science, driven by empirical and neutral approaches, aims to comprehend natural phenomena cautiously and incrementally. In contrast, regulatory policy focuses on influencing human behavior, resolving disputes, and achieving goals such as well-being, efficiency, and fairness.

While science remains open-ended, dedicated to understanding natural phenomena, regulatory policy has an episodic and normative nature. Science employs evidence-based methodologies, providing a foundation for incremental progress, whereas regulatory decisions are often shaped by legislative, political, and societal deadlines.

The disparity in timelines between scientific inquiry and regulatory decision-making presents significant challenges. Regulatory decisions must often be made within specific timeframes, potentially leading to two key issues: ① regulations may become increasingly outdated in relation to evolving scientific data and understanding; ② scientific inputs into regulatory decisions may be uncertain or underdeveloped due to time constraints.

Regulatory Agencies and Statutes

The regulation of human exposure to toxic materials represents a fundamental component in safeguarding public health and environmental integrity. In the United States, four primary federal agencies administer over two dozen statutes designed to achieve comprehensive protection. These agencies include FDA, Environmental Protection Agency (EPA), Occupational Safety and Health Administration (OSHA), and Consumer Product Safety Commission (CPSC), each employing distinct regulatory approaches and safety benchmarks as detailed in Table 11-1. This regulatory framework has evolved to address the complex challenges of toxic substance management, with each agency contributing unique expertise and authority to the overall protective strategy.

The FDA's mandate encompasses the regulation of food, drugs, medical devices, and cosmetics, with particular emphasis on establishing rigorous standards for product safety and efficacy. Through its regulatory oversight, the FDA implements comprehensive evaluation processes for new products while maintaining surveillance of existing ones to ensure ongoing safety. The EPA, with its broader environmental protection mandate, addresses toxic substances through various programs designed to safeguard air, water, and soil quality. The agency's approach integrates human health protection with ecological preservation, implementing regulations that consider both immediate and long-term environmental impacts.

OSHA's regulatory focus centers on workplace safety and health, establishing and enforcing standards that protect workers from exposure to toxic materials across diverse industrial settings. The agency's standards encompass permissible exposure limits, monitoring requirements, and protective measures necessary to maintain safe working environments. The CPSC complements these efforts by overseeing consumer product safety, with particular attention to products that may expose consumers to toxic substances during normal use. Their regulatory oversight extends to various consumer goods, from household items to children's products, ensuring appropriate safety standards are maintained throughout the consumer market.

Table 11-1 Major Legislation Involving Toxic Substances in the US

Statute	Agency, Date	Description
Clean Air Act (CAA)	EPA, 1970	Deals with control of hazardous air pollutants; sets national ambient air quality standards.
Clean Water Act (CWA)	EPA, 1970	Addresses water pollution; restricts pollution discharge into waters and streams; focus on controlling toxic pollutants.
Consumer Product Safety Act (CPSA)	CPSC, 1972	Regulates products that pose unreasonable risk of injury; establishes safety standards; promotes research on prevention of product-related injuries.
Federal Food, Drug, and Cosmetic Act (FFDCA)	FDA, 1938	Protect foods from harmful additives and pesticides; requires premarket approval of all new drugs; regulates the distribution of cosmetics which pose a risk of harm.
Federal Insecticide, Fungicide, and Rodenticide Act (FIFRA)	EPA, 1972	Regulates pesticides through registration requirements.
Food Quality Protection Act (FQPA)	EPA, 1996	Regulates safety standards (allowable level of residual pesticides on crops); provides special protection of infants and children; requires periodic re-evaluation of pesticides
Occupational Safety and Health Act (OSHA)	OSHA, 1970	Develop occupational safety standards including permissible exposure limits; requires assessment of chemical hazards and notification of workers of such hazards (material safety data sheets).
Safe Drinking Water Act (SDWA)	EPA, 1974	Sets standards for drinking water; Maximum contaminant levels (MCLs) are prescribed.
Toxic Substances Control Act (TSCA)	EPA, 1976	Regulates notification of production of a new chemical; requires testing for hazard assessment for high volume chemicals; requires reporting requirements of significant health effects.

This comprehensive regulatory framework in the United States has served as a model for many developed countries, which have established analogous environmental regulations and regulatory bodies. These international efforts reflect a global recognition of the importance of managing toxic substance exposure through systematic regulatory approaches. While specific organizational structures and regulatory mechanisms may vary among countries, the fundamental commitment to protecting public health and environmental quality through scientific-based regulation remains consistent across developed nations.

The collaborative efforts of these regulatory agencies create a multi-layered system of protection, with each agency contributing specific expertise and authority within its designated sphere. This integrated approach ensures comprehensive coverage of potential exposure scenarios while allowing for specialized attention to particular aspects of toxic substance management. Through ongoing refinement of regulatory strategies and adaptation to emerging challenges, these agencies continue to evolve their protective measures to address contemporary threats to public health and environmental safety.

China's regulatory framework for toxicology and chemical safety represents a complex multi-agency oversight system that has evolved significantly over recent decades to meet the challenges of rapid industrialization and increasing public health concerns. At the forefront of this framework is the National Medical Products Administration (NMPA), formerly known as the China Food and Drug Administration (CFDA), which operates under the State Administration for Market Regulation (SAMR). The NMPA serves as the primary regulatory authority for drugs, medical devices, and cosmetics, overseeing safety evaluations, establishing testing guidelines, and implementing GLP regulations for toxicology studies.

Working alongside the NMPA, the Ministry of Agriculture and Rural Affairs (MARA) plays a vital role in regulating pesticides, veterinary drugs, and feed additives. MARA's responsibilities encompass toxicological evaluations of agricultural chemicals, establishment of maximum residue limits, and implementation of safety standards for agricultural products. The Ministry of Ecology and Environment (MEE) complements these efforts by focusing on environmental toxicology regulations, overseeing chemical safety assessments, and implementing China's version of the Registration, Evaluation, Authorization and Restriction of Chemical Substances (REACH) regulations through Order No. 7, which mandates comprehensive toxicological data for new chemical substances.

The National Health Commission (NHC) addresses public health aspects of toxicology, including occupational exposure limits and food safety standards, while the Chinese Center for Disease Control and Prevention conducts crucial toxicological research and monitoring activities. These regulatory bodies are supported by an extensive network of research institutions and testing facilities, including the National Center for Safety Evaluation of Drugs (NCSED), the National Institute of Environmental Health, and various provincial toxicology centers.

Recent reforms in China's regulatory landscape have emphasized harmonization with international standards while maintaining unique characteristics. The system has increasingly focused on enhancing risk assessment capabilities, strengthening enforcement mechanisms, and developing alternative testing methods. There has been significant progress in integrating new approach methodologies, artificial intelligence applications, and big data analytics in toxicological assessment. The framework also emphasizes post-market surveillance and international cooperation in toxicology research and regulation.

Despite these advances, the system continues to address various challenges, including inter-agency coordination, regional standardization, and the development of technical capabilities in emerging areas of toxicology. China's regulatory landscape reflects a balanced approach between maintaining national characteristics and aligning with international standards, demonstrating the country's commitment to establishing a comprehensive and effective framework for managing chemical safety and toxicological risks. This evolving system (Table 11-2) serves China's large and diverse population while contributing to global efforts in toxicological safety assessment and regulation.

Table 11-2 **Major Legislation Involving Toxic Substances in China**

Statute	Agency, Date	Description
Environmental Protection Law	MEE, 2015	Establishes standards for hazardous substance emissions; mandates environmental impact assessments; requires pollution control and monitoring.
Regulations on the Safety Management of Hazardous Chemicals	State Council, 2011	Governs the production, storage, use, transportation, and disposal of hazardous chemicals; establishes registration and emergency response systems.
Food Safety Law	NPC, 2015	Protects food from harmful additives and pesticide residues; sets safety standards and establishes risk monitoring and assessment mechanisms.
Law on the Prevention and Control of Occupational Diseases	NPC, 2018	Sets occupational exposure limits for hazardous substances; mandates hazard assessments and worker protection measures.
Regulations on the Environmental Management of New Chemical Substances	MEE, 2020	Requires registration and risk assessment of new chemical substances; establishes reporting and monitoring requirements.
Pesticide Administration Regulations	MARA, 2017	Regulates pesticide registration, production, and use; establishes pesticide residue limits and monitoring systems.
Drug Administration Law	NMPA, 2019	Regulates drug safety, including toxicological testing and risk assessment; requires premarket approval for new drugs.
Drinking Water Quality Standards	NPC, 2006	Sets maximum contaminant levels (MCLs) for drinking water; establishes monitoring and assessment systems for water safety.
Environmental Protection Law	MEE, 2015	Establishes standards for hazardous substance emissions; mandates environmental impact assessments; requires pollution control and monitoring.

* NPC stands for National People's Congress, which is the supreme legislative body in China.

Like the US system, China's regulatory framework demonstrates comprehensiveness and systematization, while maintaining characteristics specific to China's regulatory system. These regulations are continuously updated and improved to adapt to technological advances and social needs, with an increasing emphasis on international harmonization while maintaining

Chinese characteristics.

An Overview of Regulatory Approaches

Regulatory agencies and their various programs exhibit distinct approaches in utilizing toxicological data. A crucial distinction lies in the level of premarket analysis or approval required before a new product can enter the market. While certain products necessitate premarket approval (e. g. drugs, devices, pesticides), others only require premarket notification (e. g. new chemical substances). Some products, like foods and cosmetics, have no premarket requirements before commercialization.

Another significant difference lies in determining who bears the burden of proof to demonstrate safety or hazard. For instance, the manufacturer of a new food additive must demonstrate to the FDA the lack of hazard before human exposure. Conversely, regulations like OSHA place the burden on regulators to prove a substance's hazard before imposing restrictions on exposure. The Congress's choice for a specific product or activity profoundly impacts an agency's authority to mandate comprehensive toxicological investigations before commercialization.

Regulatory agencies generally adopt one of three approaches in determining the permissible level of a substance: ① acceptable risk, ② balancing, ③ technical feasibility. Often, a combination of these approaches is employed. The selection among these approaches for a particular hazard is typically dictated by the applicable statutory framework.

The statutory framework plays a pivotal role in shaping the regulatory landscape, influencing the agency's capacity to require thorough toxicological assessments before a product is introduced to the market.

Acceptable Risk Approaches

One fundamental strategy in risk management involves assessing the level of risk associated with a substance and subsequently implementing measures to reduce it to an acceptable level when necessary. These programs primarily emphasize health evidence, with toxicological data playing a pivotal role in the assessment process.

In the pharmaceutical industry, safety metrics such as the therapeutic index and margin of safety are calculated to evaluate the risk-benefit profile of drugs. The therapeutic index represents the ratio between the toxic dose and the effective dose, while the margin of safety indicates the difference between the usual effective dose and the dose that induces adverse effects.

For environmental pollutants, food additives, and occupational exposures, regulatory agencies establish "safe" levels of exposure. Such as reference dose (RfD), acceptable daily intake (ADI), and permissible exposure limits (PEL) are determined by applying safety factors to the lowest "no observed adverse effect level (NOAEL)" from animal experiments. These safety thresholds are typically derived by applying uncertainty factors (also known as safety factors) to the lowest observed adverse effect level (LOAEL) or, preferably, the NOAEL from animal experiments. Human exposure below these thresholds is generally considered safe or acceptable. For substances without clear thresholds, such as genotoxic carcinogens, the concept of virtually safe doses (VSD) or virtually safe exposures is employed. This approach involves determining exposure levels that correspond to society's acceptable risk levels, often set at one additional cancer case per million exposed individuals over a lifetime.

A more stringent approach to risk management is the "zero" or "negligible" risk requirement. A notable example of this is the Delaney clause, enacted in 1958 as part of the Food Additives Amendment to the Federal Food, Drug, and Cosmetic Act in the United States. This clause prohibits the approval of food additives that have been shown to induce cancer in humans or animals, regardless of the dose. While this approach aims for the highest level of safety, it has been criticized for its inflexibility and potential to overlook the principle of dose-dependent toxicity.

Balancing Approaches

An alternative strategy in risk management involves balancing the health benefits of risk reduction against the associated costs. This approach, known as cost-benefit analysis (CBA) or risk-benefit analysis, requires quantifying both the health risks and the economic implications of various regulatory options. The primary goal is to identify and implement the regulatory option that offers the largest estimated net benefit to society.

In these regulatory programs, both toxicological and economic data serve as essential components in decision-making processes. Toxicological data provides the foundation for assessing potential health risks and benefits under different regulatory scenarios, while economic data enables the estimation of implementation costs for various risk reduction measures and quantifies the potential economic benefits associated with improved public health outcomes. The integration of these two data types allows regulatory agencies to develop comprehensive and balanced approaches that consider both health protection and economic feasibility in their risk management strategies.

The process typically involves the following five steps: identifying potential regulatory options, estimating the health risks and benefits associated with each option, calculating the economic costs and benefits of each option, comparing the net benefits across options, and selecting the option with the highest net benefit.

While this approach aims to maximize societal welfare, it faces challenges such as accurately monetizing health benefits and addressing ethical concerns about putting a monetary value on human life and health.

Technical Feasibility Approaches

The third major approach in risk management focuses on reducing exposures to the lowest feasible level or requiring entities (e. g. industries, companies) to implement the best available technology (BAT). Unlike risk-based approaches, this method does not explicitly rely on health data. While it simplifies the complexities and uncertainties of toxicological evidence, it may result in standards that either overprotect or underprotect health.

Regulatory Influences on Toxicology

The relationship between regulation and toxicology is bidirectional and dynamic. Regulatory programs significant influence the practice of toxicology, while toxicological data inform and shape regulatory decisions. Modern toxicology has evolved considerably in response to the information needs of contemporary regulation, resulting in a complex interplay between scientific research and policy-making. Regulatory agencies, such as the USFDA and the EPA, play a pivotal role in shaping toxicological studies. These agencies prescribe specific objectives and study designs to meet regulatory requirements, effectively steering the direction of toxicological research. Typically, they mandate a range of tests, including acute toxicity studies, subchronic toxicity studies (usually 90-day studies), chronic toxicity studies (often combined with carcinogenicity studies), reproductive and developmental toxicity studies, genotoxicity studies, and toxicokinetic studies. These agencies provide detailed guidelines for executing these tests, ensuring consistency and comparability of data across different studies and laboratories.

On an international level, organizations such as the Organization for Economic Co-operation and Development (OECD) strive to promote standardized testing guidelines and establish minimum data requirements for new chemicals. The OECD Test Guidelines Program aims to facilitate consistent approaches to toxicological testing across different regulatory jurisdictions, promoting mutual acceptance of data and reducing redundant testing.

To ensure the quality and integrity of toxicological data submitted for regulatory consideration, both the FDA and EPA have established GLP regulations. These regulations outline critical laboratory procedures and cover essential aspects of laboratory science, including: animal husbandry standards, equipment calibration and maintenance, standard operating procedures (SOPs), data collection and record-keeping practices, quality assurance and quality control measures, and personnel qualifications and training. The implementation of GLP regulations has significantly enhanced the reliability and reproducibility of toxicological studies used in regulatory decision-making.

In recent decades, growing concern for animal welfare has led to the development of laws and regulations governing the use of animals in research. Scientists conducting studies for regulatory submission must comply with animal protection provisions outlined in agency GLP regulations and other relevant legislation, such as the Animal Welfare Act in the United States. These provisions typically include requirements for adequate living conditions, veterinary treatment, and record-keeping.

The influence of regulatory on toxicology is pervasive, shaping not only the practice of toxicology but also the conduct of toxicological studies and the treatment of animals used in research. By understanding and adhering to regulatory requirements, toxicologists contribute to sound regulatory decision-making and the protection of human health and the environment.

Risk Assessment Basics

This section provides an overview of the risk assessment process, encompassing both health risk assessment and environmental risk assessment. Health risk assessment focuses on potential threats to human health, while environmental risk assessment addresses potential damage to ecosystems, wildlife, and endangered species. Although this section primarily emphasizes human health risks, we will also discuss environmental risks that have direct or indirect impacts on human health.

Risk assessment is the initial and critical step in a three-part risk analysis process, followed by risk management and risk communication. The overarching goal of risk assessment is to control situations where organisms or populations could be exposed to hazards. Before delving into the intricacies of risk assessment, it's essential to grasp fundamental concepts and terminologies.

Risk

Risk in toxicology represents a mathematical concept that quantifies the probability of adverse effects occurring in individuals or populations under specific exposure conditions to chemical agents or other hazards. This probability can be expressed quantitatively on a scale from zero (indicating no harm) to one (representing absolute certainty of harm), providing a scientific basis for risk assessment and management decisions.

In the context of toxicology and public health, risk values typically represent the excess probability of serious adverse effects, such as cancer, beyond the background incidence in the general population. For example, exposure to a chemical carcinogen might carry a risk estimate of 1×10^{-6}(one in a million), indicating the potential for one additional cancer case among one million exposed individuals over their lifetimes. To provide perspective, daily consumption of one packet of cigarettes carries a considerably higher lung cancer risk of approximately 5×10^{-3} per year (one in 200 per year). These estimates should be considered in the context of background cancer rates, where the lifetime risk of developing any type of cancer in the general population is approximately one in three.

The fundamental goal of risk analysis is to reduce risks to acceptable levels, acknowledging that complete risk elimination is often unrealistic despite public aspirations for "zero risk". Table 11-3 presents estimated risks for certain activities and natural occurrences, illustrating the wide range of risks that humans encounter in daily life.

Table 11-3 Estimated Risks for Certain Activities and Natural Occurrences

Activity	Risk*
Smoking (10 cigarettes a day)	1/400
All accidents	1/2, 000
Driving (16, 000 km/year)	1/5, 000
All traffic accidents	1/8, 000
Work in industry	1/30, 000
Natural disasters	1/50, 000
Being struck by lighting	1/1, 000, 000

* Risk is expressed as probability of death of an individual for a year of exposure.

The determination of acceptable risk involves a complex interplay of scientific evidence, societal values, and practical considerations. This acceptance threshold is influenced by multiple factors, including the quality and extent of scientific data, sociocultural perspectives, economic implications, political considerations, and the perceived benefits associated with exposure to the agent in question. Importantly, the concept of acceptable risk extends beyond pure scientific determination, incorporating value judgments and policy considerations that reflect societal priorities and trade-offs.

Risk assessment serves as a cornerstone of the risk analysis process, providing the scientific foundation necessary for effective risk management and communication. Through rigorous quantification of adverse effect probabilities associated with chemical exposures, risk assessment enables informed societal decision-making regarding acceptable risk levels and appropriate risk management strategies. This systematic approach helps bridge the gap between scientific understanding and practical risk management, facilitating the development of evidence-based policies that protect public health while acknowledging real-world constraints and considerations.

Risk Assessment

Risk assessment is a crucial process in safeguarding human health, providing a systematic approach to characterizing potential adverse effects resulting from exposure to hazardous agents or situations. This multifaceted process incorporates both qualitative and quantitative elements, offering a solid foundation for informed decision-making by risk managers.

The primary objective of risk assessment is to furnish risk managers with a rational basis for decisions regarding the management of chemical use, ensuring the protection of human health. By integrating qualitative evidence and quantitative exposure assessments, risk assessment initiates a comprehensive decision-making process that aims to balance public safety with the benefits associated with product use. While risk assessment is not research per se, it relies on the systematic collection and evaluation of existing data. It's important to note that despite its foundation in scientific principles, the assessment often involves making estimates or judgments about certain data inputs, introducing an element of uncertainty. Nevertheless, human health risk assessment remains a valuable tool for addressing fundamental questions about potential dangers from chemical exposure.

Four Steps Process for Risk Assessment

The National Research Council of the US National Academy of Science outlines four interconnected steps in risk assessment, as illustrated in Figure 11-1. These steps include hazard identification, dose-response assessment, exposure assessment, and risk characterization. Each of these components plays a pivotal role in the overall risk assessment process and will be discussed in more detail in the following sections.

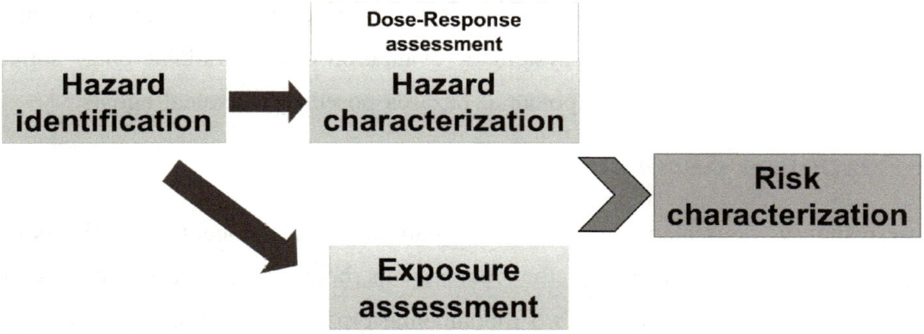

Figure 11-1 Four steps process for risk assessment

Hazard Identification

Hazard identification, the initial step in the risk assessment process, aims to evaluate whether exposure to a chemical agent, under any conditions, can lead to an increased incidence or severity of adverse health effects such as cancer, birth defects, or neurotoxicity or not. This crucial step draws upon various sources of information, including human studies (epidemiological and clinical), animal experiments, in vitro tests, computer simulations, and structural-activity relationships (SARs).

The most compelling evidence for hazard identification is derived from well-designed human epidemiological studies or statistically controlled clinical studies. However, such data are not always available, particularly for new chemicals or those with limited human exposure. In the absence of human data, reliance is placed on animal studies to infer potential hazards to humans. While animal studies provide valuable insights, extrapolation to human health effects requires careful consideration of interspecies differences.

Structural activity relationships aid in assessing the relative toxicity of chemically related compounds. This approach is based on the principle that chemicals with similar structures often exhibit similar biological activities. However, SARs have limitations and are typically used in conjunction with other data sources.

The process of hazard identification involves a degree of professional judgment, as evidence from different study types is weighed. A weight-of-evidence (WoE) approach is often employed, assessing the extent to which available biomedical data support the hypothesis that a substance causes adverse effects in humans. Factors such as the number of affected tissue sites, animal species, strains, sexes, experiments, doses showing a response, and a clear dose-response relationship increasing the weight of evidence.

To enhance transparency and reproducibility in hazard identification, formalized schemes, akin to evidence-based, medicine, have been proposed, termed evidence-based toxicology. This approach ensures a systematic evaluation of the available data, supporting a comprehensive understanding of the potential hazards posed by chemical agents.

Dose-Response Assessment

Dose-response assessment is a crucial quantitative component of risk assessment, primarily focuses on characterizing the relationship between chemical potency and the incidence of adverse health effects. Two fundamental types of dose-response relationships are recognized in risk assessment: the threshold model and the nonthreshold model.

Threshold Models

The threshold model is typically applied to noncarcinogenic chemical agents and certain nongenotoxic carcinogens. In this approach, the goal is to develop "exposure criteria" such as the reference dose or acceptable daily intake (ADI).

The Concept of Critical Effect

In the threshold model, there exists a dose below which no adverse effect is observed, termed the threshold dose. This model is based on the assumption that protective mechanisms in the body can repair or prevent damage up to a certain point. When the dose of the chemical is sufficiently high, these defense mechanisms are overwhelmed, resulting in an adverse effect.

A chemical may elicit multiple adverse effect (endpoint), each with its distinct dose-response relationship. The dose-response assessment aims to identify the most sensitive effect (the critical effect)——the one that occurs at the lowest dose. By basing the risk assessment on this critical effect, one can reasonably ensure that all other adverse effects requiring higher doses will also be prevented.

The establishment of "safe" doses for human exposure relies fundamentally on identifying threshold doses for the most sensitive adverse effects. This process traditionally employs two key approaches in toxicological assessments. The NOAEL, which represents the highest experimental dose that produces no statistically or biologically significant increases in adverse effects compared to controls, is generally considered to represent the threshold dose and serves as the preferred basis for safety assessment. When NOAEL data are unavailable, toxicologists utilize the LOAEL, which represents the lowest tested dose that produces detectable adverse effects. To address the inherent limitations of the NOAEL/LOAEL approach, such as its dependence on experimental dose selection and sample size, the BMD methodology has been developed as a more sophisticated alternative. The BMD approach employs mathematical modeling of the dose-response relationship to provide a more statistically robust estimation of threshold doses, thereby enhancing the scientific basis for establishing safety margins in human exposure guidelines.

The "Safe" Dose Derived from a Threshold Model

The "safe" dose is typically expressed as an exposure rate (mg/(kg · d)). Common terms include: RfD or RfC (developed by US EPA), and ADI (developed by World Health Organization). These values estimate the amount of a substance that can be taken in daily over a lifetime without appreciable health risk. the formula which is to calculate the RfD (or ADI) is RfD (or ADI) = NOAEL (LOAEL, BMD or BMDL)/ UFs×MF.

Application of Uncertainty Factors

The purpose of dividing the NOAEL/LOAEL or BMD/BMDL by uncertainty factors is to ensure that the "safe" dose used in the risk assessment is below the actual human threshold dose for all individuals in the exposed population, thereby avoiding any underestimation of risk. These uncertainties arise because of our inability to directly measure the actual human threshold dose. The general rationale for selecting the size of the uncertainty factor for a particular area of uncertainty is as follows:

A UF of up to 10 is used to extrapolate from animals to humans.

A UF of up to 10 is used to account for sensitive subpopulations.

A UF of up to 10 is used if dose-response data are only available for a less-than-lifetime exposure than a lifetime exposure to develop a "safe" dose.

A UF of up to 10 is used when deriving a "safe" dose from a LOAEL instead of a NOAEL.

An MF between 1 and 10 is used to reflect the quality of the toxicity database, and the default value for the MF is 1.0.

The UFs are multiplicative, meaning they are multiplied together to determine a final UF. For example, if the NOAEL for the most sensitive endpoint of a chemical is 5 mg/(kg · d) and this was derived from multiple chronic animal studies, UFs for interspecies extrapolation and for sensitive human subpopulations could be applied. If UFs of 10 were chosen for both, the total UF would be 100 (10×10). The NOAEL of 5 mg/(kg · d) is divided by the total UF (in this case 100) to arrive at the "safe" dose of 0.05 mg/(kg · d).

Nonthreshold Models

Nonthreshold models represent a fundamental approach in toxicological risk assessment, particularly applicable to certain categories of adverse effects where any level of exposure is presumed to carry some degree of risk. While these models are most commonly associated with carcinogenicity assessment, they also apply to various other toxicological endpoints, including mutagenesis, certain developmental effects, and some immunological responses where biological repair mechanisms or compensatory processes may not completely counteract the adverse effects even at very low doses.

The conceptual framework of nonthreshold models is based on the premise that the dose-response relationship extends linearly (or through other mathematical functions) toward zero, with no dose level considered entirely free of risk. This approach is particularly relevant for stochastic effects, where the probability of an adverse effect, rather than its severity, increases with dose. For genotoxic carcinogens, the assessment typically involves calculating the carcinogenic potency through the slope of the dose-response curve for tumor induction. Similarly, for mutagenic compounds, the relationship between exposure and mutation frequency often follows nonthreshold patterns.

The practical implementation of nonthreshold models faces significant methodological challenges. Conventional toxicological studies, including chronic bioassays, typically employ relatively high doses and limited sample sizes, constraining their ability to detect low-level responses. For instance, standard animal studies with approximately 50 subjects per dose group can reliably detect response rates only above about 10%. This creates a substantial challenge in assessing risks at the extraordinarily low response rates (10^{-5} to 10^{-6}) often relevant for environmental and occupational exposure standards.

Furthermore, the experimental data points usually lie several orders of magnitude above environmentally relevant exposure levels, necessitating extensive extrapolation to estimate risks at lower doses. This extrapolation process introduces considerable uncertainty, particularly in the low-dose region most pertinent to human exposure scenarios. Various mathematical models, including linear no-threshold (LNT), multistage, and other statistical approaches, have been developed to address these extrapolation challenges, each with its own assumptions and limitations.

The selection and application of nonthreshold models also consider mechanistic understanding of the toxicological process, including factors such as DNA repair capabilities, cell cycle regulation, and other biological responses that might influence the shape of the dose-response relationship at low doses. This integration of mechanistic insights with mathematical modeling helps refine risk assessments, though uncertainty remains an inherent aspect of low-dose extrapolation.

Low-Dose Extrapolation Models

The quantitative assessment of toxicological risks at environmentally relevant exposures necessitates extrapolation from high-dose bioassay data, as direct measurement of low-dose responses remains experimentally unfeasible. This creates a critical knowledge gap between the empirically observable high-dose effects and the zero-dose/zero-risk origin point, particularly in carcinogenicity assessment. To bridge this gap, sophisticated statistical methodologies, collectively termed "low-dose extrapolation models", have been developed to characterize the dose-response relationship across the full exposure spectrum.

Three primary mathematical approaches—Weibull, probit, and multistage models have emerged as standard tools for low-dose extrapolation. These models employ different mathematical functions to characterize the dose-response relationship, enabling the estimation of risks at doses substantially below those tested in experimental studies. Depending on the selected model and underlying biological assumptions, the extrapolated dose-response curve may exhibit linear, sublinear, or superlinear characteristics in the low-dose region, each carrying distinct implications for risk assessment.

In the absence of mechanistic data demonstrating nonlinear dynamics, regulatory agencies typically default to linear, nonthreshold models, particularly the linearized multistage model for carcinogen assessment. This conservative approach involves linear extrapolation from a defined point within the observed data range to the origin. The selection of this starting point for extrapolation has been standardized through the "point of departure" (POD) methodology, which typically utilizes the effective dose producing a 10% tumor response (ED_{10}) as determined by the linearized multistage model, as illustrated in Figure 11-2. This standardized approach provides a consistent framework for risk assessment while acknowledging the inherent uncertainties in low-dose extrapolation.

The selection and application of extrapolation models must consider both statistical rigor and biological plausibility, recognizing that different toxicological mechanisms may warrant different mathematical approaches to low-dose risk estimation. This systematic approach to dose-response assessment enables science-based decision-making in regulatory contexts while acknowledging the inherent uncertainties in extrapolating beyond the range of empirical observation.

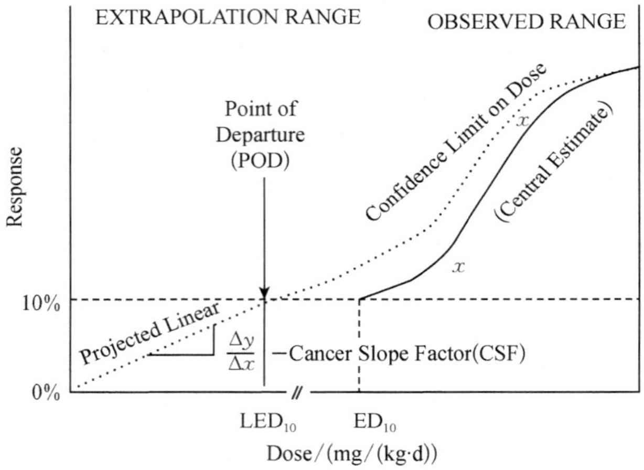

Figure 11-2 **Low dose extrapolation models**

Cancer Slope Factor Determination

The culmination of dose-response assessment using the linearized multistage model yields a quantitative measure of carcinogenic potency, designated as the cancer slope factor (CSF). This critical parameter represents the upper 95% confidence limit of the slope in the low-dose linear region of the dose-response curve. Expressed in units of (mg/(kg · d)), the CSF provides a standardized metric for comparing carcinogenic potencies across different compounds and serves as a fundamental tool in cancer risk assessment.

The derivation of the CSF employs conservative statistical approaches to account for uncertainties inherent in the extrapolation process. By utilizing the upper confidence limit rather than the central estimate, this methodology incorporates a margin of safety in subsequent risk calculations. This quantitative parameter enables risk assessors to estimate lifetime cancer risks associated with chronic exposure to carcinogenic substances across a range of environmental exposure scenarios, facilitating evidence-based regulatory decision-making and risk management strategies.

Exposure Assessment

Exposure assessment constitutes the third critical component of the risk assessment framework, representing a fundamental determinant of risk as no adverse effects can occur without exposure. This systematic process encompasses the quantification of exposure magnitude, frequency, and duration, while simultaneously characterizing the exposed population's demographics and susceptibility factors.

The comprehensive evaluation of exposure scenarios involves identifying both potential and completed exposure pathways, incorporating detailed analysis of population characteristics that may enhance or diminish risk concerns. Modern exposure assessment recognizes two critical dimensions of exposure: cumulative exposure, addressing multiple compounds sharing similar toxicological mechanisms, and aggregate exposure, which considers the totality of exposure to a single agent across various environmental media.

Environmental contamination pathways typically involve multiple media, including soil, sediment, groundwater, surface water, and air, which may become contaminated through direct releases or secondary transport mechanisms. Human exposure occurs through contact with these contaminated media, with toxic agents accessing the body via three primary routes: ingestion, inhalation, and dermal absorption. A crucial component of exposure assessment involves identifying and characterizing relevant exposure pathways for specific risk scenarios under evaluation.

The quantitative phase of exposure assessment involves systematic measurement or estimation of exposure through each identified pathway, followed by integration of pathway-specific exposures to determine overall exposure levels. This process requires careful consideration of temporal and spatial variations in exposure patterns, as well as the physicochemical properties of the agents that influence their environmental fate and bioavailability. The resulting exposure estimates, combined with information about population characteristics and activity patterns, provide the foundation for subsequent risk characterization and management decisions.

Basic Techniques for Quantifying Exposure

There are two basic methods for quantifying exposure: direct measurement and modeling. Direct measurement results in the most accurate and realistic exposure data.

Exposure can be quantified, for example, by analyzing food intake and measuring urine output of the chemical or its metabolites. However, in most situations, the exposure has occurred without the benefit of direct measurements. In these situations, exposure can be estimated through modeling. Fate and transport models use mathematical models to simulate the behavior and breakdown of chemicals in the environment and predict chemical concentrations in various media. Hundreds of models exist for these purposes, including atmospheric models, surface water models, groundwater models, and food-chain models. All of these models are based on assumptions and are often limited by a large degree of uncertainty in the results. Despite their limitations, exposure models are of value in that they can make predictions for an unlimited number of exposure scenarios and predict past and future exposures. Exposure measurement, however, is limited to the present. Another means of exposure assessment, biological monitoring of blood and air samples, may represent new ways of reducing uncertainty in this step.

Calculations for ADD or LADD

The dose can be summed across pathways to estimate the total dose per day. Time-weighted averages are commonly used when estimating dose. The period over which the dose is averaged depends upon the length of exposure and the type of adverse effect that will be used to evaluate risk. In general, for chemicals assessed using the threshold model, the average is taken over the exposure period, and an average daily dose (ADD) is used. For carcinogens assessed using the nonthreshold model, the average dose should be an average over a lifetime. If exposure occurs for less than a lifetime, the total dose the individual or population has accumulated during their entire exposure interval is first converted into a lifetime average daily dose (LADD). With this view, a dose of a chemical received every day at a given rate for a lifetime poses a cancer risk equal to the total dose at ten times that rate for a tenth of a lifetime. The following section provides example dose equations for some common exposure pathways.

$$ADD(\mathrm{mg/(kg \cdot d)}) = \frac{C \cdot IR \cdot EF \cdot ED}{BW \cdot AT}, \ and\ LADD(\mathrm{mg/(kg \cdot d)}) = \frac{C \cdot IR \cdot EF \cdot ED}{BW \cdot LT}$$

Where:

C: Concentration of the chemical in the contaminated environmental medium (soil or water) to which the person is exposed. The units are mg/kg for soil and mg/L for water.

IR: Intake rate of the contaminated environmental medium. The units are mg/d for soil and L/d for water.

BW: Body weight of the exposed person (kg).

EF: Exposure frequency (days/year). This describes how often a person is exposed to the contaminated medium for a typical year.

ED: Exposure duration (years). This describes how long a person is exposed to the contaminated medium throughout their lifetime.

AT: Average time (days). This term specifies the length of time over which the average dose is calculated.

LT: Life-time (years). This term is for quantifying cancer risk, a "lifetime" of 70 years is used (i. e. 70 years times 365 days/year).

It should be noticed that the ED is in the numerator (part of total dose estimation) and is different from the AT, which is in the denominator (part of the averaging per day). The ED and AT may be equal for some exposure scenarios to non-carcinogens but they tend to be different for exposures to carcinogens where the averaging time is always a lifetime (default = 70 years).

Risk Characterization

Risk characterization is the final and critical step of the risk assessment process. It integrates information from the three previous steps to develop risk estimates, which can be qualitative, quantitative, or both, including associated uncertainty.

Because the dose-response assessment step is performed differently for the type of adverse effects considered nonthreshold compared to those classified as threshold effects, the risk characterization process for these two kinds of effects differs as well. For threshold effects, quantitative risk characterization is expressed in terms of a ratio. Typically, it involves a comparison of the estimated dose and the results of the exposure assessment with the numerical estimate of the "safe" dose developed in the first two steps for the chemical. When a nonthreshold approach is used, the risk is expressed as a probability that the effect will occur as a result of exposure, for example, the excess cancer risk associated with exposure to a carcinogen at a specified level.

Quantifying Risk for Non-cancer Effects

Hazard Quotient

In general, the threshold approach to characterizing risk is used for chemicals with noncarcinogenic effects. For non-cancer risk assessment, the potential for non-cancer effects is instead evaluated by comparing an ADD over a specified period with a "safe" dose (RfD).

This ratio is called a hazard quotient (HQ): HQ = ADD / RfD.

If the HQ is less than one, the dose received is less than the "safe" dose and no adverse effects are expected to occur. However, if the HQ is greater than one, the possibility of adverse effects is indicated. Often, that is sufficient to stimulate regulatory action. It does not necessarily mean that toxicity is likely, however. It can only be said that the chance of toxicity increases as the HQ increases. HQ can vary among different routes of exposure. If the exposure to a chemical is by more than one route of administration, the HQ for each route would be calculated separately and summed to derive an overall ratio called a hazard index (HI). It should be noted that HI is also a ratio and is not to be interpreted as a statistical probability.

Margin of Exposure

The other meaning of expressing hazard for non-cancer effects is through the calculation of a margin of exposure (MOE). This is most often used in the context of the BMD approach. The BMD for a sensitive effect is used as an expression of the no-effect dose and divided by the estimated dose to produce the MOE. The MOE indicates the extent to which estimated exposure is above or below the no-effect level. Unlike the HQ, where numbers less than one indicate safety, low risk is conveyed by high MOEs.

Quantifying Risk for Cancer Effects

Because the dose-response relationship for most carcinogens is assumed to follow a linear, nonthreshold model, the risk is characterized in a way fundamentally different from threshold chemicals. For these carcinogens, risk is conveyed as the lifetime excess probability of developing cancer as a result of exposure. Risk (unitless) is calculated from a chemical-specific cancer slope factor [CSF(mg/(kg · d))], and an estimate of lifetime average daily dose [LADD(mg/(kg · d))] received from exposure to the chemical: Risk = CSF · LADD.

Uncertainty Analysis and Monte Carlo Simulation

A discussion of the uncertainties is a particularly important aspect of the risk characterization. Because of the extensive use of models and assumptions in calculating risks, the resulting risk values are inherently imprecise. To use these risk values effectively to assist sound risk management, it is important to describe as transparently as possible where the uncertainties lie and, if possible, the magnitude of error that may be associated with them. The uncertainty associated with the risk estimates can be considered as coming from two sources or types: type 1 uncertainty, that is, variability, and type 2 uncertainty from our lack of basic knowledge. Variability is the natural variation that as an inherent property exists within a population while type 2 uncertainty can be reduced by additional examination, study, or research.

Probabilistic risk assessment is an alternative approach for addressing the inherent problems in terms of variability and uncertainty. In probabilistic risk assessment, input variables are entered as probability density functions (PDFs) instead of single values. These PDFs are then combined in such a way as to yield a risk distribution, indicating the probability of each risk value occurring within the population. To combine PDFs, the most commonly used technique is Monte Carlo simulation. For each risk calculation, the computer program selects a value from each input PDF and calculates a numerical risk. This simulation process is repeated, usually, thousands of times, and the resulting range of risk values is tallied in the form of a distribution. From this distribution, the variability in risk among individuals can be visualized and the quantitative representation of the uncertainties in the risk calculation can also be provided. With Monte Carlo simulation, a computer program in essence creates a simulated population designed to resemble the exposed population in every key respect. As discussed above, probabilistic techniques can be used to provide a more precise quantitative expression of the uncertainties associated with risk estimates, as well as a description of variability in risks encountered in exposed populations. It is technically demanding, however, requiring much greater time, resources, and data than do the traditional risk estimation techniques.

Risk Management

Definition of Risk Management

Risk management is a comprehensive decision-making process that entails the consideration of political, social, economic, statutory, and engineering information together with risk-related information in order to develop, analyze, and compare the regulatory options and select the appropriate regulatory response to a potential health or environmental hazard. A number of options are available for risk reduction, for instance, education and communication of risk, allocation of tax dollars to safety programs, exposure monitoring and controls, limitations in the use of the substance of concern, or a total ban of the chemical, etc. The goal of risk management is to choose the scientifically sound, cost-effective, integrated action that reduces or prevents risks.

Risk assessment and risk management answer different questions: the former answers such questions as "What is the estimate of likelihood of specific harm to an exposed individual or population?", and the latter "How do we mitigate this risk?". Risk management decisions are based on the technical risk assessment information, but they also incorporate other information. Specifically, risk managers consider costs, benefits, risk of alternative actions, and risk of no actions. For example, some drugs have a very small safety margin between the level that is effective and the level that is toxic, but the benefits of the drug are judged to outweigh the risks; therefore, it is decided that these drugs can be used. At the other end of the spectrum, some food-coloring additives have very large safety margins between what is toxic and what is in the diet, but the benefits of food coloring are minimal and alternatives exist, so this risk would generally face a higher level of scrutiny in a risk management decision.

Risk Management Framework

The effective management of risks requires a systematic approach through six key stages:

(1) Problem Definition: Identify and contextualize the risk issue within relevant public health frameworks.

(2) Risk Analysis: Evaluate the nature, magnitude, and probability of potential risks.

(3) Option Assessment: Examine available strategies and interventions for risk mitigation.

(4) Decision Making: Select optimal risk management approaches based on evidence and feasibility.

(5) Implementation: Execute chosen risk management measures through coordinated action.

(6) Evaluation: Assess the effectiveness of implemented strategies and adjust as needed.

Three Elements of Risk Management

Risk management comprises three elements: risk-benefit evaluation; emission and exposure control; and risk monitoring.

Risk-benefit Evaluation

Risk-benefit evaluation is the establishing process of a qualitative or quantitative relationship between risks and benefits of exposure to an agent, involving the complex process of determining and comparing the significance of the identified hazards and estimated risks to the individual or population concerned or affected by the exposure, with the significance of the benefits brought about by the agent. Risk-benefit evaluation has the advantage of helping make choices among policies and actions with quite different benefits and risks. This evaluation, especially in the more complex situations is often conducted on behalf of society by scientific committees consisting of relevant experts [and ideally some lay ("stakeholder") participation], and their recommendations are implemented by the regulatory authority.

Emission and Exposure Control

Emission and exposure control are associated particularly with industrial hazards—the control of emissions from stacks to the atmosphere or discharges to wastewater. However, it also applies to most sources of exposure to chemicals, including drugs. Drugs are controlled by designating those authorizing the obtaining of the medicine (doctors, and so on, with prescribing rights) and through designating the outlets from which they may be obtained (e. g. pharmacy only, or any supermarket). Most other regulatory programs control emissions, for example, for foods, there are emission limits from packaging and allowable residue levels for additives and contaminants in foodstuffs.

Risk Monitoring

Monitoring includes inspection to ensure that conditions of control are being met in the field. It also includes procedures, such as those associated with pharmacovigilance, designed to ensure that previously unidentified effects do not go unrecorded. The process, which involves measuring risk reduction concerning a particular hazard, can also help to make decisions concerning a reassessment of the risk and further control actions.

General Principles of Decision-Making

Some of the principles proposed to guide risk management decision-making. Firstly, non-maleficence—the ultimate goal of good risk management is to prevent or minimize risk, or to "do good" as much as possible; secondly, fairness, natural justice, equity, utility, and honesty; thirdly, the Golden Rule (Impose no more risk that you would tolerate yourself)—it forces decision makers to abandon complete detachment from their decisions so they may understand the perspectives of those affected; fourthly, be cautious in the face of uncertainty; fifthly, autonomy—fostering autonomous decision making involves both providing people with the opportunity to participate, and full and honest disclosure of all the information required for informed decisions; lastly, the risk management is a flexible, evolutionary, and iterative process.

The principles are mainly based on fundamental ethical principles and values and are intended to be aspirational rather than prescriptive. Their application requires flexibility and practical judgment, and trade-offs may sometimes have to be made between seemingly conflicting principles.

Risk Communication

Concept of Risk Communication

Risk communication is an area that draws from several disciplines in the natural and social sciences. Because of its short history, the concept of risk communication is still evolving. It can be defined as an interactive two-way process involving the exchange among individuals, groups, and institutions of information and expert opinion about the nature, severity, and acceptability of risks and the decisions taken to combat them. The people that may involve in this process are risk assessors and managers, the general public, news media, interested groups, etc. (also known as "stakeholders"). The components of the process are the risk communicator or source, the message, the message channel, and the recipient of the message.

Risk Perception

Risk perception of the recipient can play a critical role in the process and is an aspect of risk communication that has been studied very intensively. Risk perception is the apprehension or opinion of the likelihood of risk(s) associated with performing a certain activity or living a certain lifestyle and needs to be considered for developing effective risk communication. Each individual has their way of thinking and decision-making ability, which can make risk communication a challenge.

Psychologists have identified a set of affective characteristics (outrage, anxiety, fear, etc.) that make some risks seem larger and some smaller, the scientific data notwithstanding. By understanding the biology and psychology of how humans perceive risk, we can understand why and how "estimated" and "perceived" risks are not aligned with "actual" risks. An increasing amount of research done in the area of risk perception has identified a number of attributes that make certain risks seem more worrisome than others. These "risk perception factors" are essentially the personality traits of potential threats that help us subconsciously decide what to be afraid of and how afraid to be. Some of the main factors that affect the perception of risk are indicated in Table 11-4. The factors work in such a manner that, for example, an action voluntarily undertaken by an individual is perceived as posing a smaller risk than one imposed upon that individual, all else being equal. Knowledge of these perception factors can be used to guide more effective risk communication. The results of research on the factors that influence successful risk communication are the basis for sets of risk communication principles that have been developed.

Table 11-4 **Risk Perception Factors**

Less Risky	More Risky
Natural	Artificial
Familiar	Unfamiliar
Controlled by self	Controlled by others
Voluntary	Involuntary
Uninteresting and forgettable	Dramatic and memorable
Associated with a trusted source	Related to an untrusted source
Certainty	Uncertainty
Common, everyday risks	Seldom occurring events
Not dreaded	Dreaded
Risks only affect adults	Risks affect children or pregnant women

Key Principles of Effective Risk Communication

Effective risk communication is built upon fundamental principles that foster meaningful dialogue between stakeholders and enhance public understanding of risks. At its core, this approach recognizes the public as an essential partner in risk management, actively engaging communities in the decision-making process while valuing their perspectives and contributions.

Successful risk communication requires careful planning and evaluation to ensure messages are both accessible and relevant to their intended audience. The content must be strategically designed to match the audience's comprehension level while maintaining cultural sensitivity and clarity. Beyond technical accuracy, the establishment of trust and credibility stands as a paramount concern, as these elements often carry more weight with communities than statistical data or scientific details. Once lost, such trust becomes exceptionally difficult to restore.

The manner and tone of communication frequently supersede the actual content in importance, highlighting the critical role of non-verbal elements in message delivery. Risk communicators must ensure that information remains accurate and consistent across different agencies while avoiding speculative statements that could undermine credibility. This comprehensive approach enables government and industry to better understand and anticipate public responses while increasing the effectiveness of risk management actions.

While current understanding of risk communication continues to evolve, these core principles provide a foundation for effective stakeholder engagement. Ongoing research in this field promises to further enhance our understanding of communication processes and strengthen the bridge between technical expertise and public comprehension.

International Harmonization and Collaboration on Regulatory Toxicology

The concept of "harmonization" plays a crucial role in various global and regional programs aimed at improving the assessment and management of potential risks associated with toxic substances. Notably, the International Programme on Chemical Safety (IPCS) Harmonization Project is a major effort working towards the development, harmonization, and promotion of scientifically sound methodologies for evaluating risks to human health and the environment from chemical exposure. The IPCS's work, including the publication of Environmental Health Criteria, focuses on addressing uncertainties and challenges related to emerging scientific issues like toxicogenomics, fostering mutual acceptance of risk assessment products.

Numerous national regulatory authorities and international organizations are actively involved in processes that encourage harmonization of regulatory testing requirements and test protocols. The Organization for Economic Cooperation and Development (OECD), comprising 30 member countries from Europe, is a prominent player in this arena. The OECD Health Effects Test Guidelines serve as a global reference for key toxicity tests, ensuring that different countries and regions adhere to the same data requirements for regulatory decisions, contributing to a streamlined and consistent approach.

In the realm of drug regulations, the International Conference on Harmonization (ICH) of Technical Requirements for Registration of Pharmaceuticals for Human Use plays a significant role. Collaborative efforts by experts from regulatory authorities and pharmaceutical industry trade associations in the US, Europe, and Japan within the ICH framework have led to the harmonization of technical requirements for human drug product registration. ICH's establishment of internationally recognized safety guidelines further contributes to the uniformity of toxicity testing approaches on a global scale.

An essential milestone in harmonization efforts is the development of the Globally Harmonized System for the Classification and Labeling of Chemicals. Recognizing the need for a unified global system, the Globally Harmonized System for the Classfication and Labding of Chemicals was formulated to provide a harmonized approach to classification and labeling. This international effort is crucial in laying the foundation for all countries to create comprehensive national programs ensuring the safe use of chemicals. The Inter-Organization Program for the Sound Management of Chemicals (IOPSMC), comprising seven participating organizations, including WHO, plays a vital role in supporting the establishment and implementation of Globally Harmonized System for the Classfication and Labding of

Chemicals through technical assistance, guidance, training, and capacity building for countries. The collaborative goal of International Organization for Medical Cooperation (IOMC) is to strengthen cooperation and coordination in the field of chemical safety.

Specific Regulatory Programs Utilizing Toxicological Data

Within the legislative framework, it is traditional to have separate regimes for different end uses, for example, food additives, human drugs, veterinary products, medical devices, cosmetics, foods and contaminants, and pesticides. For all of these programs, there is an identifiable entity seeking to place the chemical on the market and it is usually possible to insist that they accept the costs of premarketing and postmarketing testing and, sometimes, postmarketing monitoring and surveillance. Additional regulatory programs deal with indoor and outdoor air quality, water quality (drinking and environmental), and soil contamination. Generally, it is difficult to identify a nongovernmental entity to underwrite testing and controlling risk when dealing with these latter programs. Consequently, in such circumstances, the government is frequently both a regulator and provider of research funds to acquire new knowledge. Another group of substances where it may be more difficult to identify an entity other than the government to underwrite testing is food contaminants such as aflatoxins.

Food Additives

The 1958 Food Additives Amendments require the safety of food additives to be demonstrated before marketing. The manufacturer of a food additive must submit a petition demonstrating that the substance is "reasonably certain to be safe"; no inquiry into the benefits of an additive is undertaken or authorized. Two categories of nonnatural food ingredients were exempted from this food additive requirement: ① Generally Recognized As Safe(GRAS) substances (substances generally recognized as safe among experts qualified by scientific training and experience to evaluate safety); ② so-called "prior sanction" substances (substances that either FDA or the US Department of Agriculture had sanctioned for use in food before 1958).

Human Drugs

The current law requires premarket approval, for both safety and efficacy, of all "new" drugs. Premarket approval of therapeutic agents for commercial use primarily relies on randomized controlled trials in human subjects to establish safety and efficacy. However, animal and in vitro studies are the primary source of information about a substance's biological effects before human trials are begun, and their results influence not only the decision of whether to expose human subjects but also the design of clinical protocols. The FDA reviews the clinical evidence before authorizing human clinical trials through a review of an Investigational New Drug (IND) application.

Cosmetics

The statutory provisions governing cosmetics do not require premarket approval of any ingredient or demand that manufacturers test their products for safety, though many manufacturers routinely do so. The basic safety standard for cosmetics is similar to that for food ingredients: no product may be marketed if it contains "a poisonous or deleterious substance, which may render it injurious to health".

Pesticides

Pesticides are subject to two types of regulation: ① registration under the Federal Insecticide Fungicide and Rodenticide Act (FIFRA), which is required for a pesticide to be marketed; ② tolerance under the Federal Food, Drug, and Cosmetic Act (FFDCA), which sets the allowable level of pesticide residue in food for human consumption. A 1954 amendment to the FFDCA allowed the regulatory agency to consider in setting tolerances both the potential adverse health effects of residues and the benefits of pesticide use. And, if the pesticide was a carcinogen, the Delaney clause prohibited its approval for that use. This framework was revised by Congress in 1996 by the Food Quality Protection Act (FQPA) to exempt pesticide residues from the operation of the Delaney clause but also restricted the consideration of pesticide benefits in setting tolerances. The 1996 amendments also introduced some additional novel elements to the tolerance process by requiring EPA: ① to determine the safe level of a pesticide residue in a cumulative context; ② to give special consideration to the health of infants and children; ③ to develop a program to test for endocrine disrupting effects of pesticides.

Industrial Chemicals

The Toxic Substances Control Act (TSCA) was promulgated to regulate chemical substances and it gives the EPA three main powers. First, the agency is empowered to restrict or even ban the manufacturing, processing, distribution, use, or disposal of a chemical substance when there is a reasonable basis to conclude any such activity poses an "unreasonable risk of injury to health or environment". In determining whether a chemical substance presents an unreasonable risk, the agency is instructed to balance the costs of restricting the substance against the health benefits of the proposed regulation. Second, if the

EPA suspects that a chemical may pose an unreasonable risk but lacks sufficient data to take action, TSCA empowers the agency to require testing to develop the necessary data. Third, to enable the EPA to evaluate chemicals before humans are exposed, TSCA requires the manufacturer of a new chemical substance to notify the agency prior to production or distribution (called a pre-manufacturing notice or PMN).

In contrast, the European Union (EU) is implementing a much more aggressive regulatory program for chemical substances, known as REACH program. REACH puts the responsibility for ensuring the safety of chemicals on the companies that produce, import, and use chemicals. REACH employs a tiered testing approach, with the amount of initial testing determined by production volume. A technical dossier is required for all registered chemicals; however, only chemicals with a production volume of 10 or more tons per year require a chemical safety assessment documented in a chemical safety report.

Toxic Water and Air Pollutants

Under the Federal Water Pollution Control Act, the EPA had developed health-based "water quality criteria" for 126 compounds it had identified as toxic. These criteria essentially described desirable maximum contamination levels. As the law required, the EPA adopted standards for toxic water pollutants that provided an "ample margin of safety". One example of an "acceptable" risk-regulatory program is the national ambient air quality program under the CAA. Under this program, EPA must set standards for air pollutants such as particulate matter, ozone, and carbon monoxide that protect against "adverse effects" in the most susceptible subgroup with an adequate margin of safety. EPA may only consider risk data in setting these standards; no consideration of costs or feasibility is permitted.

Drinking Water

The SDWA was enacted to ensure that public water supply systems "meet minimum national standards for the protection of public health". Under the SDWA, the EPA is required to regulate any contaminants "which may have an adverse effect on human health". Over time and several Congressional amendments, this system has evolved into a two-tier system in which EPA adopts for each contaminant a maximum contaminant level goal (MCLG) that represents the optimal level to be achieved to ensure safety and the usually less stringent, feasibility-based maximum contaminant level (MCL). Only the MCL is legally enforceable.

Occupational Agents

A program using a hybrid feasibility/acceptable risk approach is the Occupational Safety and Health Act, which directs the Occupational Safety and Health Administration (OSHA) to set workplace standards for hazardous exposures to the level "which most adequately assures... that no employee will suffer material impairment of health or functional capacity". This language has been interpreted by OSHA and the courts as requiring the agency to set occupational healthy standards at the lowest exposure level that is technologically and economically feasible, to the extent necessary to reduce a "significant" risk.

(Li Jianxiang)

CHAPTER 12

Immunotoxicology

Introduction

Immunotoxicology is an emerging field within toxicology that gained recognition in the early 1970s. It was during this period that scientists began to understand how exposure to environmental chemicals and therapeutic drugs could alter immune functions, subsequently increasing susceptibility to infections and cancer. Early interest in immunosuppression within the toxicological community was primarily driven by studies showing that exposure to exogenous compounds could reduce resistance to infections, underscoring significant implications for human health.

In recent years, both the scientific community and the public have directed greater attention toward identifying and modulating exogenous substances that inadvertently alter the immune system and consequently impact human health. Given the immune system's complexity and its indispensable role in maintaining health, the study of immunotoxicity is of paramount importance.

Within the context of immunotoxicity, it is critical to recognize that toxins can exert differential effects on innate and adaptive immunity. Certain chemicals may blunt the innate immune response, thus increasing vulnerability to initial infections. Conversely, others may disrupt the development or function of key adaptive immune cells, thereby compromising the ability of the body to respond to specific pathogens or to retain immunological memory.

The Structure and Functions of Immune System

The Structure of Immune System

The immune system is a complex system which is dependent on the integration and orchestrated cooperation among several types of organs, tissues, immune cells, and immune molecules. Components of the immune system are distributed throughout the body.

Immune Organs and Tissues

The immune system comprises several organs and tissues, including the bone marrow, thymus, spleen, lymph nodes, a network of lymphatic vessels, and various mucosal surfaces.

The bone marrow serves as the primary site of origin for all immune cells, acting as the immune system's "nursery" where these cells originate and initiate their maturation processes. The thymus, a small organ situated superior to the heart, is where T cells, or T-lymphocytes, mature. These cells are central to the adaptive immune response, which is characterized by a tailored attack against specific pathogens. The spleen, a blood-filtering organ, performs the dual function of recycling aged red blood cells and housing white blood cells, which are capable of attacking foreign invaders. Lymph nodes, small bean-shaped structures strategically distributed throughout the body, serve as critical junctures where immune cells encounter foreign invaders. These nodes also act as hubs for immune cell communication and the execution of defense strategies. Mucosal-associated lymphoid tissue (MALT), located on mucosal surfaces such as the gastrointestinal and respiratory tracts, plays a crucial role in safeguarding the body from the entry of foreign agents at these key sites.

Immune Cells

Immune cells, akin to vigilant sentinels, each possess distinct roles and responsibilities, working in concert to repel unwanted invaders and thereby protect well-being.

T cells are the strategic regulators of the immune response. Originating in the bone marrow, these cells mature within the thymus, the origin of their designation as "T" cells. T cells are central to directly attacking infected cells and orchestrating the immune response. These cells exist in diverse forms, including cytotoxic T cells, which destroy compromised cells; the helper T cells, which manage and direct the immune response; and regulatory T cells, which serve to modulate the response, thereby preventing excessive activation and resultant tissue damage.

B cells function as the body's antibody producers. These cells produce antibodies, highly specific proteins that neutralize pathogens. B cells are also capable of developing immunological memory, which is pivotal for long-term protection, as exemplified by the principle underlying vaccination. Upon subsequent exposure to a known pathogen, memory B cells facilitate the body to mount a rapid and potent response.

Macrophages are a key component of the immune system, playing an essential role in engulfing and digesting pathogens, dead cells, and cellular debris, thus contributing to the maintenance of overall health and function. These cells are not only responsible for clearing debris but also act as alarm signals, alerting other immune cells when an invader is encountered.

Dendritic cells are critical antigen-presenting cells. These cells capture antigens derived from pathogens, process them, and present them to T cells, thereby linking the innate and adaptive immune responses. These cells act like scouts, conveying information from the frontlines back to the command center in order to initiate a strategic defense.

Natural killer (NK) cells are rapid responders within the immune system. They possess an innate ability to recognize and destroy cells that fail to display proper molecular signals, particularly those that are infected by viruses or have become cancerous.

Neutrophils are the most abundant type of white blood cell and are among the first responders to microbial invasion. Their primary function is to rapidly migrate to sites of infection and eliminate pathogens through phagocytosis, degranulation, and NETosis—a process by which they expel their DNA to trap pathogens.

Eosinophils and basophils, though less numerous, fulfill essential roles in combating multicellular parasites and orchestrating allergic reactions. Eosinophils are particularly effective against parasites, whereas basophils release histamine, which contributes to the inflammation observed in allergic reactions. Mast cells, located at strategic points throughout the body, such as the skin and mucous membranes, serve as surveillance sentinels. These cells release histamine and other mediators, contributing to inflammation and alerting the immune system to the presence of an invader. These various immune cells, and their roles in innate and adaptive immunity, are visually summarized in Figure 12-1.

Immune Molecules

Immune molecules are fine-tuned instruments of the body's defense system and play a pivotal role in identifying, neutralizing, and eliminating foreign threats. Like highly trained special force units, they are precise, vigilant, and incredibly specialized.

Immunoglobulins, also known as antibodies, serve as the scouts of the immune system. Produced by B cells, these Y-shaped proteins exhibit a remarkable ability to identify and bind to specific antigens—unique molecules found on pathogens. Antibodies can be thought of as the body's custom-designed lock-picking sets; each immunoglobulin is specifically tailored to

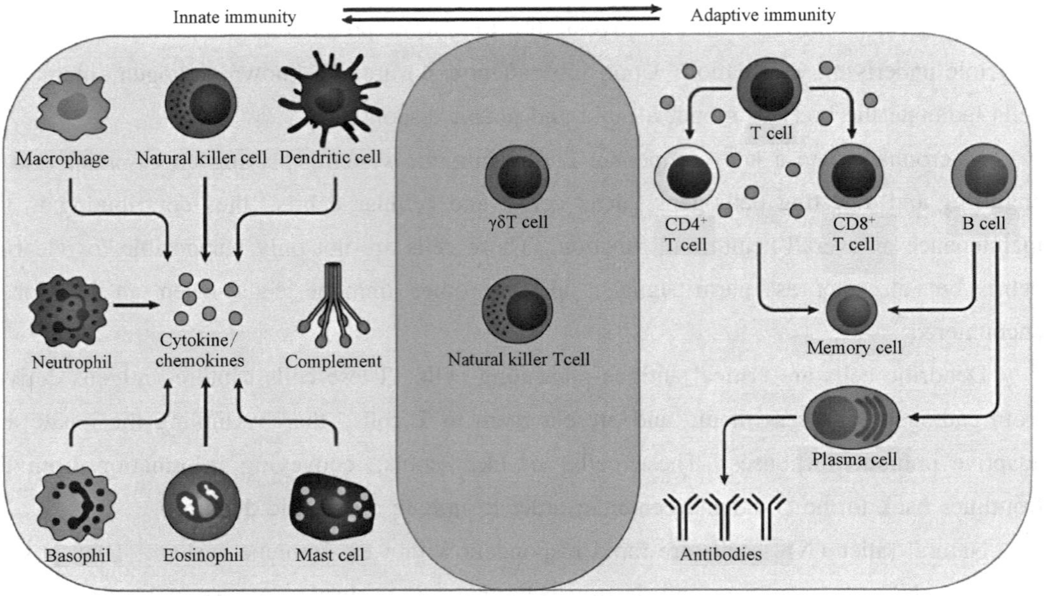

Figure 12-1 **Immune cells in innate and adaptive immunity**

bind to a particular antigen, much like a key fitting a lock. Once bound, they can neutralize the pathogen or mark it for destruction by other immune cells.

Cytokines act as communicators within the immune system; these small proteins are secreted by immune cells and function as signals that alert other cells to sites of infection or inflammation. Cytokines can mobilize reinforcements, increase the defensive response, and even signal the resolution of the response, thus preventing excessive damage to the body's own tissues.

The complement system is analogous to the immune system's demolition crew. Once activated, this group of proteins works in concert to disrupt and breaks down the cell walls of invading pathogens, ultimately resulting in their destruction. This system also assists antibodies and phagocytic cells in clearing microbes and damaged cells from the organism, promotes inflammation, and attacks the pathogen's cell membrane.

Major histocompatibility complex (MHC) molecules serve as the identity markers present on the surface of every cell in the body. These molecules present fragments of proteins from within the cell on the cell surface. If the cell is healthy, the immune system recognizes these proteins as "self" and leaves the cell undisturbed. If a cell is infected, for example by a virus, it will display fragments of the viral proteins on its MHC molecules, essentially signaling a "red flag" to the immune system that something is amiss.

Cluster differentiation (CD) molecules are analogous to the specialized equipment carried by a soldier. Located on the surfaces of immune cells, these proteins aid in various cell functions. For example, CD4 facilitates the binding of helper T cells to MHC class II molecules, which is essential for T cells to receive necessary signals to combat infection.

The T-cell receptor (TCR), located on the surface of T cells, functions as a highly sophisticated sensor. It is designed to recognize and bind to antigens presented by the MHC on other cells. Upon binding to an antigen-MHC complex, the TCR triggers the T cell to activate and proliferate, initiating a cascade of events that leads to the destruction of the infected cell or the production of antibodies.

These immune molecules are versatile and adaptive tools that enable the immune system to respond to a broad spectrum of pathogens and other threats with precision. Immunoglobulins provide specificity to directly target pathogens, cytokines send signals to mobilize and regulate the immune response, complement proteins work to destroy invaders, MHC molecules present internal snapshots for immune surveillance, CD molecules facilitate varied immune functions, and TCRs enable T cells to detect and respond to infected cells.

Immune System Functions

The primary function of the immune system is to defend the body against infectious organisms and other invaders through a series of coordinated events collectively known as the immune response. Immunity can be classified into two principal functional divisions: innate immunity and acquired (adaptive) immunity. This system, acting as the body's natural defense mechanism, is equipped not only to combat invaders but also to retain a record of each encounter. This immunological memory ensures that, upon subsequent exposure to the same pathogen, the body can respond more rapidly and efficiently. Beyond simply fighting infections, the immune system also monitors and clears old and damaged cells, contributing to overall health and longevity.

Immune response

The body's initial line of defense against adverse environmental effects consists of mechanical barriers such as the skin and mucous membranes. When pathogens penetrate these barriers, they interact with the mechanisms of innate and acquired immunity. Innate immunity, which is present even prior to exposure to a pathogen, is characterized by a non-specific, generalized response. Conversely, acquired immunity is absent or of low potency at the initial encounter but increases sharply with repeated exposure. The immune system combats pathogens through a diverse array of immune responses, broadly categorized into innate and adaptive immunity.

Innate Immunity: The First Line of Defense

Innate immunity represents the body's initial line of defense, a non-specific barrier that responds to pathogens in a rapid manner. This form of immunity is inherited and active from birth, thus providing immediate defenses against infection. The innate immune system encompasses physical barriers, such as the skin and mucous membranes, chemical barriers, such as stomach acid and enzymes in saliva, and cellular defenses that include various white blood cells. The cells essential to this defense layer consist of macrophages, neutrophils, dendritic cells, and natural killer cells. These cells respond promptly upon contact with pathogens, performing tasks such as engulfing foreign particles via phagocytosis, releasing enzymes that degrade pathogens, and initiating inflammation, which serves to attract additional immune cells to the affected area.

Adaptive Immunity: The Tailored Response

While innate immunity provides a rapid and broad response, adaptive immunity employs a more calculated and targeted approach. Although it is slower to initiate, adaptive immunity is highly specific to the invading pathogen and possesses a memory component, which ensures a rapid and robust response upon subsequent exposure to the same pathogen.

Adaptive immunity can be divided into two main types: humoral immunity and cellular immunity.

Humoral immunity is characterized by the production of antibodies by B cells. Antibodies are specialized proteins that specifically recognize antigens, which are unique molecules found on pathogens. When an unknown antigen is encountered, B cells transform into plasma cells, which secrete antibodies. These antibodies circulate in the blood and lymph, binding to antigens, neutralizing pathogens, and facilitating destruction by other immune cells.

Cellular immunity, in contrast, is mediated by T cells. These cells do not produce antibodies but instead execute their protective functions through other mechanisms. Cytotoxic T cells directly attack and kill infected cells. helper T cells orchestrate the immune response through the release of signaling molecules known as cytokines, which direct the activity of other immune cells, including B cells and macrophages. Regulatory T cells play a crucial role in modulating the immune response after the clearance of an infection, preventing excessive damage to the body's own tissues.

The adaptive immune response unfolds in several basic steps.

(1) Antigen Presentation: Before T cells can effectively respond, they must be alerted to the presence of an invader. Dendritic cells play a crucial role in this process by capturing antigens from pathogens, processing them, and presenting them on their surface in a form that T cells can recognize.

(2) Lymphocyte Activation: Upon presentation of an antigen by an antigen-presenting

cell, T cells with receptors that match the antigen become activated. This activation induces the proliferation of T cells, and their differentiation into various types of helper, cytotoxic, or regulatory T cells, depending on the nature of the threat.

(3) B Cell Activation and Antibody Production: Helper T cells also contribute to the activation of B cells. When B cells encounter their specific antigen and receive the necessary signals from helper T cells, they undergo division and differentiation into plasma cells, which secrete antibodies.

(4) Elimination of Pathogens: Antibodies bind to antigens to neutralize pathogens and make them more accessible to other immune cells. Cytotoxic T cells and other immune components then function to destroy infected cells.

(5) Development of Immunological Memory: Following the initial encounter with a pathogen, the majority of activated B and T cells undergo apoptosis, while a select few persist as memory cells. These long-lived cells remain poised for years, ready to initiate a swifter and more robust defense in the event of a subsequent encounter with the same pathogen.

Types of Immunotoxic Responses

Immunostimulation

Immunostimulation occurs when an agent induces an overactivation of the immune system. This heightened activity can manifest as an excessive inflammatory response or an inappropriate immune reaction against typically harmless entities, such as allergens or even the body's own tissues. While a robust immune response is necessary to protect against infections, an overstimulated immune system can cause tissue damage and contribute to the development of inflammatory diseases. For example, certain bacterial toxins can act as superantigens, which amplify the immune response to dangerous levels, potentially resulting in severe conditions such as toxic shock syndrome. Immunostimulatory effects are not limited to infections; certain drugs and environmental chemicals can also trigger similar reactions, leading to a state of chronic inflammation that predisposes individuals to various diseases.

Immunosuppression

Immunosuppression, also referred to as immunodepression, represents a reduction in the activity of the immune system. This can be induced by a variety of factors, including exposure to certain chemicals, stress, aging, or adverse effects of immunosuppressive drugs used to prevent organ transplant rejection. When the immune system is suppressed, the body becomes more vulnerable to infections, the healing process may be delayed, and there is an increased risk of cancer development, given the immune system's crucial role in surveilling and eliminating cancerous cells. Immunotoxic agents that cause immunosuppression can disrupt the maturation, function, or communication of immune cells. For example, pesticides such as organophosphates have been shown to impair the function of immune cells, thereby reducing resistance to infectious diseases.

Hypersensitivity

Hypersensitivity is an exaggerated immune response to an antigen that is normally harmless, such as pollen, pet dander, or certain foods. This inappropriate immune reaction can range from mildly irritating, such as in cases of allergic rhinitis, to life-threatening, such as in anaphylaxis. Hypersensitivity is classified into four types: Type I hypersensitivity, also termed immediate hypersensitivity, encompasses common allergic reactions and asthma. Type Ⅱ hypersensitivity involves antibody-mediated responses against the body's own cells or tissues. Type Ⅲ hypersensitivity is caused by the deposition of immune complexes, which can lead to conditions such as systemic lupus erythematosus. Type IV hypersensitivity, or called delayed-type hypersensitivity, involves T-cell-mediated responses and includes contact dermatitis resulting from exposure to specific chemicals or metals. Agents that induce hypersensitivity reactions may be biological, such as proteins that act as allergens, or chemical, such as certain drugs that induce serum sickness or drug allergies.

Autoimmunity

Autoimmunity refers to a condition in which the immune system erroneously targets and attacks the body's own tissues, perceiving them as foreign entities. This aberrant attack can lead to autoimmune diseases such as rheumatoid arthritis, type 1 diabetes, and multiple sclerosis. The causes of autoimmunity can be genetic, environmental, or a combination of both. Certain drugs and chemicals can induce autoimmune responses by disrupting the normal function of immune cells or by altering the structure of self-antigens in a manner that renders them unrecognizable to the immune system. Autoimmunity can be systemic, affecting multiple organs, or organ-specific, and can target a single organ or tissue. Environmental factors such as heavy metals, solvents, and other pollutants have been implicated in both the development and exacerbation of autoimmune diseases.

Mechanisms of Immunotoxicity

Direct Effects on Immune Cells

Certain toxic agents can directly damage immune cells, resulting in a compromised immune system. For example, chemotherapeutic drugs are known to have cytotoxic effects on rapidly dividing cells, including immune cells. This direct cytotoxic action can significantly reduce the population of white blood cells, such as lymphocytes, weakening the body's capacity to combat infections and surveil for malignant cells. Another example is benzene, a chemical component of cigarette smoke and industrial emissions, which can induce direct bone marrow toxicity. Given that the bone marrow is the primary site of blood cell production, including immune cells, exposure to benzene can result in a reduction in the number of these cells, leading to immunosuppression.

Modulation of Immune Signaling Pathways

The immune system's signaling pathways represent complex networks that maintain a delicate balance between the activation and suppression of immune responses. Immunotoxic agents can disrupt these pathways, resulting in altered immune responses. For example, certain environmental pollutants, such as dioxins, can bind to the aryl hydrocarbon receptor (AHR) in immune cells. This interaction can alter the expression of various genes that regulate immune cell function and immune tolerance, potentially leading to heightened susceptibility to infections or autoimmune diseases. Similarly, certain medications used to treat autoimmune conditions or prevent transplant rejection operated by precisely modulating these pathways. While therapeutic in specific contexts, these drugs can have unintended immunotoxic effects if not carefully managed, such as an increased risk of opportunistic infections due to a suppressed immune response.

Alteration of Immune Cell Development

The development of immune cells is a meticulously regulated process, originating from stem cells in the bone marrow and culminating in a diverse array of specialized cells that constitute the immune system. Toxic substances can disrupt the normal development of immune cells at various stages. For instance, exposure to heavy metals such as lead can impede the maturation and differentiation of immune cells, thereby impairing the body's defense mechanisms. Pesticides and other chemical agents can also affect the thymus, the organ in which T cells mature. Alterations in T cell development can exert widespread effects on the immune response, impacting the capacity to mount effective defenses against pathogens and regulate immune tolerance, potentially predisposing individuals to hypersensitivity or autoimmune disorders.

Key Research Areas in Immunotoxicology

To evaluate immunotoxic effects, researchers can conduct studies in both laboratory and clinical settings, focusing on the following key areas:

(1) Immunosuppression: Characterized by a weakened immune response.

(2) Immunostimulation: Characterized by an excessively activated immune response.

(3) Developmental Immunotoxicology: Explores the impact of harmful substances on the immune system during early life.

(4) Immunosenescence: Refers to the weakening of the immune system associated with advanced age.

(5) Molecular Immunotoxicology: Focuses on investigating how toxic substances interfere with immune processes at the molecular level, with specific emphasis on the mechanisms of intercellular communication via cytokines.

(6) In Silico Immunotoxicology: Utilizes computational modeling and in vitro laboratory assays to forecast immune responses.

Immunotoxicology Testing Methods

In the field of immunotoxicology, a tiered approach is utilized to assess the potential impact of chemicals on the immune system. This method is analogous to climbing a ladder, where each successive step provides increasingly detailed insights.

Tier Ⅰ commences with basic laboratory tests. These are straightforward assessments designed to count blood cells, measure the weights of organs associated with the immune system, and evaluate tissue samples for any overt signs of damage. This stage can be likened to a general health screening. Tier Ⅱ is initiated if any unusual findings arise from Tier Ⅰ. Here, more specific tests are conducted to determine the functionality of immune cells. For instance, an assessment is made to determine if an individual can effectively combat pathogens. This situation is analogous to a focused health check-up where a physician orders tests to investigate a particular symptom. If significant changes be detected, Tier Ⅲ is initiated. This tier entails complex tests designed to elucidate the mechanisms behind these changes and their potential implications for health. This stage is akin to a specialist conducting a thorough investigation to determine the underlying issue.

In addition to this tiered approach, it is essential to understand the three main types of immune dysfunction that can arise due to toxic exposures:

Immunosuppression: This condition occurs when the immune system's capacity to respond to pathogens is diminished. Testing for immunosuppression typically involves evaluating the functionality of lymphocytes, measuring serum immunoglobulin levels, and conducting assays to determine the response to vaccines or specific antigens. A significant reduction in immune response can signal potential risks associated with chemical exposure.

Hypersensitivity: This term refers to excessive immune responses to antigens that can precipitate allergic reactions. Testing for hypersensitivity may involve skin prick tests, patch tests, or in vitro assays to measure specific IgE levels. Understanding hypersensitivity reactions is essential due to their potential to progress into chronic inflammatory conditions and other health complications.

Autoimmunity: Autoimmune responses manifest when the immune system inappropriately targets the body's own tissues. Testing in this category often involves the detection of autoantibodies through serological assays, as well as functional assessments of immune cell activity. Identifying autoimmune markers is essential for elucidating how chemical exposures can trigger or exacerbate autoimmune diseases.

In Vivo Testing Methods

Animal Models

Animal models serve as essential proxies for human immune responses in the assessment of immunotoxicity. These models provide a complex, whole-organism context within which to observe the interaction of various immune system components in response to external agents. Rodents are commonly utilized due to their genetic and physiological similarities to humans. Through controlled exposures to substances, it is possible to monitor changes in organ weights, cell counts, and behavior, which can indicate compromised immune function.

Biomarkers of Immunotoxicity

Biomarkers are quantifiable indicators that can reflect the state of an organism's immune system. For example, an increase in specific antibodies may signify an allergenic response, while altered levels of white blood cells may suggest either an enhancement or suppression of the immune system. The monitoring of these biomarkers is critical for early detection of immunotoxic effects and can guide further testing and risk assessment procedures.

In Vitro Testing Methods

Cell-based Assays

These assays facilitate the examination of how individual cells respond to a specific substance. By isolating and culturing immune cells in the laboratory and then exposing them to a test agent, changes in cell viability, proliferation, and signaling can be observed. This detailed analysis allows for the identification of specific immune functions that may be altered due to exposure to the substance in question.

Cytokine Release Assays

Cytokines are crucial to signal molecules of the immune system, coordinating the body's response to both infection and inflammation. Cytokine release assays measure the quantity and type of cytokines released following cellular exposure to a substance. This is particularly important for evaluating the potential of a substance to induce an overreaction of the immune system, such as a cytokine storm, which can have detrimental consequences for health.

Additional In Vitro Testing Methods

In addition to cell-based and cytokine release assays, other in vitro methods are crucial. These include:

(1) Lymphocyte Proliferation Assays are commonly used in research to evaluate the impact of substances on the multiplication of lymphocytes, a type of white blood cell, in response to an invader.

(2) Natural Killer Cell Activity: A critical role is played by NK cells as they attack tumor cells or virally infected cells. Testing for changes in their activity can indicate immunosuppression.

(3) Mixed Lymphocyte Reaction is a laboratory test used to observe the function of immune cells in a simulated environment. In this test, immune cells are "introduced" to foreign cells, mimicking a transplant scenario.

(4) Macrophage Function Tests: Since macrophages are involved in engulfing and digesting cellular debris and pathogens, determining their function helps researchers understand phagocytic activity and the overall integrity of the innate immune response.

(5) Comet Assay: This assay is used to detect DNA damage in individual cells, which can be an indicator of genotoxicity and potential immunotoxicity.

Risk Assessment in Immunotoxicology

Immunotoxicology risk assessment is a detailed process in which we carefully analyze biological information to determine the potential harm a substance may cause to our immune system. This includes evaluating the nature of the effect (qualitative) and its intensity (quantitative). When examining the immune system, our body's defense against illness, we discover that it is resilient and capable of adapting to minor changes with ease. Therefore, a slight alteration in one aspect of the immune system does not automatically indicate a problem. It looks like to see a single leaf drop from a tree, which could just be a natural part of the tree's life, not a sign of disease.

Now, if we notice changes in several parts of the immune system and these changes lined up with each other, that is when we pay close attention. Think of the immune system as a sports team, with each player having a specific role. If only one player is off their game, the team might still play well. However, if multiple players start to falter and their poor performance is linked, the team's overall game will suffer. This finding is similar to how we observed changes in immune parameters. If various indicators of immune function begin to show a consistent pattern of disturbance, several teammates may play poorly in a coordinated way. This pattern suggests that the agent in question may indeed weaken the immune defense and thus could be considered immunotoxic.

Common Immunotoxicants

Metals and Metalloids

Metals and metalloids are elements that can interfere with biological processes and are commonly found in the environment, arising from both natural and anthropogenic activities.

Lead is a heavy metal that has been widely used in various industries but is now known for its potential to compromise immune function. Even at low levels, lead exposure can affect both innate and adaptive immune responses, potentially leading to increased susceptibility to infections and possibly influencing the development of autoimmune diseases.

Mercury is another heavy metal that can have profound effects on the immune system. Mercury exposure has been linked to alterations in the quantity and functionality of various immune cells, including lymphocytes and macrophages, and can also skew immune responses, which can lead to imbalances and autoimmune phenomena.

Arsenic, while naturally occurring, can be highly toxic and has been shown to affect immune responses. Chronic exposure to arsenic can suppress the immune system and has been associated with an increased risk of infections and possibly some forms of cancer due to its impact on cellular immunity.

Cadmium is a metal often found in industrial environments. It can accumulate in the body over time and has been shown to cause a decrease in the production of certain cytokines, which are critical for cell signaling in the immune system and impair the function of immune cells, such as T cells and macrophages.

Organic Compounds

Organic compounds are carbon-based chemicals that are prevalent in many daily products and may pose risks to the immune system.

Polychlorinated Biphenyls (PCBs) are a group of synthetic organic chemicals that can be found in electrical equipment, hydraulic fluids, and plasticizers, among other products. Although their production has been banned in many countries, PCBs persist in the environment. They can alter immune cell function, which may reduce the ability to combat infections.

Dioxins and furans are byproducts of industrial processes and are recognized as some of the most potent toxicants. Even at very low levels, they can induce immunosuppression and disrupt thymus function, which is essential for the development of T cells and the establishment of immune tolerance.

Pesticides, such as organophosphates and carbamates, are commonly utilized to control pests in agriculture; however, they can have unintended effects on human health. These compounds can inhibit enzymes that are crucial for proper functioning of the nervous system and can also affect the immune system, leading to altered immune responses and a reduced capacity to combat diseases.

Solvents

Solvents are commonly employed in industrial and laboratory settings and can exert deleterious effects on immune health.

Benzene is utilized in the manufacture of plastics, resins, and synthetic fibers. Chronic exposure to benzene has been shown to induce bone marrow suppression, which can lead to immunosuppression and an elevated risk of infection.

Toluene is used in paint thinners, adhesives, and some personal care products. It can affect the central nervous system and may also have subtle effects on immune function, although the specific immunotoxic effects remain less well characterized.

Xylene, another solvent utilized in the printing, rubber, and leather industries, has been associated with alterations in immune function, including changes in white blood cell counts and the immune response.

Biological Agents

Biological agents are living entities or derivatives of living organisms that can cause adverse effects on the immune system.

Bacterial toxins, such as those produced by Staphylococcus aureus (e. g. toxic shock syndrome toxin), can act as superantigens that overstimulate immune cells, leading to massive cytokine release and potentially fatal outcomes.

Mycotoxins are toxic compounds produced by certain types of fungi. These toxins can contaminate food supplies and have been shown to suppress the immune system, thereby making the body more susceptible to infectious diseases.

Viruses, such as human immunodeficiency virus (HIV), directly target immune cells, resulting in severe immunosuppression. Other viruses may exert more subtle or transient immunotoxic effects but can still have significant health implications.

Drugs and Immune System Interaction

Immunosuppressive Drugs

Immunosuppressive drugs are agents specifically designed to inhibit or prevent activity within the immune system. They are primarily used to reduce the risk of organ transplant rejection and to manage autoimmune disorders.

Corticosteroids are among the most frequently utilized immunosuppressive drugs. They function through mimicking the actions of cortisol, a hormone that naturally suppresses inflammation and modulates the immune response. Corticosteroids can reduce the production of inflammatory molecules and inhibit the function of various immune cells. Although they are highly effective, their long-term use can lead to adverse effects, such as an increased risk of infection, bone loss, and metabolic alterations.

Cyclosporine is a calcineurin inhibitor that specifically suppresses T cells function, which is a type of white blood cell that is essential to the immune response. It is commonly administered to organ transplant recipients to prevent rejection. Cyclosporine binds to the cytosolic protein cyclophilin in T cells and inhibits calcineurin, which is critical for activating the transcription of interleukin-2, a key cytokine in the proliferation and activity of T cells. Adverse effects may include nephrotoxicity, hypertension, and an elevated risk of infections and malignancies.

Methotrexate is a chemotherapeutic agent that also possesses immunosuppressive properties. It is frequently used in lower doses to treat rheumatoid arthritis and psoriasis. Methotrexate inhibits dihydrofolate reductase, resulting in a decrease in DNA synthesis and cellular replication. This action particularly affects rapidly dividing cells, including those of the immune system, hence its immunosuppressive properties. Potential adverse effects include liver toxicity, bone marrow suppression, and pulmonary disease.

Immunomodulating Drugs

Immunomodulating drugs can augment or modify the immune response and are used to treat cancer, chronic infections, and immune-mediated diseases.

Interferons are a group of signaling proteins generated and released by host cells in response to the presence of pathogens, such as viruses, bacteria, or tumor cells. They function to modulate the activity of the immune system. As pharmaceutical agents, interferons are used to treat conditions such as multiple sclerosis, hepatitis C, and certain cancers. They can enhance the immune response by improving the capacity of immune cells to process and present antigens, resulting in improved targeting of pathogens or cancer cells. Adverse effects can include flu-like symptoms, fatigue, and mood alterations.

Monoclonal antibodies are laboratory-produced molecules specifically engineered to act as substitute antibodies that can restore, enhance, or mimic the immune system's attack on cells. They are designed to bind to specific targets and can induce an immune response that specifically targets cells or proteins. Their applications range from cancer therapies (e. g. rituximab) to the management of autoimmune diseases (e. g. adalimumab). While generally effective, they may sometimes induce immune-related adverse effects, such as triggering an immune response against normal tissues or infusion reactions.

Immune checkpoint inhibitors represent a class of drugs that inhibit proteins produced by certain types of immune cells, such as T cells, and some cancer cells. These proteins are crucial for maintaining immune responses and preventing T cells from destroying cancer cells. By inhibiting these proteins, checkpoint inhibitors allow immune cells to respond more robustly to cancer. Examples include CTLA-4, PD-1, and PD-L1 inhibitors. Potential adverse effects, such as colitis, hepatitis, endocrinopathies, and pneumonitis, are associated with autoimmune reactions and may affect any organ system.

Vaccines are biological formulations that provide active acquired immunity to a specific infectious disease. Adjuvants are substances that enhance the body's immune response to antigens. Vaccinations are generally safe and efficacious. However, as with any medical intervention, they can sometimes elicit adverse reactions. Most of these effects, such as a sore arm or mild fever, are minor and transient. More serious reactions are rare but can include allergic responses (e. g. anaphylaxis), and very rare neurological conditions (e. g. Guillain-Barré syndrome). It is important to note that the risk of adverse reactions from vaccines is significantly lower than the risk of serious complications from the diseases they prevent.

Advances in Immunotoxicology Research

Continuous advancements in research are broadening our understanding of how toxins affect immune homeostasis and resistance to disease. Cutting-edge in vitro and in silico models complement traditional in vivo studies, providing deeper insights while also addressing ethical concerns about animal testing. These models aid in analyzing intricate immune responses to toxins and can be utilized to screen chemicals more effectively and predict potential human immunotoxic effects with higher precision.

The genetic and proteomic underpinnings of the immune response to toxins are being elucidated with remarkable precision. Genomics, the study of an organism's complete set of DNA, allows researchers to identify genetic variations that confer susceptibility or resistance to the toxic effects of chemicals. Proteomics, the large-scale study of proteins, helps to elucidate the intricate network of signaling pathways and immune responses induced by toxicants. These disciplines are revolutionizing the field of immunotoxicology, providing molecular fingerprints that can be used to predict adverse immune outcomes.

The potential of personalized medicine is particularly promising in the context of immunotoxicology. Each individual's genetic makeup can influence their susceptibility to immunotoxicants. Therefore, understanding these genetic factors provides a foundation for more tailored risk assessments and interventions. Personalized medicine in immunotoxicology may involve the use of biomarkers to monitor individual exposures and immune status, leading to customized advice on environmental and occupational health risks, as well as personalized treatment strategies for those affected by immunotoxicity.

Global Challenges, Opportunities and Prospect

Immunotoxicity does not occur in isolation; it is intricately linked to global health challenges, such as emerging infectious diseases, climate change, and the widespread distribution of environmental pollutants. The international community is facing the challenge of balancing industrial development with the preservation of environmental and human health. Immunotoxicology presents opportunities to engage in this balancing act by contributing to the design of safer chemicals and informing public policy to protect vulnerable populations.

Technological advances are empowering researchers to investigate immunotoxic effects in diverse populations across the globe, resulting in more inclusive and representative data. This global perspective is vital for identifying and mitigating the risks posed by both legacy pollutants and novel chemical entities that accompany technological progress and industrialization. The future of immunotoxicology is also likely to be shaped by interdisciplinary collaboration. Integrating knowledge from fields such as epidemiology, molecular biology, environmental science, and public health policy is essential for developing a comprehensive understanding of how toxic exposures impact immune health at both the individual and population levels. Moreover, the advent of big data analytics and machine learning offers a powerful toolkit for processing large datasets, identifying patterns, and predicting outcomes. These tools can enhance our ability to assess risk and develop preventive strategies against immunotoxic exposure.

In conclusion, the future of immunotoxicology is a tapestry of promise woven with new technologies, personalized healthcare, and global interconnectedness. It is a field on the cusp of transformative change, embracing a holistic and integrative approach that is poised to unlock deeper understandings and deliver solutions to some of the most pressing health challenges of our time. Our journey forward is one of cautious optimism, as we leverage our expanding toolkit to protect and enhance immune health in an ever-changing world.

(Wang Jing　Li Jianxiang)

CHAPTER 13

Toxicology of the Liver

Introduction

Toxicology of the liver, which is also called hepatotoxicology, is a crucial field within target organ toxicology. It applies fundamental principles and methods of toxicology to study the harmful effects of exogenous harmful factors on the liver, elucidating the underlying mechanisms, and developing strategies for diagnosis, treatment, and prevention of liver injury. To distinguish from liver diseases caused by biological pathogens (such as viruses, histolytic amoeba), various acute and chronic liver injuries caused by foreign chemicals are usually collectively referred to as "chemical-induced liver injury". All the major liver functions can be detrimentally altered by acute or chronic exposure to toxicants (Table 13-1).

The liver is an organ that is closely connected with the blood circulatory system and is filled with blood. Due to its unique anatomical position in the body, as well as its special organizational structure and physiological and biochemical functions, the liver is often the primary target organ for the toxic effects of foreign chemicals. The liver has two sets of hepatic vessels, the portal vein and the hepatic artery, which can receive the blood from the gastrointestinal vein and the arterial blood from the systemic circulation, respectively. No matter how the foreign chemicals enter the body, they eventually reach the liver quickly through the blood circulation system, especially those absorbed from the digestive tract, which encounter the liver before entering the systemic circulation. Therefore, the liver is an important organ for the biological transformation of nutrients and also the main organ for the metabolism and excretion of chemical toxicants, including certain medications. Under specific conditions, chemical toxicants are easy to cause damage to the liver, when toxic metabolites formed during the liver's metabolic processes can inflict primary damage to the liver. Additionally, toxic chemicals or their metabolites excreted into the bile can be reabsorbed into the liver via the enterohepatic circulation, prolonging their toxic effects.

Table 13-1 **Major Functions of Liver and Consequences of Impaired Hepatic Functions**

Type of Function	Examples	Consequences of Impaired Functions
Nutrient homeostasis	Glucose storage and synthesis Cholesterol uptake	Hypoglycemia Hypercholesterolemia
Filtration of particulates	Products of intestinal bacteria (e. g. endotoxin)	Endotoxemia
Protein synthesis	Clotting factors Albumin Transport proteins (e. g. very low density lipoproteins)	Excess bleeding Hypoalbuminemia, ascites Fatty liver
Bioactivation and detoxification	Bilirubin and ammonia Steroid hormones Xenobiotics	Jaundice, hyperammonemia-related coma Loss of secondary male sex characteristics Diminished drug metabolism, inadequate detoxification
Formation of bile and biliary secretion	Bile acid-dependent uptake of dietary lipids and vitamins Bilirubin and cholesterol Metals (e. g. Cu and Mn) Xenobiotics	Fatty diarrhea, malnutrition, Vitamin E Deficiency Jaundice, gallstones, hypercholesterolemia Mn-induced neurotoxicity Delayed drug clearance

Numerous foreign chemicals can lead to liver dysfunction and even organ failure. Therefore, studying the hepatotoxicity of these chemicals is essential for preventive medicine to safeguard public health. For example, if an industrial chemical such as carbon tetrachloride, bromobenzene, or vinyl chloride is identified as hepatotoxic, its usage should be strictly controlled, and individuals handling it should be advised to wear protective clothing and masks to reduce exposure. Efforts should also be made to find safer alternatives. In the pharmaceutical industry, hepatotoxicity is often a common reason for discontinuing the development of drugs. If significant liver toxicity is detected post-marketing, it is generally agreed that the drug should be withdrawn. Given the rapid pace of drug development, the early identification of hepatotoxic substances remains a significant challenge in toxicology.

Structure and Functions of the Liver

Morphologic Considerations

The liver, or hepar, is the largest glandular organs of the body, situated under the diaphragm. It has a large right lobe and a somewhat smaller left lobe, as well as two other lesser lobes. The liver is essentially a large mass of cells surrounding vascular trees of arteries and veins. Terminal branches of the hepatic artery and portal vein, along with the bile duct are found together, forming the portal triad in cross-section.

Dual Blood Supply of the Liver

The liver's blood supply is derived from two major sources. The portal vein, which drains the capillary beds of the intestines and spleen, provides approximately 75% of the liver's blood flow, delivering about 1, 100 mL per minute. The remaining 25% is supplied by the hepatic artery, which carries about 350 mL of oxygenated arterial blood per minute. These vessels, along with the bile duct, enter the liver at the porta hepatis and distribute blood to the hepatic sinusoids. Venous outflow from the liver occurs via the hepatic veins, which drain into the inferior vena cava near the heart.

intestinal vasculature→portal vein↘
sinusoids→hepatic veins→inferior vena cava
hepatic artery↗

Unique Structure of Hepatic Sinusoids

Hepatic sinusoids are specialized capillaries characterized by a larger and more variable diameter compared to typical capillaries. They are lined with endothelial cells and Kupffer cells, the latter being actively phagocytic and critical for clearing microorganisms and foreign particles from the blood. Unlike conventional blood vessels, hepatic sinusoids feature discontinuous endothelial linings with gaps up to one micrometer wide. These gaps allow blood plasma, including plasma proteins, to freely pass into the space of Disse, where it directly interacts with liver cells.

Cellular Composition of the Liver

The liver is predominantly composed of hepatocytes, which make up approximately 75% of the organ's cellular mass. Hepatocytes play a central role in metabolism and detoxification and are primary targets for hepatotoxic chemicals. The sinusoidal lining contains numerous small endothelial cells, while Kupffer cells, though less numerous, perform essential immune and phagocytic functions. Ito cells (also known as stellate or fat-storing cells) are involved in collagen production, vitamin A metabolism, and storage.

Functional Unit of Liver

The liver's functional microanatomy can be viewed as either the classic liver lobule or the Hepatic acinus.

(1) Liver Lobule: The liver lobule is a hexagonal structural unit centered around a

central vein, with portal triads positioned at each corner. Morphologically, the lobule can be divided into distinct regions: centrilobular, midzonal, and periportal regions. These regions exhibit variations in glycogen and fat deposition, reflecting their functional differentiation.

(2) Hepatic Acinus: The hepatic acinus is the liver's smallest functional unit, organized around the terminal branches of the portal vein and hepatic artery. It is divided into three zones: Zone 1, located closest to the blood inflow near the portal triad; Zone 2, the intermediary region; and Zone 3, situated nearest to the terminal hepatic vein. Each zone performs specialized metabolic and physiological functions, with Zone 3 hepatocytes being particularly prone to damage due to their high concentration of cytochrome P450 enzymes, which are involved in xenobiotic metabolism.

(3) Relationships Between the Liver Lobule and the Hepatic Acinus: Zone 3 of the hepatic acinus aligns with the centrilobular region of the liver lobule, forming a star-shaped pattern around the central vein. Zone 1, adjacent to the portal triad, corresponds to the periportal region, while Zone 2 occupies the midzonal area. Hepatocytes in Zone 1, which are closer to the arterial blood supply, receive higher concentrations of oxygen and nutrients, supporting processes like bile acid uptake and biliary secretion. Conversely, Zone 3 hepatocytes, enriched with cytochrome P450 enzymes, are more vulnerable to the harmful effects of bioactivated toxic metabolites due to lower oxygen availability and their role in xenobiotic metabolism.

Physiologic Considerations

The liver performs four essential functions that are crucial for the maintenance of homeostasis and integration of metabolism:

(1) Storage: Serves as a reservoir for blood, glycogen, fats, fat-soluble vitamins, and other nutrients.

(2) Metabolism: Metabolizes xenobiotics, nutrients, and endogenous compounds such as bile acids, fatty acids, and hormones.

(3) Secretion and Excretion: Produces and secretes bile, destroys senescent erythrocytes, converts hemoglobin into bile pigments, forms urea from amino acids, and detoxifies absorbed intestinal toxins.

(4) Biosynthesis: Synthesizes plasma proteins, such as fibrinogen and albumin, and produces heparin and other constituents of blood plasma.

Factors Contributing to Liver Susceptibility to Chemical Injury

The liver is particularly susceptible to chemical-induced tissue injury due to several underlying factors. Firstly, the liver holds a distinctive position within the circulatory system.

As most xenobiotics enter the body via the gastrointestinal (GI) tract, they are absorbed and transported by the hepatic portal vein to the liver, making it the first organ to be perfused by gut-absorbed chemicals. Even if a chemical is successfully excreted in the bile, it can still return to the liver through the enterohepatic circulation. Moreover, the liver has a high concentration of binding sites, which contributes to its tendency to accumulate certain xenobiotics.

Secondly, once a chemical reaches the general circulation, regardless of the route of absorption, it is still subject to extraction and metabolism by the liver. The liver receives nearly 30% of the cardiac output, and at any given time, 10% - 15% of the total blood volume is present in the liver.

Lastly, the liver has a high concentration of xenobiotic metabolizing enzymes, particularly the cytochrome P450-dependent monooxygenase system, primarily located in the centrilobular region. Although most biotransformations are detoxication reactions, many oxidative reactions produce toxic reactive metabolites that can induce lesions within the liver.

Types and Mechanisms of Toxic Liver Injury

Toxic liver injury encompasses a wide range of pathological manifestations driven by the nature of chemical exposure, its duration, and host-specific factors, particularly the activity of hepatic metabolic enzymes. The liver's central role in metabolism and detoxification renders it vulnerable to biochemical disruptions and damage. Toxic liver injuries can lead to various forms of dysfunction, including steatosis, necrosis, cholestasis, fibrosis, apoptosis, and carcinogenesis. Below, we examine these types and their underlying mechanisms. Some types of injury are the result of acute toxicity to the liver, while others appear only after chronic exposure or treatment (Table 13-2).

Table 13-2 **Morphologic Types of Toxic Hepatic Injury**

Type of Injury	Representative Toxicants
Acute	
Cytotoxic	
Necrosis	
(1) Zonal	
Central (Zone 3)	CCl_4, halothane, acetaminophen, bromobenzene, pyrrolizidine alkaloids (PA)
Mid (Zone 2)	Beryllium, ngaione, furosemide, paraquat
Peripheral (Zone 1)	Allyl formate, albitocin, manganese Compounds, aflatoxin (AF)
(2) Massive	Trinitrotoluene (TNT), some drugs
(3) Diffuse (panlobular)	Some drugs
(4) Focal	Some drugs

(continue)

Type of Injury	Representative Toxicants
Steatosis	
(1) Microvesicular	Ethionine, tetracycline, phosphorus
(2) Macrovesicular	Ethanol, methotrexate (MTX)
Cholestatic	
Hepatocanalicular ("pericholangitic")	Chlorpromazine (CPZ), erythromycin estolate, organic arsenicals
Canalicular ("bland")	C-17 alkylated anabolic and contraceptive steroids
Chronic	
Cirrhosis	
Macronodular	CCl_4
Micronodular	CCl_4, AF
Congestive ("cardiac" type)	PA
Biliary	CPZ
Steatosis	Ethanol, MTX
Neoplasm	
Carcinoma	
(1) Hepatocellular	AFB_1, CCl_4, PA, azo dyes, dimethylnitrosamine (DMN)
(2) Cholangiocellular	Rare (thorotrast)
Angiosarcoma	Vinyl chloride, thorotrast, inorganic arsenic
Sarcoma	DMN (some species)
Adenoma	Anabolic and contraceptive steroids

Hepatic Steatosis (Fatty Liver)

Hepatic steatosis, or fatty liver, is a frequent response to toxic liver injury, characterized by the abnormal accumulation of triglycerides within hepatocytes. This condition arises from disruptions in lipid metabolism, including an oversupply of free fatty acids, increased triglyceride synthesis, impaired fatty acid oxidation, and reduced secretion of very low-density lipoproteins (VLDL). Lipid accumulation manifests as large droplets (macrovesicular steatosis) or numerous small droplets (microvesicular steatosis). For example, ethanol induces macrovesicular steatosis, while tetracycline is associated with microvesicular steatosis. Although steatosis is often reversible and non-lethal, it signals significant metabolic dysfunction and may progress under chronic exposure or in individuals with pre-existing metabolic conditions such as obesity.

Liver Necrosis

Hepatocyte necrosis involves cell death due to mechanisms such as lipid peroxidation, mitochondrial dysfunction, cytoskeletal damage, and immune-mediated injury. The pattern of necrosis—focal, zonal (e. g. centrilobular or periportal), or panacinar—depends on the toxicant's target site. For instance, carbon tetrachloride and acetaminophen primarily cause centrilobular necrosis due to their bioactivation by cytochrome P450 enzymes. Necrosis can lead to life-threatening liver failure if extensive, though localized injuries may resolve without significant functional loss. Biomarkers such as alanine aminotransferase (ALT) and lactate dehydrogenase (LDH) indicate necrosis, as these enzymes leak into the bloodstream following hepatocyte membrane disruption.

Cholestasis

Cholestasis, defined as impaired bile formation or flow, results from toxicant-induced disruptions at multiple levels. These include hepatocellular dysfunction, bile canalicular damage, or biliary obstruction. Toxicants such as α-naphthylisothiocyanate disrupt bile canalicular tight junctions, while anabolic steroids interfere with bile salt transport. Consequently, bile components, including bilirubin, accumulate in the bloodstream, leading to jaundice when plasma bilirubin levels exceed 2 mg/100 mL. Cholestasis is also frequently a secondary consequence of severe liver injury, as structural and functional damage impair normal bile secretion.

Hepatocyte Apoptosis

Apoptosis, or programmed cell death, is another critical mechanism of toxic liver injury. Unlike necrosis, apoptosis is a highly regulated process involving mitochondrial pathways (intrinsic) and death receptor pathways (extrinsic). Toxicants such as ethanol, acetaminophen, and certain pharmaceuticals trigger apoptosis by inducing oxidative stress, mitochondrial dysfunction, or activation of death receptors (e. g. Fas and TNF receptor). Morphological features include cell shrinkage, chromatin condensation, and the formation of apoptotic bodies. Apoptosis plays a dual role in liver injury: it may mitigate inflammation by removing damaged cells in a controlled manner but can also exacerbate hepatotoxicity under sustained exposure.

Fibrosis and Cirrhosis

Fibrosis is a chronic response to repeated hepatocyte injury, characterized by excessive deposition of extracellular matrix (ECM) proteins, especially collagen. This disrupts liver architecture, impairs hepatocyte function, and may progress to cirrhosis, an irreversible condition defined by regenerative nodules and extensive scarring. Cirrhosis leads to complications such as portal hypertension, hepatic encephalopathy, and eventual liver failure. Hepatotoxicants like carbon tetrachloride, vinyl chloride, and chronic alcohol intake are well-known inducers of fibrosis. The activation of hepatic stellate cells (HSCs) plays a central role, as these cells transition into myofibroblasts that secrete ECM proteins in response to inflammatory signals.

Liver Carcinogenesis

Chronic exposure to hepatocarcinogens can lead to liver cancers, including hepatocellular carcinoma (HCC), cholangiocarcinoma, and angiosarcoma. The mechanisms of liver carcinogenesis involve both genotoxic and nongenotoxic pathways. Genotoxic agents, such as aflatoxins and nitrosamines, cause direct DNA damage, leading to mutations. Non-genotoxic mechanisms include chronic inflammation, oxidative stress, and compensatory hepatocyte proliferation. Environmental and occupational exposures to chemicals like vinyl chloride and arsenic are strongly linked to specific liver cancers. Additionally, synergistic interactions among risk factors, such as hepatitis B virus infection and aflatoxins, significantly enhance carcinogenic potential.

Toxicants and Their Effects

Classification of Hepatotoxicants According to Xenobiotic Sources

Many chemicals are hepatotoxic, including thousands of synthetic drugs and chemicals, as well as numerous natural compounds such as bacterial, fungal, plant, and animal toxins. Some examples of chemicals causing liver injury are shown in Table 13-3. Chemical hepatic injury is encountered in a variety of circumstances. Some natural toxicants, such as the pyrrolizidine alkaloids and the toxicant of the cycad nut, are taken as food or as folk medicine, in ignorance of their toxicity. Others, such as mycotoxins, are ingested because climatic conditions and cultural practices in some parts of the world favor their presence as unsuspected food contaminants. Hepatotoxic chemicals also may be ingested as accidental contaminants of food. Exposure to hepatotoxicants also may result from the accidental or suicidal inhalation or ingestion of known toxicants (e. g. CCl_4, elemental phosphorus, or copper salts). Hepatotoxic agents have been encountered in industrial operations (e. g. chlorinated hydrocarbons, nitroaromatic compounds, inorganic arsenicals, vinyl chloride). Among the industrial by-products, wastes and pesticides that contaminate the environment, there are known hepatotoxicants, although the magnitude of the hepatotoxic threat remains to be defined. Hepatic injury due to medicinal agents is the facet of hepatotoxicity of most interest to clinicians. There are a large number of drugs that can produce liver damage as the result of a therapeutic misadventure or large overdoses.

Table 13-3 Types of Hepatotoxic Agents

Types of Hepatotoxic Agents	Representative Toxicants
Inorganic agents	
Metals and metalloids	Antimony, arsenic, beryllium, bismuth, boron, cadmium, chromium, copper, iron, lead, manganese, mercury, gold, phosphorus, rare earths, selenium, tellurium, thallium
Hydrazine derivatives	
Iodides	
Organic agents Natural	
Plant toxicants	Albitocin, cycasin, cytochalasin, icterogenin, indospicine, lantana, ngaione, nutmeg, pyrrolizidines, safrole, tannic acid
Mycotoxins	Aflatoxins, cyclochlorotine, ethanol, luteoskyrin, ochratoxins, rubratoxins, sterigmatocystins, griseofulvin, sporidesmin, tetracycline, and other antibiotics
Bacterial toxicants	Exotoxins, endotoxins, ethionine
Synthetic	
Nonmedicinal agents	Azo compounds, Haloalkanes and haloolephins, haloaromatic compounds, nitroalkanes, nitroaromatic compounds, organic amines, phenol and derivatives, and various other organic compounds
Medicinal agents	Over 100 drugs used for treatment and diagnosis

Classification of Hepatotoxicants According to Host Response

Another classification system refers to the nature of the host response to the causative agent. Clinical and experimental observations have led to general agreement that there are two main categories of substances that produce hepatic injury. One group consists of intrinsically toxic agents; i. e. their hepatotoxicity is a fundamental property to which most exposed individuals are susceptible. These are called intrinsic, true, or predictable. The other group consists of agents that produce hepatic injury only in unusually susceptible individuals; i. e. their toxic effects result from the special vulnerability of the affected individual rather than from their intrinsic toxicity. This form of chemical hepatic injury is called idiosyncratic or unpredictable. The hepatic injury caused by most drugs (chlorpromazine, phenytoin, penicillin) is idiosyncratic, although some drugs are intrinsic hepatotoxicants. Chemicals that produce hepatic injury as the result of occupational or accidental exposure or large overdose are intrinsic hepatotoxicants.

Two main types of intrinsic hepatotoxicants are termed direct and indirect. Direct (toxipathic) hepatotoxicants (e. g. CCl_4) produce direct injury to the plasma membrane, endoplasmic reticulum (ER), and other organelles of the hepatocyte. Indirect (trophopathic) hepatotoxicants (e. g. ethionine) are antimetabolites that produce hepatic injury by interfering with a specific metabolic pathway or by distorting individual cell molecules.

Examples of Liver Toxicants Causing Specific Types of Injury

Acetaminophen (APAP): Acetaminophen, a widely used analgesic, is safe at therapeutic doses but can cause severe liver injury or failure with overdose. In humans and mice, overdose leads to centrilobular hepatocellular necrosis. At therapeutic doses, approximately 90% of APAP is conjugated with sulfate or glucuronide and excreted, limiting the formation of its toxic metabolite, N-acetyl-p-benzoquinone imine (NAPQI). NAPQI is detoxified by conjugation with glutathione (GSH), preventing cellular protein binding, which is critical to hepatocellular damage.

Murine models have been instrumental in understanding APAP-induced hepatotoxicity. Key mechanisms, such as GSH depletion, mitochondrial dysfunction, and necrotic cell death, have also been demonstrated in metabolically competent human hepatoma cells (HepaRG) and primary human hepatocytes (HPCs). These studies confirm that APAP toxicity involves reactive metabolite formation, oxidative stress, and JNK activation.

Ethanol: Chronic alcohol abuse is a major cause of liver disease, progressing from hepatic lipid accumulation (steatosis) to inflammation (steatohepatitis), cirrhosis, and ultimately liver failure. Ethanol metabolism primarily occurs in the liver through three pathways, with alcohol dehydrogenase (ADH) being the most significant. ADH oxidizes ethanol to acetaldehyde, which is further metabolized to acetate by acetaldehyde dehydrogenase (ALDH). Excess NADH production and acetaldehyde toxicity disrupt fatty acid metabolism, promote oxidative stress, and impair liver functions such as detoxification and protein synthesis.

Ethanol also induces inflammation via gut-derived endotoxins and cytokine production, which exacerbate liver injury. CYP2E1 contributes to oxidative stress by generating reactive oxygen species. Kupffer cell activation further amplifies damage by producing TNF-α, which promotes hepatocyte death and fibrosis.

Allyl Alcohol: Allyl alcohol is metabolized by ADH to acrolein, a highly reactive aldehyde responsible for its periportal hepatotoxicity. Acrolein depletes hepatic GSH, forming adducts with cellular proteins and inducing lipid peroxidation under oxidative stress conditions. Toxicity is modulated by variations in ADH and ALDH activity, as well as antioxidant status.

Carbon Tetrachloride (CCl4): CCl4 causes centrilobular necrosis through CYP2E1-mediated bioactivation, forming trichloromethyl free radicals that initiate lipid peroxidation and disrupt calcium homeostasis. Resultant mitochondrial damage and Kupffer cell activation exacerbate injury. Protective strategies include CYP inhibition and antioxidant therapy.

Aflatoxins: Aflatoxins, produced by Aspergillus molds, are potent hepatotoxins and carcinogens. Aflatoxin B1 (AFB1), the most toxic, undergoes bioactivation by CYPs to a reactive epoxide that forms DNA and protein adducts, leading to acute toxicity and hepatocellular carcinoma. Co-exposure to hepatitis B virus synergistically increases cancer risk.

Pyrrolizidine Alkaloids: Pyrrolizidine alkaloids, derived from certain plants, cause hepatotoxicity through CYP-mediated bioactivation to reactive pyrrole metabolites. These metabolites form DNA and protein adducts, inducing hepatocyte injury and fibrosis.

Cyanobacterial Toxins: Microcystins, primarily microcystin-LR, target the liver by disrupting cytoskeletal and cellular integrity, leading to necrosis and fibrosis. Transported by organic anion transporters, microcystins are detoxified via GSH conjugation.

Mushroom Toxins: Cyclic peptides like phallotoxins and amatoxins from Amanita phalloides inhibit RNA polymerase II, causing severe hepatic necrosis and potentially fatal liver failure.

Testing Procedure and Evaluation

Morphologic Evaluation

For laboratory animal studies of hepatotoxicity, morphologic observation provides important clues and is an integral part of any comprehensive study of the potential hepatotoxicity of a chemical. Histopathologic analysis can provide information on the nature of the lesion and the regions of the liver affected, which, in turn, can provide insight into the mechanism of toxicity. For example, the presence of a fatty liver would suggest that the chemical may interfere with triglyceride metabolism and/or lipoprotein secretion by the liver.

Gross Pathology: The liver's color and appearance can provide valuable diagnostic clues, such as identifying fatty liver or cirrhosis. Organ weight is a particularly sensitive indicator of hepatic effects and can reflect the severity of toxicity.

Microscopic Examination: Light microscopy is essential for detecting histologic abnormalities, including fatty changes, necrosis, cirrhosis, hyperplastic nodules, and neoplasia. For example, carbon tetrachloride (CCl_4) induces liver damage at doses lower than those required to alter serum enzyme levels. Electron microscopy offers a deeper view, uncovering subcellular changes that, combined with biochemical findings, are instrumental in elucidating toxicant mechanisms.

Biochemical Tests

The liver is involved in the metabolism of carbohydrates, lipid, and protein, as well as in the formation of prothrombin and the excretion of bilirubin and certain xenobiotics. It is also the major site of the biotransformation of toxicants. Thus, tests have been devised to determine these hepatic functions.

Measurement of the Functional Capabilities of the Liver

Excretion Function (Dye Clearance Tests): Dye clearance tests assess the liver's excretion function by tracking the rate at which an intravenously administered dye is removed from the bloodstream. Delayed clearance signals potential hepatic dysfunction. Sulfobromophthalein (BSP), historically used in such tests, depends on active transport into liver cells, glutathione conjugation, and biliary excretion. Disruption of any step, particularly biliary excretion, can impair clearance. Indocyanine green (ICG), another dye, bypasses conjugation and allows noninvasive measurement via ear densitometry. Although these tests are well-established, they are rarely used in clinical practice today.

Drug Metabolism (Drug Clearance Tests): Liver injury often leads to impaired drug biotransformation, which can be evaluated by tracking the elimination rate of a test drug predominantly cleared through hepatic metabolism. Drugs like antipyrine, aminopyrine, or caffeine are commonly used in this context. Serial blood samples are analyzed to compare clearance rates against normal values. Additional tests, such as barbiturate-induced sleeping time and zoxazolamine paralysis duration, also provide indirect measures of hepatic function.

Measurement of Hepatic Enzymes in Serum: Serum enzyme levels are critical markers of liver damage. Hepatocyte injury causes the release of intracellular enzymes into the bloodstream. Alanine aminotransferase (ALT) levels correlate strongly with histologically confirmed hepatic necrosis, making it the preferred marker. Other enzymes, such as ornithine carbamoyltransferase (OCT) and sorbitol dehydrogenase (SDH), are more sensitive but less specific than ALT. In cholestatic lesions, both alkaline phosphatase (AP) and ALT show significant elevation.

Alterations in Chemical Constituents of the Liver

Biochemical analyses of liver tissue itself can provide additional insights, such as: ① content of triglycerides, ② activity of glucose-6-phosphatase, ③ measurement of lipid peroxidation, ④ covalent binding of reactive metabolites to tissue macromolecules.

In Vitro Tests

In vitro models provide valuable tools for investigating the mechanisms of liver toxicity and screening for potential hepatotoxicants. These models offer a controlled and simplified system to study specific aspects of liver function and toxicity, complementing in vivo studies.

Isolated Perfused Liver: The isolated perfused rat liver is a valuable model for studying hepatotoxicant effects, such as CCl4-induced disruptions in triglyceride and fatty acid metabolism.

Isolated Hepatocytes: Isolated rats and human hepatocytes, in suspension or culture, have been used in a variety of biochemical studies. The isolated hepatocytes can be used to determine the nature of various toxic effects: Membrane damage, changes in cellular macromolecules, and changes in the activity and growth of the hepatocytes.

Other In Vitro Systems: Additional in vitro models utilized in liver toxicity testing include these three kinds.

① Tissue Homogenates and Slices: These preparations provide a readily accessible source of liver enzymes and metabolic pathways for studying specific biochemical reactions and toxicological endpoints. ② Suspension Cultures of Hepatocytes: This method allows for the long-term maintenance and propagation of hepatocytes, facilitating chronic toxicity studies. ③ Organelle Suspensions: Isolating specific organelles, such as mitochondria or microsomes, allows for targeted investigations into organelle-specific toxicity.

(Yang Qianlei An Yan)

CHAPTER 14

Toxicology of the Kidney

Introduction

Toxicology of the kidney, also called renaltoxicology, is a critical subfield of target organ toxicology. It applies fundamental principles and methods of toxicology to study the harmful effects of exogenous chemicals, physical and biological factors on the kidney, elucidate the underlying mechanisms, and develop strategies for diagnosis, treatment, and prevention of kidney injury. Numerous chemicals and their metabolites, such as heavy metals, some antibiotics, antipyretic and analgesic drugs, excreted primarily via the kidneys and urine, are known to cause renal damage.

The mammalian kidney is an anatomically and physiologically complex organ. Its proper function is essential for maintaining systemic homeostasis. The kidneys play a pivotal role in waste excretion, regulation of extracellular fluid volume, electrolyte and acid-base balance, and are also involved in the synthesis and release of hormones such as renin and erythropoietin, as well as in the activation of vitamin D. Toxicants can directly impair renal function or indirectly disrupt these critical physiological processes.

Despite its robust compensatory and detoxification capabilities, the kidney is highly susceptible to injury. Renal damage often lacks specific clinical manifestations, and the availability of sensitive monitoring methods remains limited. Symptoms of kidney injury are frequently masked by systemic toxic reactions, making it a hidden and underrecognized condition that demands greater attention. Consequently, in toxicology, the kidney is recognized as a major target organ for various toxicants.

Structure and Functions of the Kidney

The Structure of the Kidney

The nephron, the functional unit of the kidney, consists of several components, each with distinct roles in maintaining renal function.

(1) Glomerulus: A network of capillaries that mechanically filters blood.

(2) Bowman's Capsule: Surrounds the glomerulus and collects the filtrate.

(3) Proximal Tubule: Reabsorbs essential substances such as water, salts, glucose, and amino acids back into the bloodstream.

(4) Loop of Henle: Establishes concentration gradients through a countercurrent exchange mechanism, crucial for water and salt balance.

(5) Distal Tubule: Actively secretes hydrogen ions, potassium, and specific drugs into the filtrate.

The human kidney contains approximately 1.3 million nephrons. Blood filtration begins at the glomerulus, where an ultrafiltrate is formed. This filtrate traverses the various segments of the nephron, undergoing reabsorption and secretion processes, before being excreted as urine.

The Functions of the Kidney

The kidney plays a pivotal role in maintaining overall homeostasis and detoxification. Substances can be excreted in the urine through two primary mechanisms: glomerular filtration and tubular secretion. However, once a substance enters the renal tubule, it may not necessarily be excreted, as reabsorption can occur. The amount of a substance ultimately excreted in the urine is determined by the following equation:

Amount excreted = Amount filtered + Amount secreted − Amount reabsorbed.

The kidney's primary functions include the excretion of waste products and xenobiotics through urine formation, as well as the regulation of critical physiological parameters. Additionally, the kidneys function as endocrine organs, producing hormones and activating vitamin D.

Key functions of the kidney include:

Regulation of extracellular fluid: Kidney controls volume, pH, and osmotic concentration within the internal environment.

Maintenance of ionic balance: Kidney ensures the stability of ions such as sodium, potassium, and calcium in extracellular fluid.

Excretion of metabolic waste: Kidney eliminates toxic by-products, including urea, ammonia, and uric acid.

Detoxification and excretion of foreign substances: Removes xenobiotics such as drugs, pesticides, food additives, and their metabolites through urine.

Endocrine functions: Firstly, kidney secretes hormones like erythropoietin (stimulates red blood cell production) and renin (regulates blood pressure); Secondly, kidney converts vitamin D into its active form, 1, 25-dihydroxy vitamin D_3, essential for calcium homeostasis.

Reasons for the Susceptibility of the Renal System to Toxicity

The kidneys are highly susceptible to toxicants due to their unique physiological and metabolic characteristics. Although they constitute only about 0.5% of total body mass, the kidneys receive an exceptionally large proportion of the resting cardiac output—approximately 20%-25%. This substantial blood flow exposes them to high concentrations of systemic chemicals, making them a primary target for toxicants circulating in the body.

In addition, the process of urine formation further enhances the risk of toxicity. As the kidneys filter blood and concentrate substances in the tubular fluid, chemicals that are relatively harmless at plasma concentrations can accumulate to toxic levels within the renal tubules. Furthermore, the kidneys actively transport, accumulate, and metabolize xenobiotics, a process that may transform certain pro-toxicants into reactive and potentially harmful compounds. These combined factors—high renal blood flow, the concentrating effect of the tubular system, and metabolic activation of toxicants—make the kidneys particularly vulnerable to toxic injury.

Mechanisms of Renal Cell Injury

Mediators of Toxicity

The pathogenesis of toxic renal injury involves multiple interconnected cellular mechanisms. Toxicants can initiate cellular damage through direct chemical reactivity with cellular macromolecules, biotransformation to reactive intermediates either within or outside the kidney, or generation of oxidative stress. The resulting reactive oxygen species (ROS) and reactive nitrogen species can cause extensive damage to cellular proteins, lipids, and DNA, compromising cellular function and integrity.

Cell Death

Cell death in renal tissue manifests through two primary pathways: necrosis and apoptosis. While apoptosis represents a controlled process affecting individual cells with minimal inflammatory response, necrosis involves cellular rupture and subsequent inflammation. The concentration of nephrotoxicants often determines the mode of cell death, with lower doses typically triggering apoptosis and higher doses leading to necrosis.

Cell Volume and Ion Homeostasis

Toxicants disrupt cell volume and ion homeostasis by altering ion permeability or inhibiting energy production, often leading to loss of ATP and membrane transporter function.

Cytoskeleton and Cell Polarity

The cellular cytoskeleton and polarity are similarly vulnerable to toxic injury, with toxicants capable of disrupting cytoskeletal architecture and disturbing the normal polarized distribution of transporters and enzymes. A notable example occurs during ischemic conditions, where ATP depletion leads to the redistribution of Na^+/ K^+-ATPase from its normal basolateral location to the apical membrane domain in proximal tubule cells.

Mitochondria

Mitochondrial dysfunction is a common result of exposure to nephrotoxicants, affecting respiration and ATP production. The mitochondrial permeability transition (MPT) can lead to apoptosis if ATP levels are sufficient or necrosis if ATP is depleted. Release of cytochrome C from mitochondria activates downstream caspases, leading to apoptosis.

Lysosomes

Lysosomal integrity can be compromised by the accumulation of toxic substances, resulting in the release of hydrolytic enzymes into the cytoplasm and exacerbating cellular injury.

Ca^{2+} Homeostasis

The distribution of Ca^{2+} in renal cells is complex, involving binding to anionic sites on macromolecules and compartmentalization within subcellular organelles. The critical cellular Ca^{2+} pool for regulation is the free Ca^{2+} present in the cytosol at a concentration of approximately 100 nmol. This level is maintained by a series of pumps and channels located on the plasma membrane and the endoplasmic reticulum (ER). Disruption of calcium homeostasis can activate degradative enzymes, leading to structural and functional abnormalities in cytoskeletal elements.

Sites and Types of Toxic Responses of the Kidney

The kidney exhibits distinct patterns of toxic injury across its anatomical segments, with each region demonstrating unique susceptibilities based on its structural and functional characteristics.

Glomerular Injury

The glomerulus, as the initial site of chemical exposure in the nephron, demonstrates specific vulnerability to nephrotoxicants through alterations in both structural integrity and functional capacity. Nephrotoxicants can alter glomerular permeability to proteins by changing size and charge selectivity. The decrease in charge selectivity is thought to result from a decrease in negatively charged sites, while the loss of size selectivity is thought to result from the focal detachment of podocytes from the glomerular basement membrane.

Cyclosporine, amphotericin B, and gentamicin impair glomerular filtration rate (GFR) through different mechanisms, often involving vasoconstriction and interactions with anionic sites on endothelial cells. Cyclosporin, amphotericin B, and gentamicin impair glomerular ultrafiltration, often without significant loss of structural integrity, and decreased GFR. Amphotericin B decreases GFR by causing renal vasoconstriction and decreasing the glomerular capillary ultrafiltration coefficient (K_f). Gentamicin interacts with the anion sites on the endothelial cells, decreasing K_f and GFR. Finally, cyclosporine not only causes renal vasoconstriction and vascular damage but also is detrimental to the glomerular endothelial cell.

Chemically induced glomerular injury also may be mediated by extrarenal factors. Circulating immune complexes may be trapped within the glomeruli. Neutrophils and macrophages are commonly observed within glomeruli in membranous glomerulonephritis, and the local release of cytokines and ROS may contribute to glomerular injury. Heavy metals, hydrocarbons, penicillamine, and captopril can produce this type of glomerular injury. A chemical may function as a hapten attached to a native protein or as a complete antigen and may elicit an antibody, leading to immune deposit formation within the glomeruli, mediator activation, and subsequent injury to glomerular tissue.

Proximal Tubular Injury

The proximal tubule exhibits particularly high susceptibility to toxic injury due to several distinctive characteristics. Its extensive absorptive and secretory functions, abundant cytochrome P450 expression, and specialized transport systems create multiple pathways for toxicant-induced damage. The segment's relatively leaky epithelium, combined with its concentrated transport systems for organic compounds, proteins, and heavy metals, results in preferential accumulation of toxic substances. This selective vulnerability is evident in the toxicity patterns of various compounds, including cisplatin, ochratoxin, and heavy metals. Furthermore, the proximal tubule's high concentration of biotransformation enzymes, particularly cytochrome P450 and cysteine conjugate β-lyase, enhances its susceptibility to toxicants requiring metabolic activation. The segment's heightened sensitivity to ischemic injury further compounds its vulnerability to compounds that disturb renal blood flow or cellular energetics.

Loop of Henle /Distal Tubule/Collecting Duct Injury

The loop of Henle, distal tubule, and collecting duct, while less frequently targeted, can sustain significant functional impairment when injured. Toxicants affecting these segments typically manifest as defects in urinary concentration and acidification capabilities. Amphotericin B exemplifies such toxicity through its formation of transmembrane channels that compromise the normally tight epithelial barrier, while methoxyflurane's metabolite fluoride interferes with solute transport and ADH-mediated water reabsorption through specific molecular mechanisms.

Papillary Injury

Papillary injury, particularly associated with chronic analgesic use, represents a distinct pattern of renal toxicity. This injury pattern typically involves progressive changes in medullary interstitial cells, capillaries, and collecting ducts, often exacerbated by the high local concentration of toxicants and compromised regional blood flow in this anatomical region.

Pathophysiologic Responses of the Kidney

Acute Renal Failure (ARF)

ARF is a common outcome of nephrotoxic damage, marked by an abrupt decline in GFR and azotemia. Various chemicals can cause ARF through different mechanisms, such as prerenal factors, vasoconstriction, crystalluria, tubular toxicity, endothelial injury, and glomerulopathy. Table 14-1 provides a partial list of chemicals that produce ARF through different mechanisms.

The maintenance of tubular integrity is dependent on cell-to-cell and cell-to-matrix adhesion. It has been hypothesized that after a chemical or hypoxic insult, adhesion of nonlethally damaged, apoptotic, and oncotic cells to the basement membrane is compromised, leading to gaps in the epithelial cell lining, potentially resulting in back leak of filtrate and diminished GFR. These detached cells may aggregate in the tubular lumen (cell-to-cell adhesion) and/or adhere or reattach to adherent epithelial cells downstream, resulting in tubular obstruction.

Table 14-1 **Classified Mechanisms of Chemically Induced Acute Renal Failure**

Mechanisms	Chemicals
Prerenal factors	Diuretic; interleukin-2; angiotensin-converting enzyme inhibitors; anti-hypertensive agents
Vasoconstriction	Nonsteroidal anti-inflammatory drugs; radiocontrast agents; cyclosporine; tacrolimus; amphotericin B
Crystalluria	Sulfonamides; methotrexate; acyclovir; triamterene; ethylene glycol; protease inhibitors
Tubular toxicity	Aminoglycosides; cisplatin; vancomycin; pentamidine; radiocontrast agents; heavy metals; haloalkene and haloalkene-cysteine conjugates
Endothelial injury	Cyclosporine; mitomycin C; tacrolimus; cocaine; conjugated estrogens; quinine
Glomerulopathy	Gold; penicillaminc; nonsteroidal anti-inflammatory drugs

Adaptation After a Toxic Insult

The kidney possesses an extraordinary capacity to compensate for the loss of renal functional mass. Following unilateral nephrectomy, GFR of the remaining kidney undergoes a compensatory increase by approximately 40% to 60%. This elevation in single-nephron GFR is paralleled by a proportional augmentation in the proximal tubular reabsorption of water and solutes; consequently, glomerulotubular balance is preserved, and overall renal function remains within normal limits on standard clinical evaluations. This compensatory mechanism can effectively mask chemically-induced renal dysfunction until significant nephron loss or damage surpasses the adaptive capabilities of these mechanisms.

The cellular response to toxic insults encompasses a complex spectrum of processes, including cell death, repair, adaptation, and compensatory hypertrophy. Among the most significant adaptive responses are the induction of stress proteins and metallothioneins. The stress response system, particularly the expression of heat-shock proteins (Hsps) and glucose-regulated proteins (Grps), demonstrates distinct patterns of distribution across different renal cell types and subcellular compartments. These molecular chaperones serve crucial functions in maintaining protein homeostasis by facilitating proper protein folding, mediating the degradation of damaged proteins, and orchestrating cellular repair mechanisms. This sophisticated protein quality control system represents a fundamental defense mechanism against toxic injury, enhancing cellular resilience and promoting recovery through the preservation of essential cellular functions and the facilitation of repair processes.

Chronic Renal Failure

Long-term exposure to chemicals can lead to chronic renal failure, characterized by progressive nephron loss, glomerulosclerosis, tubular atrophy, and interstitial fibrosis. Compensatory mechanisms initially maintain kidney function but eventually contribute to further damage. After nephron loss, adaptive increases in glomerular pressures and flows increase the single-nephron GFR of remnant viable nephrons, which serve to maintain whole-kidney GFR. However, these compensatory mechanisms prove maladaptive over time, as the sustained elevation in glomerular pressures and flows subjects the remnant glomerular capillaries to mechanical stress, leading to altered capillary permeability and structural integrity. This vicious cycle promotes the development of focal glomerulosclerosis, which subsequently triggers a cascade of pathological changes including tubular atrophy and interstitial fibrosis. This progressive deterioration exemplifies how initially beneficial adaptive responses can transform into detrimental processes, ultimately contributing to the inexorable progression of chronic renal failure.

Assessment of Renal Toxicity

Evaluation of nephrotoxicity involves both in vivo and in vitro methods. Initial assessments include serum and urine chemical substabces, measuring urine volume, osmolality, pH, and composition (Table 14 - 2). Chemical-induced changes in urine composition can indicate specific types of renal injury.

Toxicant-induced polyuria accompanied by decreased urinary osmolality typically suggests impairment of renal concentrating capacity, potentially reflecting disruptions in antidiuretic hormone (ADH) synthesis, secretion, or target organ responsiveness. The presence of glucosuria may indicate either direct chemical interference with proximal tubular glucose reabsorption mechanisms or manifest as a secondary consequence of systemic hyperglycemia. The urinary excretion pattern of proteins provides valuable diagnostic insights: elevated levels of high-molecular-weight proteins such as albumin generally indicate glomerular dysfunction, while increased excretion of low-molecular-weight proteins, exemplified by β2-microglobulin, typically suggests proximal tubular injury. The appearance of brush border enzymes, including alkaline phosphatase and γ-glutamyl transferase, in the urine often reflects more extensive cellular damage. However, it is crucial to note that enzymuria frequently presents as a transient phenomenon, as initial chemical injury may result in rapid depletion of available cellular enzymes. Consequently, the absence of enzymatic markers in urine should not be interpreted as definitive evidence for the absence of renal injury.

Table 14-2 **The Type of Method of Renal Function**

Method Type	Examples
Urinalysis	Urine volume and osmolarity Urine pH Amount of proteins Amount of glucose Enzymes
Blood analysis	Blood urea nitrogen (BUN) Creatinine
Renal clearance-GFR	Renal clearance of *p*-aminohippuric acid (PAH) PSP excretion test
Morphologic examinations	Gross examination Light and electron microscopy
In vitro studies	Renal cortex slices Isolated perfused renal tubule Isolated nephrons

Specific Nephrotoxicants

Heavy Metals

Various metals, such as cadmium, chromium, lead, mercury, platinum, and uranium, are known nephrotoxicants. The form of the metal significantly affects the type and severity of renal injury. A prime example is mercury, where inorganic salts induce more severe kidney damage compared to organic compounds. Metals often bind to sulfhydryl groups in critical cellular proteins, disrupting their functions. In addition, different metals have different primary targets within the kidney. For example, potassium dichromate and cadmium primarily affect the S1 and S2 segments of the proximal tubule, whereas mercuric chloride affects the S2 and S3 segments.

Mercury

The kidneys are the primary target organs for the accumulation of Hg^{2+}. The acute nephrotoxicity induced by $HgCl_2$ is characterized by proximal tubular necrosis and acute renal failure (ARF) within 24 to 48 hours after administration. Early markers of $HgCl_2$-induced renal dysfunction include an increase in the urinary excretion of brush border enzymes such as alkaline phosphatase and gamma-glutamyl transpeptidase (γ-GT). Subsequently, when tubular injury becomes severe, intracellular enzymes such as lactate dehydrogenase and aspartate aminotransferase increase in the urine. As injury progresses, tubular reabsorption of solutes and water decreases.

Mitochondrial alterations in morphology and function are very early events after $HgCl_2$ administration, supporting the hypothesis that mitochondrial dysfunction is an early and important contributor to inorganic mercury-induced cell death along the proximal tubule.

Cadmium

Cadmium has a half-life of more than 10 years in humans and thus accumulates in the body over time. Approximately 50% of the body burden of cadmium can be found in the kidney. Cadmium produces proximal tubule dysfunction and injury that may progress to chronic interstitial nephritis.

Halogenated Hydrocarbons

Halogenated hydrocarbons are a diverse class of compounds and are used extensively as chemical intermediates, solvents, and pesticides. Consequently, humans are exposed to these compounds not only in the workplace but also through the environment. Numerous toxic effects have been associated with acute and chronic exposure to halogenated hydrocarbons, including nephrotoxicity.

Chloroform

The primary cellular target of chloroform is the proximal tubule, with no primary damage to the glomerulus or the distal tubule. Proteinuria, glucosuria, and increased blood urea nitrogen (BUN) levels are all characteristic of chloroform-induced nephrotoxicity. The nephrotoxicity produced by chloroform is linked to its metabolism by renal cytochrome P450, which biotransforms chloroform to trichloromethanol, which is unstable and releases HCl to form phosgene, which reacts injuriously with cellular macromolecules.

Tetrafluoroethylene

Tetrafluoroethylene (TFE) is metabolized in the liver to a glutathione conjugate, which is then converted to a cysteine S-conjugate (TFEC) in the bile and small intestine. This conjugate is reabsorbed and transported to the kidneys, where it can also form mercapturic acid. In the kidneys, the cysteine S-conjugate, the main nephrotoxic species, is transported into proximal tubule cells. Here, it undergoes further transformation by the enzyme β-lyase, producing reactive thiols that can covalently bind to cellular proteins, leading to kidney damage. Notably, these reactive thiols interact with mitochondrial proteins, potentially affecting heat shock proteins and resulting in cellular dysfunction. Overall, the metabolic conversion of TFEC leads to significant nephrotoxic effects by targeting kidney cells.

Fungal Toxins and Aristolochic Acid

Nephrotoxic compounds derived from natural and pharmaceutical sources demonstrate diverse mechanisms of renal injury. Among these, mycotoxins produced by various molds and fungi represent significant nephrotoxic agents, including aflatoxin B1, citrinin, ochratoxins, fumonisins, and patulin. Citrinin exemplifies the complexity of mycotoxin-induced nephrotoxicity, manifesting through decreased urine osmolality, reduced GFR and renal blood flow (RBF), glycosuria, and elevated urinary enzyme excretion. The compound enters cells via organic anion transporters, inducing mitochondrial dysfunction, though species-specific variations exist in the localization of tubular damage.

Aristolochic acids (AAs) and aristolactams, derived from Aristolochia and Asarum genera, gained significant attention following the 1993 recognition of their human nephrotoxicity, despite millennia of traditional medicinal use. These compounds have been implicated in both Balkan endemic nephropathy and Chinese herb nephropathy (now termed AA nephropathy), characterized by tubular dysfunction, proteinuria, and interstitial fibrosis.

Pharmaceutical Agents

Pharmaceutical agents exhibit diverse nephrotoxic profiles. APAP induces proximal tubular necrosis, manifesting through elevated BUN and plasma creatinine, decreased GFR, and altered urinary parameters, with both cytochrome P450-mediated activation and glutathione conjugation contributing to its nephrotoxicity. Aminoglycoside nephrotoxicity presents as nonoliguric renal failure with characteristic phospholipidosis through lysosomal hydrolase inhibition. Amphotericin B causes complex nephrotoxicity including ADH-resistant polyuria and renal tubular acidosis, while cyclosporine demonstrates three distinct patterns of nephrotoxicity: acute reversible dysfunction, acute vasculopathy, and chronic nephropathy with interstitial fibrosis.

Cisplatin-induced nephrotoxicity manifests in both acute and chronic forms, characterized by magnesium wasting and polyuria, with primary effects on proximal tubular function through DNA synthesis inhibition and transport dysfunction. Radiocontrast agents, particularly iodinated contrast media, present significant nephrotoxic risk, especially in vulnerable populations with pre-existing conditions. Modern nonionic contrast agents demonstrate improved safety profiles, though their nephrotoxicity still operates through dual mechanisms of vasoconstriction and direct tubular injury.

(Yang Qianlei An Yan)

CHAPTER 15

Neurotoxicology

Introduction

Most multicellular animals possess a nervous system. In every case the function of the nervous system is to receive information about the external and internal environment, integrate the information, and then coordinate a response appropriate to the environmental stimulus. In addition to these basic vital functions, the nervous systems of higher organisms are responsible for feeling, thinking, and learning. All of the other organ systems of the body are subject to control by the nervous system; thus, damage to this "master" system by toxicants can have far-reaching and even devastating effects.

Neurotoxicology is a specialized branch of toxicology that focuses on studying the adverse effects of chemical substances, biological toxins, and environmental agents on the nervous system, encompassing both the central and peripheral nervous systems. This discipline investigates the mechanisms by which toxicants enter and interact with neural tissues, their distribution and metabolism within the nervous system, and the resulting structural and functional alterations. It examines the dose-response relationships, temporal patterns of neurotoxicity, and the behavioral manifestations of neural dysfunction. The field also encompasses the investigation of protective mechanisms, therapeutic interventions, and the development of biomarkers for early detection of neurotoxic effects. This interdisciplinary science integrates principles from toxicology, neuroscience, pharmacology, and behavioral sciences to understand how various agents can impair neural development, function, and maintenance throughout the lifespan.

In recent decades, human exposure to neurotoxic substances has escalated significantly, presenting a critical public health concern that demands our immediate attention. Lead exposure from environmental sources continues to be a persistent threat, particularly in urban and industrial settings, affecting both occupational workers and the general population, especially vulnerable groups such as children. The widespread use of volatile organic compounds (VOCs) in industrial processes, consumer products, and building materials has created numerous exposure pathways through inhalation and dermal contact. Additionally, the extensive application of organophosphate pesticides in agriculture, coupled with their occasional misuse, has led to both acute and chronic poisoning incidents among agricultural workers and nearby communities. These mounting challenges underscore the paramount importance of neurotoxicological research in contemporary toxicology. Scientists and researchers must intensify their efforts to understand the mechanisms of neurotoxicity, establish more effective preventive measures, and develop improved therapeutic interventions. The expanding field of neurotoxicology has become an indispensable area of study for toxicologists, as it directly addresses these pressing public health challenges and seeks to protect human neurological health in an increasingly chemically complex world.

Structure and Functions of the Nervous System

In vertebrates there are two major components of the nervous system. Although these two systems are anatomically separable, they are contiguous and they function interactively. The brain and spinal cord comprise the central nervous system (CNS), and the nervous tissue (ganglia and peripheral nerves) outside the brain and spinal cord comprise the peripheral nervous system (PNS). The PNS can be further divided into the somatic and autonomic nervous systems. Somatic afferents carry sensory information from the skin, muscle, and joints to the CNS, while motor efferents innervate skeletal muscle to cause contractive movement. The autonomic nervous system can be thought of as a motor system for visceral organs, since it projects to these organs to innervate and control the function of smooth muscle, cardiac muscle, and endocrine and exocrine glands. The autonomic nervous system is further divided anatomically and functionally into the sympathetic and parasympathetic subdivisions. Most organs are innervated by both subdivisions, and their influences generally oppose one another. For example, stimulation of sympathetic nerves increases heart rate, while stimulation of the vagus nerve, the primary parasympathetic innervation of the heart, slows its rate of contraction.

The Neurons

A neuron, or nerve cell, is the structural and functional unit of the nervous system. It transmits impulses, receives stimuli, and integrates information. Structurally, a neuron comprises a cell body and protrusions, specifically dendrites and axons. Neuronal cell bodies are concentrated in regions such as the brain's cortex, cerebellum, brainstem, spinal cord, and ganglia. Dendrites branch out from the cell body and often feature tiny protrusions called dendritic spines, which serve as synapse formation sites. A neuron typically has a single, elongated axon with minimal branching, ending in synaptic vesicles that form synapses with other neurons.

Neurons' fundamental functions include synthesizing and secreting neurotransmitters, sensing various stimuli to induce excitation or inhibition, integrating information, and exerting physiological regulation through efferent pathways. Some neurons, especially those in the hypothalamus, can synthesize and secrete hormones, providing neuroendocrine functions.

Neurotransmitter and Their Receptors

Neurotransmitters bind to specific receptors located on postsynaptic membranes of neurons, neuromuscular junctions, or effector organs. Receptor binding initiates signaling, the nature of which depends on the receptor type. Ionotropic receptors, such as the nicotinic acetylcholine receptor at neuromuscular junctions, are ligand-gated ion channels. Acetylcholine binding directly opens the channel, permitting sodium influx and rapid depolarization. This contrasts with metabotropic receptors, primarily G protein-coupled receptors (GPCRs), which trigger slower, more sustained intracellular signaling cascades. These cascades modulate ion channel activity, alter gene expression, and influence cell survival. Most neurotransmitters interact with both ionotropic and metabotropic receptors; however, some, such as dopamine and norepinephrine, exclusively bind to GPCRs. The postsynaptic response to neurotransmitter binding can be either excitatory or inhibitory. For example, glutamate binding to its receptors generally excites the postsynaptic neuron, while GABA binding typically inhibits it.

Glial Cells

Neuroglial cells, which outnumber neurons by 5 – 10 fold, comprise astrocytes, oligodendrocytes, microglia, and Schwann cells. These cells occupy the interstitial spaces surrounding neuronal cell bodies, dendrites, and axons, serving critical functions in structural support, neuroprotection, metabolic regulation, phagocytosis, and myelination.

Astrocytes, the most abundant and morphologically diverse glial cells, are distributed throughout the central nervous system (CNS) gray and white matter. They are classified into protoplasmic and fibrous subtypes based on their structural characteristics. Their specialized processes, termed perivascular end feet, form connections with meningeal tissues and encircle cerebral blood vessels. Oligodendrocytes are responsible for CNS myelination, creating multilayered myelin sheaths by spirally enwrapping axons. Microglia, which derive from mesodermal embryonic monocytes, migrate and differentiate within the brain parenchyma after traversing the cerebrovascular wall. In the peripheral nervous system, Schwann cells envelope peripheral nerve axons and facilitate saltatory conduction.

Glial cells perform diverse essential functions, including structural support, electrical insulation, blood-brain barrier maintenance, neuroprotection, tissue repair, neuroregeneration, metabolic regulation, nutritional support, ionic homeostasis, immune surveillance, neurotransmitter modulation, and synthesis of neuroactive compounds. Within brain tissue, astrocytic perivascular end feet establish a neurovascular interface, facilitating bidirectional transport of nutrients and metabolites between neurons and the vasculature. Additionally, neuroglia synthesize and secrete various neurotrophic factors crucial for neuronal growth, development, and functional maintenance.

Blood-brain Barrier

The blood-brain barrier (BBB) is a highly specialized interface separating the circulating blood from the CNS, encompassing both brain and spinal cord parenchyma. This barrier is composed of tightly interconnected capillary endothelial cells, characterized by the presence of tight junctions, a basement membrane, and surrounding astrocytic end-feet. This intricate structure restricts the passage of large molecules, including proteins and viruses, thereby maintaining the CNS's homeostatic environment and protecting it from circulating toxins and pathogens. However, the integrity of BBB can be compromised under various pathophysiological conditions, including infection, stroke, brain tumors, and traumatic brain injury, leading to increased permeability and potentially harmful consequences.

Brain-cerebrospinal Fluid Barrier

The brain-cerebrospinal fluid barrier (CSFB) is located between the cerebrospinal fluid (CSF) and the brain parenchyma, specifically in the ventricles and subarachnoid space. Unlike the BBB, the CSFB is less restrictive and does not efficiently limit the exchange of substances. As a result, changes in the composition or pressure of the CSF can rapidly affect the environment surrounding neurons, impacting their function and the overall homeostasis of the brain.

Toxicant Effects on the Nervous System

Neurotoxicants can affect the nervous system through diverse mechanisms. These effects range from selective damage to axon terminals, to complete neuronal death, to disruption of neural signaling without apparent structural damage. The diversity of neurotoxic effects reflects the complex organization and specialized functions of different neuronal and glial populations.

Neurons may exhibit selective vulnerability to specific neurotoxicants based on their functional characteristics. A classic example is 1-methyl-4-phenyl-1, 2, 3, 6-tetrahydrophridine (MPTP)-induced Parkinsonism. MPTP's active metabolite, MPP^+, specifically targets dopaminergic neurons in the substantia nigra. These neurons, which project to the striatum and regulate movement control, possess specialized dopamine transporters that inadvertently transport MPP^+ into the cell. Once inside, MPP^+ disrupts mitochondrial function and generates free radicals, ultimately causing neuronal death. The resulting dopamine deficiency in the striatum produces characteristic Parkinsonian symptoms: bradykinesia, rigidity, and tremor. Epidemiological evidence linking pesticide exposure to Parkinsonism suggests that environmental toxicants targeting mitochondria may contribute to some cases of Parkinson's disease.

Neurotoxic effects encompass both structural and functional alterations in the nervous system. Structural effects include disruption of myelin formation, axonal degeneration, and direct neuronal death. Functional changes often involve disruption of neurotransmission, altered cellular homeostasis, and secondary damage through glial cell dysfunction. While MPTP exemplifies direct structural neurotoxicity, many compounds act through multiple mechanisms or target supporting cells rather than neurons directly. Some toxicants primarily affect synaptic transmission without causing obvious structural damage, while others may induce secondary neuronal damage by disrupting glial cell function and homeostatic mechanisms. Understanding these diverse mechanisms of neurotoxicity is crucial for identifying potential neurotoxicants and developing protective strategies against nervous system damage.

Structural Effects of Toxicants on Neurons

Demyelination

Myelin serves as a critical electrical insulator in the nervous system, facilitating efficient signal transmission through saltatory conduction. When toxicants compromise myelin integrity, they can produce distinct pathological patterns in the peripheral and central nervous systems. In peripheral nerves, myelin damage manifests as muscle weakness, impaired coordination, and potential paralysis. In the brain, toxicant-induced destruction of white matter tracts connecting neurons within and between hemispheres results in toxic leukoencephalopathy, characterized by mental deterioration, vision loss, speech disturbances, ataxia, and paralysis.

While demyelination commonly occurs secondary to axonal degeneration, certain neurotoxicants can cause primary demyelination through two main mechanisms. The first mechanism involves direct disruption of myelin sheath integrity without initial damage to myelinating cells. Compounds such as hexachlorophene, isoniazid, and organotins exemplify this mechanism, causing reversible edema between myelin layers through processes that remain incompletely understood. Notably, different regions of the nervous system show selective vulnerability to specific compounds. The optic nerve demonstrates particular sensitivity to hexachlorophene and organic solvents, while cranial nerves such as the trigeminal and vestibulocochlear nerves are especially vulnerable to styrene, xylene, and trichloroethylene. Tellurium represents a unique case, damaging myelin by inhibiting cholesterol synthesis, a crucial component of myelin formation. The second mechanism involves direct injury to myelin-producing cells. Chronic exposure to cyanide and carbon monoxide can directly damage Schwann cells in the peripheral nervous system and oligodendrocytes in the central nervous system. Inorganic lead presents a particularly concerning case, showing selective toxicity toward oligodendrocytes compared to astrocytes or neurons. This selective vulnerability may explain lead's devastating developmental effects, as it preferentially inhibits the differentiation of oligodendrocyte precursor cells, potentially disrupting normal myelination during critical developmental periods.

Axonopathy

Axonopathy represents a distinct form of neuronal damage, characterized by the degeneration of axons while the cell body remains intact. This distinctive injury frequently results in secondary myelin degradation. However, in certain instances, Schwann cells may endure and potentially facilitate axonal regeneration.

Neurotoxicants can induce axonopathy through two primary mechanisms: direct targeting of axons and impairment of neuronal metabolic processes. In cases of metabolic disruption, the distal segments of axons are typically the first to degenerate, as they are critically dependent on energy-dependent axonal transport. Toxicants such as Vacor, a nicotinamide analogue that disrupts ATP production, or vinca alkaloids, which disturb tubulin-based transport mechanisms, serve as prime examples of this phenomenon. The resulting "dying back neuropathy" progresses in a proximal direction, predominantly affecting the longest and largest diameter neurons. While peripheral nervous system axons have the potential to regenerate if exposure to the toxicant ceases before complete proximal axonal demise, central nervous system axons lack this regenerative ability. The success of peripheral regeneration hinges on the presence of Schwann cells, which proliferate and direct the regenerating axon tips towards their target tissues.

The process of toxicant-induced axonal degeneration frequently exhibits similarities to Wallerian degeneration, which was initially delineated by Augustus Waller in the 1850s. This pattern is characterized by axonal swelling at the proximal end of the injury, distal axonal dissolution, inflammatory cell-mediated phagocytosis, and myelin breakdown, while maintaining Schwann cell viability. Some toxicants, such as hexane, form covalent bonds with neurofilament proteins, thereby chemically "transecting" axons. The formation of crosslinks between neurofilaments results in axonal swelling, which obstructs axonal transport and ultimately leads to the death of distal regions through Wallerian degeneration.

The clinical manifestation of axonopathy typically commences with sensory deficits, followed by progressive motor dysfunction. A historic example illustrating this progression is the "Ginger Jake" epidemic during Prohibition. This incident occurred when bootleggers adulterated ginger tonics with triorthocresyl phosphate (TOCP), causing widespread poisoning. Affected individuals initially experienced peripheral sensory symptoms like tingling and numbness, progressing to muscle weakness and ataxia. While some patients recovered, thousands suffered permanent paralysis. This incident led to the recognition of organophosphate-induced delayed neuropathy (OPIDN), a syndrome now known to involve the inhibition of neuropathy target esterase (NTE) rather than acetylcholinesterase. The precise physiological role of NTE and the complete mechanism of OPIDN remain subjects of ongoing research.

Neuronopathy

Neuronopathy represents generalized damage to nerve cell bodies, leading to secondary degeneration of axons and dendrites. Neurons typically die through two main processes: necrosis and apoptosis, though the distinction between these processes often blurs depending on exposure conditions. For instance, methylmercury demonstrates dose-dependent effects: high acute doses trigger widespread necrosis, while lower chronic doses induce selective apoptosis, particularly in cerebellar granule cells.

Necrotic death typically results from severe disruption of cellular energy production and membrane integrity, causing cellular contents to spill into surrounding tissue and trigger inflammatory responses. In contrast, apoptosis represents a programmed cell death characterized by cell shrinkage, nuclear fragmentation, and membrane budding. Apoptotic cells form membrane-bound fragments that are efficiently removed by phagocytosis, minimizing collateral damage. These death mechanisms often occur simultaneously or sequentially, reflecting a spectrum of responses based on toxicant dose and neuronal subtype sensitivity.

Neurotoxicant-induced cell death has been implicated in various neurodegenerative disorders, including Alzheimer's disease, Parkinson's disease, and amyotrophic lateral sclerosis (ALS). One area of intense research focus has been the toxic effects of excessive signaling by glutamate and other excitatory amino acids (EAAs), and the role that EAAs may play in neurodegenerative disorders. When overactivated, glutamate receptors trigger calcium influx and subsequent oxidative stress, ultimately leading to programmed cell death. This mechanism is exemplified by domoic acid poisoning, as demonstrated in the 1987 Prince Edward Island incident where contaminated mussels caused human casualties and neurological symptoms. Similar toxic effects have been observed in marine wildlife along the California coast, highlighting the environmental significance of such neurotoxic mechanisms.

Glial Cell Vulnerability and Toxicant Interactions

Glial cells exhibit unique vulnerabilities to toxicants due to their specialized functions and structural characteristics. Myelinating glial cells, with their continuous synthesis of lipid components and distinctive membrane architecture, are particularly susceptible to compounds that disrupt lipid metabolism. Their hydrophobic myelin structures can also accumulate lipophilic toxicants, creating persistent exposure scenarios.

The intricate relationship between neurons and glia makes it challenging to determine primary targets of toxicant action, as injury to one cell type typically affects the other. Various metals, including lead, cadmium, and aluminum, can induce glial cell death, while methylmercury shows preferential accumulation in astrocytes and microglia, causing cellular swelling through ion channel disruption. This swelling can trigger a cascade of adverse effects: astrocytes release excess glutamate, potentially causing excitotoxicity, and their enlarged end-feet can compromise cerebral blood flow and metabolite exchange.

Brain injury, whether from trauma or toxicants, triggers reactive gliosis, characterized by astrocyte hypertrophy and hyperplasia. This response, marked by increased glial fibrillary acidic protein (GFAP) production, serves as a valuable biomarker for neurotoxic injury. While glial cells typically protect neurons through phagocytosis and neurotrophic factor production, they can sometimes contribute to toxicity through xenobiotic metabolism. A classic example is MPTP toxicity, where astrocytes convert MPTP to its toxic metabolite MPP+ via monoamine oxidase B. Though harmless to astrocytes, MPP+ selectively destroys dopaminergic neurons after release into synapses, inducing Parkinsonian symptoms. This mechanism, discovered following accidental MPTP exposure in the 1980s, has significantly advanced our understanding of Parkinson's disease pathogenesis.

Functional Neurotoxicity: Mechanisms and Clinical Manifestations

Neurotoxicants can significantly impair nervous system function without causing structural damage, primarily by interfering with neurotransmitter signaling. A classic example is the disruption of cholinergic transmission by organophosphates and carbamates through acetylcholinesterase inhibition. Organophosphates create a stable, phosphorylated inactive enzyme that persists for extended periods, while carbamates form less stable carbamylated complexes that reverse more rapidly. In severe cases, organophosphate inhibition can become permanent through "aging", where dealkylation prevents enzyme reactivation.

Acetylcholinesterase inhibition produces diverse effects due to acetylcholine accumulation throughout the nervous system. The resulting hypercholinergic state affects both nicotinic and muscarinic receptors. Nicotinic effects include muscle fasciculations, weakness, and eventual paralysis, while muscarinic effects manifest as the "SLUDGE" (salivation, lacrimation, urination, defecation, GI upset, emesis) syndrome along with bronchospasm and bradycardia. Central effects include confusion, seizures, and potentially fatal respiratory failure. Treatment involves atropine to block muscarinic effects and oxime compounds to reactivate the enzyme, though oximes are ineffective against aged enzymes or carbamate poisoning.

Other neurotoxic mechanisms involve direct receptor interactions or disruption of neurotransmitter release. Clostridial toxins exemplify the latter: botulinum toxin prevents acetylcholine release at motor end-plates, causing flaccid paralysis, while tetanus toxin blocks inhibitory neurotransmitter release in the spinal cord, resulting in spastic paralysis. Despite their different clinical presentations, both conditions typically show complete recovery through the nervous system's remarkable ability to form new synaptic connections. This plasticity demonstrates the nervous system's capacity to adapt and recover from various toxic insults, provided the initial damage is not too severe.

Many biological toxins also act through direct receptor activation or inhibition, while some neurotoxicants, particularly metals, may influence intracellular signaling pathways. Understanding these diverse mechanisms of neurotoxicity is crucial for developing effective therapeutic strategies and preventive measures.

Neurotoxicity Testing: Methods and Approaches

The assessment of chemical compounds for potential neurotoxic effects remains a critical challenge in toxicology. With approximately 2, 000 new chemicals introduced annually, systematic evaluation methods are essential. Testing typically follows the first tiered approach, which begins with preliminary screening and progressing to more detailed analyses when warranted. The initial screening phase focuses on identifying acute risks through general toxicological tests. These preliminary screenings examine changes in motor activity and conduct neuropathological assessments to detect early signs of neurological damage. The second tier approach often involves more specialized testing, such as examining the effects of repeated exposures, behavioral modifications, developmental neurotoxicity, or specific delayed neurological responses. When necessary, a third tier of testing delves deeper into understanding the molecular mechanisms underlying neurotoxicant-induced neural injury. A truly comprehensive neurotoxicity evaluation requires integrating data from multiple sources, ranging from molecular-level interactions to whole-animal studies and human exposure analyses. This multi-dimensional approach ensures a thorough and nuanced understanding of potential neurological risks, allowing researchers to characterize the complex ways in which toxic substances may impact the nervous system.

In Vivo Tests of Human Exposure

Human exposure studies primarily derive from two sources: case reports of accidental exposures and systematic epidemiological investigations. While case reports often provide limited exposure data, they can signal potential neurotoxic effects. Epidemiological studies employ standardized tools like the WHO/NIOSH Neurobehavioral Core Test Battery (NCTB, Table 15-1) and the Neurobehavioral Evaluation System (NES) to assess cognitive and psychomotor functions. These are complemented by neurophysiological measurements and advanced imaging techniques such as MRI, PET, and SPECT.

Table 15-1 **The WHO Neurobehavioral Core Test Battery (NCTB)**

Domain	Analysis	Test	Task
Psychomotor performance	Motor speed, motor steadiness	Pursuit aiming	Follow a pattern of small circles, placing a dot in each circle around a pattern; subject's score is number of taps in circle within one minute
Perceptual coding and perceptual motor speed	Mannal dexterity, hand-eye coordination	Santa Ana Dexterity Test Wechsler Digit Symbot Test	Perform skilful movements with hands and arms Each number in a list is associated with a simple symbol. On a list of random digits with blank spaces below them, write the correct symbols in blank spaces as fast as possible
Attention and short-term memory	Attention and response speed Visual perception and memory Auditory memory	Simple reaction time Benton Visual Retention Test Wechsler Digit Span Test	Test reactions of hands or feet from visual and auditory signals Recall and reproduce figures Recall digits in series forwards and backwards immediately after hearing them
Mood and affect		Profile of Mood States	Evaluate, by questionnaire, anger, tension, confusion, depression, etc

In Vivo Tests of Animal Exposure

Neurotoxicant detection and characterization predominantly rely on animal model research, with rodents serving as the primary experimental subjects. Researchers employ comprehensive behavioral and neurophysiological assessments that closely mirror human testing protocols. While certain higher-order cognitive functions like verbal abilities cannot be fully replicated in animal models, multiple neurobehavioral outcomes such as memory loss, motivational deficits, sensory impairments, and motor dysfunction can be effectively studied.

The Functional Observational Battery (FOB), a standardized screening tool developed by environmental regulatory agencies, provides a systematic approach to evaluating neurotoxicant exposure. This comprehensive examination involves detailed observations of animal appearance, physiological responses, and behavioral characteristics. Researchers meticulously document behaviors in the cage, handle the animals to assess physical responses, and conduct open-field observations to evaluate exploratory behaviors, motor capabilities, and sensory integration.

Motor activity tests complement the FOB by offering quantitative assessments of nervous system processing, including sensory input integration and motor output. Specific neurotoxic agents can demonstrate distinctive effects on motor activity that are independent of general animal health, providing valuable insights into potential neurological mechanisms.

When initial screening tests reveal dose-related toxicant effects, more specialized behavioral assessments become necessary. These advanced investigations focus on neuromotor function, sensory processing, cognitive capabilities, and motivational responses. Such detailed examinations not only help identify specific neurological lesion sites but also aid in classifying neurotoxicants and understanding their potential action mechanisms. Some advanced tests, particularly those evaluating cognitive function, require sophisticated animal training and extensive researcher interaction.

While rodent models remain the primary research platform, researchers also utilize birds and primates to create more comprehensive models of potential human neurological responses, thereby enhancing the translational potential of neurotoxicological research.

In Vitro Neurochemical and Histopathological End Points

In vitro methodologies represent a critical approach to understanding neurotoxicant mechanisms, providing researchers with valuable supplementary insights that complement whole-animal and human studies. These techniques not only enhance scientific understanding but also contribute to reducing animal testing requirements. Researchers typically collect neurochemical and histopathological data concurrently with behavioral assessments, utilizing various analytical techniques such as measuring acetylcholinesterase activity, neurotransmitter concentrations, and toxicant metabolite detection in bodily fluids and tissues.

Postmortem tissue analysis offers comprehensive insights into neurotoxicant-induced damage, revealing morphological changes at multiple levels of investigation. Microscopic examinations using specialized staining techniques—including cresyl violet (Nissl Staining) for neuronal bodies, and silver stains for axons—enable detailed evaluation of cellular morphology, damage patterns, and cell death mechanisms. Researchers can distinguish between different types of neurological injury, such as axonopathic or demyelinating lesions, and determine whether cell death occurs through necrosis or apoptosis.

Immunohistochemical techniques provide sophisticated molecular-level insights into neurological damage. Markers like glial fibrillary acidic protein (GFAP) help identify reactive astrocyte responses to tissue injury, while stress proteins and immediate early genes offer additional perspectives on neuronal activity and damage. Specific protein markers, such as tyrosine hydroxylase, enable precise identification of neuron types and quantification of selective cell death induced by neurotoxicants.

Tissue homogenization techniques allow for mechanistic investigations at the molecular level, enabling researchers to analyze neurotransmitter levels, signaling proteins, and receptor interactions. These methods reveal complex cellular responses to toxicant exposure, including mitochondrial dysfunction, protein activation changes, and oxidative stress mechanisms.

Cell culture protocols represent a sophisticated complementary approach to neurotoxicity research. By utilizing various cell lines—including primary neuronal and glial cultures—researchers can investigate selective cellular and molecular toxicity mechanisms. While these techniques offer unprecedented detailed insights into toxicant-cellular interactions, they cannot fully replicate the complex systemic and neurological interactions observed in living organisms.

The methodology's strength lies in its ability to provide granular, mechanistic understanding of neurotoxicant effects, bridging the gap between observational studies and comprehensive molecular-level comprehension of neurological damage processes.

The nervous system's unique structure and extraordinary complexity, coupled with its exquisite sensitivity and remarkable adaptability, present significant challenges to neurotoxicology. Consequently, the neurotoxic potential of many agents, and even more so their underlying mechanisms, remains largely unknown. This is particularly concerning given the potential for chronic, low-level chemical exposure to subtly impact children's behavioral development and contribute to neurodegenerative diseases in the elderly. Recent advances, including the development of comprehensive behavioral testing, improvements in pathological and biochemical techniques, and increased regulatory focus, have facilitated the immense task of assessing the neurotoxic effects of both natural and synthetic chemicals.

(Song Xiaoyao Zhang Jie)

CHAPTER 16

Reproductive Toxicology

Introduction

Reproductive toxicology represents a critical domain within the field of toxicological sciences, focusing on the adverse effects of xenobiotics on reproductive health across multiple generations. This discipline encompasses the study of toxicant-induced alterations in male and female reproductive structures, functions, and fertility, as well as effects on lactation and offspring viability.

As an interdisciplinary field bridging reproductive medicine and toxicology, reproductive toxicology employs sophisticated methodologies to elucidate the mechanisms, pathways, and consequences of reproductive system perturbation by environmental agents. The scope extends beyond direct effects on reproductive organs to encompass disruptions in endocrine signaling, pregnancy outcomes, and developmental processes. This comprehensive approach reflects the complex interplay between toxicant exposure and reproductive health across multiple biological systems and temporal scales.

Historical events have dramatically illustrated the devastating impact of reproductive toxicants, particularly chemical agents, on human health. The thalidomide catastrophe (1956—1961) served as a pivotal moment in reproductive toxicology, revealing the profound teratogenic potential of pharmaceutical agents and leading to fundamental changes in drug safety assessment. Subsequent incidents, including the polychlorinated biphenyl (PCB) contamination in Asia (Yusho and Yu-Cheng incidents, 1960s–1980s) and the Belgian dioxin crisis involving TCDD in the late 1990s, further demonstrated the far-reaching consequences of environmental reproductive toxicants. These events catalyzed the development of more rigorous regulatory frameworks and emphasized the essential role of reproductive toxicology in protecting public health and environmental safety.

Male Reproductive Toxicity

The male reproductive system operates under precise neuroendocrine control through the hypothalamic-pituitary-gonadal (HPG) axis, which orchestrates reproductive function and sexual behavior through a complex cascade of hormonal signals. This regulatory network begins with hypothalamic secretion of gonadotropin-releasing hormone (GnRH), which stimulates the anterior pituitary to release luteinizing hormone (LH) and follicle-stimulating hormone (FSH). These gonadotropins exert specific actions on the testes: FSH targets Sertoli cells to support spermatogenesis, while LH stimulates Leydig cells to produce androgens. The resultant steroid hormones complete a feedback loop by modulating hypothalamic and pituitary function (Figure 16-1).

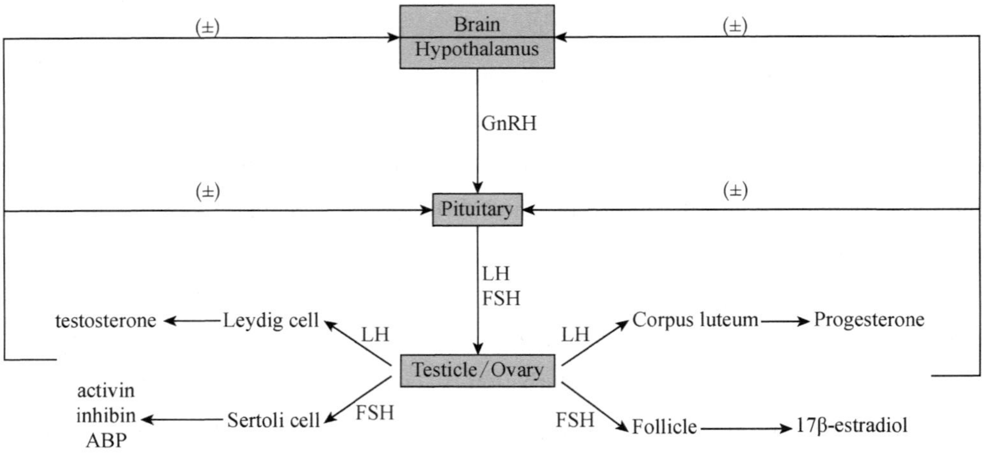

Figure 16-1 **Hypothalamic-pituitary-gonadal (HPG) axis, including a diagram illustrating this pathway**

The structural and functional organization of the testes reflects their dual roles in spermatogenesis and steroidogenesis. The seminiferous tubules, containing germ cells and sertoli cells, provide the specialized environment required for sperm development. Sertoli cells serve multiple essential functions, including physical and nutritional support of developing germ cells, production of androgen-binding protein (ABP), secretion of inhibins, and formation of the blood-testis barrier. The interstitial compartment houses the Leydig cells, which are responsible for androgen production crucial for both spermatogenesis and maintenance of secondary sexual characteristics.

A critical protective feature of male reproductive physiology is the blood-testis barrier, a complex structural interface comprising vascular endothelium, basement membranes, peritubular myoid cells, and tight junctional complexes between adjacent Sertoli cells. This barrier maintains the unique microenvironment required for germ cell development, provides immunological privilege to developing gametes, and regulates the selective transport of molecules into the seminiferous tubules.

Spermatogenesis, occurring within the seminiferous tubules over approximately 74 days in humans, represents a precisely coordinated developmental sequence involving spermatogonial proliferation, meiotic division, and spermatogenic transformation. This process is regulated by both endocrine signals from the HPG axis and local paracrine factors within the testicular microenvironment. The complexity of these regulatory mechanisms and the selective permeability of the blood-testis barrier render male reproductive function particularly vulnerable to toxicant exposure, which can disrupt multiple aspects of reproductive physiology and fertility.

Male Reproductive System Damage

Male Infertility

Male infertility, characterized by impaired reproductive capacity due to deficiencies in sperm production, function, or delivery, can be induced by various environmental and occupational toxicants through distinct mechanistic pathways. These pathways primarily involve disruption of the hypothalamic-pituitary-testicular (HPT) axis, where toxicants interfere with the complex hormonal signaling essential for normal spermatogenesis, and direct cytotoxic effects on the germinal epithelium, resulting in compromised spermatogenic function. These perturbations manifest as quantifiable alterations in semen parameters, including reduced sperm density, impaired motility, abnormal morphology, and in severe cases, azoospermia.

Epidemiological and experimental evidences have identified several classes of reproductive toxicants that significantly impact male fertility. Heavy metals, including mercury (Hg), cadmium (Cd), and lead (Pb), demonstrate particular potency in disrupting spermatogenesis, leading to reduced semen quality and compromised fertility outcomes. Organic solvents, notably benzene compounds, exhibit similar detrimental effects on male reproductive parameters. The agricultural sector presents significant risks through pesticide exposure, with documented cases of reproductive toxicity associated with dichlorodiphenyltrichloroethane (DDT) and organochlorine pesticides, manifesting as decreased sperm counts, reduced libido, and impotence among occupationally exposed individuals. Of particular concern are endocrine-disrupting chemicals, especially organic chlorinated compounds, which have been linked to developmental reproductive disorders, increased risk of cryptorchidism, and an elevated incidence of testicular cancer.

These well-documented associations between environmental toxicants and male reproductive dysfunction underscore the critical importance of rigorous occupational safety protocols and continued surveillance of emerging chemical threats to male reproductive health. The evaluation of sperm parameters serves as a valuable tool in both clinical assessment and toxicological research, providing quantifiable endpoints for assessing the impact of reproductive toxicants on male fertility.

Sexual Dysfunction

Male sexual dysfunction represents a complex spectrum of disorders affecting reproductive health, encompassing impaired libido, erectile dysfunction, ejaculatory disorders (including premature ejaculation, anejaculation, and retrograde ejaculation), and altered nocturnal emissions. The etiology of chemically-induced sexual dysfunction frequently involves disruption of testosterone biosynthesis or signaling pathways, leading to compromised androgenic function and subsequent alterations in sexual performance. A diverse array of environmental and pharmaceutical agents has been identified as potential mediators of male sexual dysfunction, including antipsychotics (such as hydroxyfluphenazine), agricultural chemicals (dicarboximide herbicides), persistent organic pollutants (TCDD, PCBs), synthetic estrogens (diethylstilbestrol), and certain antihypertensive medications. Of particular significance is the emerging evidence regarding bisphenol A (BPA), where occupational exposure studies have revealed a clear dose-dependent relationship between urinary BPA concentrations and the severity of sexual dysfunction parameters, highlighting the importance of biomonitoring and exposure assessment in occupational settings where endocrine-disrupting chemicals are present.

Other Effects

The impact of paternal exposure to reproductive toxicants extends beyond direct effects on male fertility to encompass a broad spectrum of adverse developmental outcomes in offspring. Compromised sperm quality, resulting from exposure to environmental toxicants, can contribute to significant developmental perturbations when combined with normal ova, manifesting as increased rates of spontaneous abortion, stillbirth, intrauterine growth restriction leading to low birth weight, congenital malformations, and functional developmental disorders. Of particular concern is the potential association between paternal exposures and increased risk of childhood neoplasia. Epidemiological studies have identified several high-risk populations, including men with significant exposure to tobacco smoke, chronic alcohol consumption, and occupational exposure to heavy metals (particularly lead and cadmium) and industrial chemicals such as 1, 2-Dibromo-3-chloropropane (DBCP). These findings emphasize the critical importance of considering paternal exposures in reproductive risk assessment and highlight the transgenerational implications of male reproductive toxicity.

Mechanisms and Targets of Male Reproductive Toxicants

Endocrine Disruption

The hypothalamic-pituitary-testicular (HPT) axis represents an intricately regulated neuroendocrine system that governs male reproductive function through precise hormonal signaling cascades. Environmental toxicants can perturb this delicate system through various mechanisms, potentially compromising reproductive health. This endocrine disruption occurs primarily through receptor-mediated interactions and perturbations of hormone homeostasis. The specificity of normal hormonal signaling depends on precise ligand-receptor interactions, occurring through both nuclear (intracellular) and membrane-bound receptors, making these pathways vulnerable to xenobiotic interference.

Receptor-Mediated Mechanisms: Clinical and epidemiological evidences have revealed significant endocrine-disrupting effects of various environmental and pharmaceutical compounds. A classic example is the development of gynecomastia in males occupationally exposed to oral contraceptives, primarily attributed to the compounds' estrogenic activity. Numerous environmental contaminants and their metabolites demonstrate the capacity to interact with hormone receptors. These include ethinylestradiol metabolites (M1 and M2), p, p'-DDE (a DDT metabolite), 2, 2-bis(p-hydroxyphenyl)-1, 1, 1-trichloroethane (HPTE), and levonorgestrel. These compounds typically exhibit anti-androgenic properties through competitive binding to the androgen receptor (AR), potentially compromising normal reproductive function.

Contemporary research has identified alternative flame retardants as significant modulators of multiple nuclear receptors crucial for reproduction, including estrogen receptor (ER), androgen receptor (AR), glucocorticoid receptor (GR), progesterone receptor (PR), and aryl hydrocarbon receptor (AHR). These interactions can precipitate complex alterations in gene expression patterns and cellular function, potentially leading to adverse reproductive outcomes.

Disruption of Hormone Homeostasis: Beyond direct receptor interactions, xenobiotics can disrupt hormone homeostasis through multiple mechanisms, including altered synthesis, modified secretion patterns, perturbed metabolism, impaired excretion, and changes in bioavailability. These disruptions can manifest at various levels of the HPT axis and in peripheral tissues. For instance, TCDD demonstrates the capacity to suppress testosterone synthesis in adult male rats through interference with steroidogenic enzyme function. Organochlorine pesticides like endosulfan can induce comprehensive endocrine disruption, reducing circulating levels of testosterone, FSH, and LH in experimental models.

The mechanisms of disruption can be quite specific, such as the blockade of LH receptors on Leydig cells or interference with cAMP-dependent signaling cascades, leading to rapid alterations in testosterone secretion. Additionally, metal toxicants including lead, cadmium, and zinc can perturb pituitary hormone release through disruption of calcium-dependent secretory mechanisms, potentially affecting the entire HPT axis function.

Sperm Toxicity

The complex process of spermatogenesis, requiring precise temporal and spatial regulation, exhibits particular vulnerability to xenobiotic insult. Recent advances in reproductive toxicology have elucidated several key mechanisms through which environmental toxicants can compromise sperm production and function.

Nanoparticle-mediated reproductive toxicity has emerged as a significant concern, with engineered nanoparticles demonstrating the capacity to induce adverse effects on reproductive cells through multiple pathways, including oxidative stress, inflammatory cascades, and DNA damage. Their unique ability to cross biological barriers makes them particularly concerning as reproductive toxicants.

Phthalate exposure represents another significant threat to male reproductive health. Compounds such as dibutyl phthalate (DBP) and di- (2-ethylhexyl) phthalate (DEHP) have been causally linked to impairment of sperm parameters, including alterations in morphology, reduced concentration, decreased motility, and increased DNA fragmentation. The ubiquitous presence of these compounds in consumer products raises particular concern for population-level reproductive health.

Direct mutagenic effects on male germ cells constitute another mechanism of reproductive toxicity. Chemicals such as ethylnitrosourea can directly induce mutations in spermatogonial stem cells, potentially leading to transgenerational effects on fertility and development.

The disruption of programmed cell death pathways represents an additional mechanism of reproductive toxicity. Carbon disulfide (CS_2) exposure has been shown to perturb normal apoptotic processes in testicular germ cells through modulation of the mitochondrial pathway, involving alterations in cytochrome c levels, Caspase-3 and AIF mRNA expression, and suppression of Bcl-2 gene expression, ultimately affecting the balance of cell survival during spermatogenesis.

Testicular Toxicity

The testis, as a complex organ system comprising multiple specialized cell types and functions, presents numerous potential targets for xenobiotic-induced toxicity. Understanding these diverse mechanisms of testicular injury is crucial for assessing reproductive risk and developing protective strategies. The testis possesses significant metabolic capacity through various enzyme systems, including cytochrome P450, epoxide hydrolase, and aryl hydrocarbon hydroxylase (AHH). This metabolic capability, while essential for normal function, can also contribute to toxicant activation and subsequent tissue injury through the generation of reactive intermediates. Testosterone biosynthesis in Leydig cells involves a complex cascade of enzymatic reactions, each representing a potential target for toxicant interference. Disruption of any component of this steroidogenic pathway can result in altered hormone production, with consequent effects on reproductive function and development. The blood-testis barrier, crucial for maintaining the specialized microenvironment required for spermatogenesis, can be compromised by various toxicants. Notably, cadmium, cisplatin, and methoxychlor have demonstrated the ability to disrupt this protective barrier, potentially exposing developing germ cells in the adluminal compartment to toxic insult. Phthalate esters (PAEs) exemplify compounds that can induce oxidative stress in testicular tissue, leading to multiple adverse outcomes, including the induction of apoptotic and autophagic pathways in Leydig cells, disruption of Sertoli cell cycle regulation, and consequent impairment of spermatogenesis. The developmental effects of testicular toxicants can be particularly severe when exposure occurs during critical windows of reproductive development. Prenatal exposure to DBP can result in male reproductive organ malformation, reduced testosterone production, and altered pituitary hormone secretion. Similarly, DEHP exposure can impair fetal Leydig cell function, leading to reduced adult fertility. Certain industrial chemicals, including formaldehyde and ortho-xylene, demonstrate direct testicular toxicity, with high-level xylene exposure through inhalation shown to adversely affect reproductive performance in experimental models, highlighting the importance of occupational exposure assessment and control in protecting male reproductive health.

Effects on Sexual Function and Behavioral Toxicity

Chemical and pharmaceutical agents can exert profound influences on male sexual function and behavior through both direct and indirect mechanisms. Anabolic steroids, structurally analogous to testosterone, demonstrate complex effects on male sexuality, potentially enhancing libido while simultaneously compromising erectile function through disruption of the hypothalamic-pituitary-gonadal axis. Psychoactive pharmaceuticals, particularly selective serotonin reuptake inhibitors (SSRIs) such as fluoxetine, are well-documented to induce sexual dysfunction through modulation of neurotransmitter systems, manifesting as delayed ejaculation, anorgasmia, and diminished libido. Substances of abuse demonstrate diverse effects on sexual function, potentially affecting multiple aspects including sexual drive, performance capacity, and ejaculatory function through various neurological and endocrine pathways. The critical role of testosterone in male sexual function and behavior cannot be overstated, as it serves as a central mediator of sexual response and behavior. Consequently, xenobiotics that interfere with testosterone biosynthesis, metabolism, or signaling pathways can indirectly impair sexual function through disruption of this essential androgenic regulation. This understanding of the complex interplay between chemical exposures and male sexual function highlights the importance of considering both direct neuroendocrine effects and indirect hormonal mechanisms when evaluating reproductive toxicants.

Female Reproductive Toxicity

Female reproductive toxicity represents a critical field investigating xenobiotic effects on the intricate female reproductive system. The complex interplay of hormonal regulation and cellular development in female reproduction provides multiple targets for potential toxicant interference. The hypothalamic-pituitary-ovarian axis serves as the primary regulatory system, with FSH and LH exerting precise control over ovarian function. LH specifically targets theca cells within ovarian follicles, initiating steroidogenesis to produce progesterone and estrogen, which are subsequently transferred to granulosa cells. Complementarily, FSH stimulates these granulosa cells to synthesize estradiol, establishing a sophisticated hormonal feedback system.

The process of oogenesis exemplifies the temporal complexity of female reproduction, initiating during early embryonic development and extending through multiple life stages. This developmental sequence begins with primordial germ cells undergoing mitotic division in fetal ovaries to generate oogonia. These cells then transition into primary oocytes through meiotic initiation, remaining arrested in prophase until puberty onset. Hormonal shifts at puberty activate selective primary oocyte development, typically resulting in the maturation and ovulation of a single oocyte per menstrual cycle. The final stages of oocyte development involve the completion of the first meiotic division just prior to ovulation, with the second meiotic division occurring only upon fertilization.

The menstrual cycle represents a sophisticated orchestration of hormonal and physiological changes within the female reproductive system, particularly affecting ovarian and uterine function. This cyclical process depends on the precise coordination of FSH, LH, estrogen, and progesterone. These hormones function synergistically to regulate follicular development, trigger ovulation, and prepare the uterine environment for potential implantation, demonstrating the intricate nature of female reproductive physiology and its vulnerability to toxicological disruption.

Female Reproductive System Damage

Menstrual Cycle Disruption

Menstrual cycle homeostasis, a critical indicator of female reproductive health, can be significantly disrupted by exposure to various environmental and occupational toxicants. These disrupting agents include heavy metals (particularly lead and mercury), industrial solvents (benzene and carbon disulfide), petroleum products (gasoline), agricultural chemicals (various classes of pesticides), and persistent organic pollutants (POPs). These compounds can interfere with the complex neuroendocrine signaling pathways that regulate menstrual cyclicity, resulting in a spectrum of menstrual disorders. Clinical manifestations include dysmenorrhea, alterations in menstrual flow volume (menorrhagia or hypomenorrhea), and perturbations in cycle characteristics (oligomenorrhea, polymenorrhea, or irregular cycling patterns). The mechanism of action frequently involves disruption of the hypothalamic-pituitary-ovarian axis, with POPs being particularly noteworthy due to their environmental persistence and documented ability to interfere with reproductive endocrine function. These menstrual cycle irregularities serve as sensitive biomarkers of reproductive toxicity and underscore the importance of environmental and occupational exposure assessment in women's reproductive health monitoring.

Female Infertility

Female infertility induced by environmental and occupational toxicants manifests through multiple mechanistic pathways that disrupt the complex processes essential for successful reproduction. These mechanisms include neuroendocrine disruption affecting ovulation, direct ovarian cytotoxicity, interference with gamete interaction, perturbation of steroidogenesis, and alteration of the intrauterine environment. Agricultural chemicals represent significant reproductive toxicants, as exemplified by linuron's disruption of estrous cyclicity in lagomorphs, organochlorine pesticides' estrogenic effects on ovarian development and oocyte maturation, and methoxychlor's alteration of embryo transport leading to pre-implantation loss in rodent models. These diverse mechanisms of reproductive toxicity underscore the vulnerability of female reproductive function to environmental chemical exposures and emphasize the importance of comprehensive safety assessment in occupational and environmental health protection.

Adverse Pregnancy Outcomes

Environmental and occupational exposure to chemical toxicants during pregnancy represents a significant risk factor for adverse reproductive outcomes. These exposures can precipitate a spectrum of developmental perturbations, ranging from early pregnancy loss to congenital malformations, intrauterine fetal demise, and impaired fetal growth. Women in occupational settings with frequent exposure to toxic substances demonstrate heightened susceptibility to reproductive toxicants, particularly organic solvents and heavy metals, resulting in an increased incidence of adverse pregnancy outcomes.

The mechanistic pathways underlying chemical-induced developmental toxicity have been elucidated through both epidemiological studies and experimental models. Organic solvents, including aromatic hydrocarbons, carbon disulfide, and petroleum distillates, have been consistently associated with elevated rates of spontaneous abortion. Organochlorine and carbamate pesticides exhibit significant transplacental transfer capabilities, potentially leading to fetal toxicity and death. DDT exposure demonstrates a dose-dependent relationship with pregnancy loss, as evidenced by the strong correlation between maternal DDT burden and the occurrence of spontaneous abortion and stillbirth. TCDD exemplifies the complexity of endocrine-disrupting chemicals, capable of perturbing pregnancy-associated hormonal homeostasis and inducing pregnancy loss in non-human primates through disruption of endocrine signaling pathways.

Mechanisms and Targets of Female Reproductive Toxicants

Endocrine Disruption

Environmental chemicals can profoundly disrupt female reproductive endocrine function through multiple interconnected mechanisms. At the hypothalamic-pituitary-gonadal (HPG) axis level, certain pesticides such as methoxychlor and endosulfan demonstrate dose-dependent biphasic effects on gonadotropin-releasing hormone (GnRH) secretion, exhibiting stimulatory effects at low doses while inhibitory at higher concentrations. These compounds significantly alter hypothalamic GnRH gene expression patterns in female rats, demonstrating their capacity to disrupt central reproductive control mechanisms.

Ovarian steroidogenesis represents another critical target for reproductive toxicants. The DDT metabolite p, p'-DDE enhances aromatase (P450 arom) activity, leading to increased estradiol (E2) synthesis. Similarly, perfluorochemicals (PFCs), including perfluorooctanoic acid (PFOA) and perfluorooctane sulfonic acid (PFOS), significantly modulate sex hormone levels by increasing intracellular E2 while suppressing testosterone production. These compounds also demonstrate complex effects on steroidogenic gene expression, with PFOA upregulating 17βHSD1, 3βHSD2, CYP11B2, and CYP19 while downregulating CYP17, 17βHSD4, and CYP11A. PFOS exposure similarly alters the expression of key steroidogenic enzymes, affecting HMGR, StAR, and various CYP genes, while also reducing the expression of steroidogenic factor-1 (SF-1), a crucial regulator of steroid synthesis.

Many environmental compounds exhibit estrogenic or anti-estrogenic properties through direct interaction with estrogen receptors (ERs). Chemicals such as methoxychlor, genistein, DBP, diethylstilbestrol (DES), and bisphenol A (BPA) demonstrate weak estrogenic activity compared to endogenous 17β-estradiol. While these effects may be minimal in adult females with normal estradiol levels, they can significantly impact males, developing individuals, and embryos, potentially causing reproductive malformations and developmental abnormalities.

The modulation of hormone receptor expression and function represents another significant mechanism of reproductive toxicity. Arsenic trioxide (As_2O_3) exemplifies this through its ability to inhibit transcription, downregulate ER mRNA expression, reduce cell viability, and suppress ER protein expression, collectively altering endogenous hormone secretion. Various pesticides and industrial chemicals, including cypermethrin, triflumuron, bromoxynil, and polychlorinated biphenyls, can bind to ERs and disrupt estrous cyclicity, ultimately compromising female reproductive capacity. These diverse mechanisms of endocrine disruption highlight the complexity of reproductive toxicity and emphasize the importance of comprehensive toxicological evaluation considering both direct hormonal effects and receptor-mediated responses.

Oocyte Toxicity

Mature oocytes have different DNA repair capabilities compared to mature sperm, but their repair capacity diminishes during meiotic division. Treatment with BPA can severely suppress meiotic division in mouse oocytes. The mechanism of action may involve disruption of spindle microtubule assembly by promoting centrosomal protein degradation, leading to chromosomal segregation impairment. The alkylating agent busulfan, when administered as a single intraperitoneal injection, can cause destruction of mouse primordial follicles and may be associated with mutagenic effects. Epidemiological evidence suggests an increase in spontaneous miscarriage in wives of vinyl chloride workers.

Ovarian and Uterine Toxicity

The developmental progression of ovarian follicles presents multiple vulnerable targets for xenobiotic-induced damage throughout their lifespan. Primordial follicles demonstrate particular sensitivity to polycyclic aromatic hydrocarbons, including 9, 10-dimethylbenz [a] anthracene (DMBA), 3-methylcholanthrene (3-MC), and benzo [a] pyrene (BaP), with documented toxicity across human and rodent models. Primary follicles similarly exhibit vulnerability to 3-MC and BaP exposure, often resulting in compromised fertility. Secondary follicular development can be disrupted by various compounds including DMBA, 3-MC, DEHP, and cyclophosphamide, potentially leading to premature ovarian failure, amenorrhea, and infertility. At the final stages of follicular development, antral and preovulatory follicles show susceptibility to phthalate esters (PAEs), which can impair follicular biochemistry and interfere with oocyte maturation and release.

The ovarian tissue's substantial xenobiotic metabolic capacity, coupled with its complex steroidogenic enzyme systems, creates multiple pathways for toxicant-induced dysfunction. DEHP and its metabolite mono(2-ethylhexyl) phthalate (MEHP) exemplify this complexity through their activation of peroxisome proliferator-activated receptor (PPAR) and subsequent inhibition of aromatase activity in granulosa cells and ovarian tissue. This inhibition reduces aromatase gene transcription and estradiol production through mechanisms independent of FSH-cAMP signaling, ultimately manifesting as polycystic ovarian changes. BPA demonstrates particularly broad reproductive toxicity, disrupting multiple aspects of ovarian and uterine function. In ovarian tissue, BPA interferes with meiotic initiation, germ cell nest breakdown, and follicular transition, while also compromising steroidogenesis and oocyte quality across various experimental models including animal studies, in vitro systems, and human observations. Its effects extend to the uterus, where it impairs endometrial proliferation and reduces uterine receptivity, contributing to implantation failure. While epidemiological evidence suggests associations between BPA exposure and various reproductive disorders, including altered androgen levels, sexual dysfunction, and adverse pregnancy outcomes, additional research is needed to fully elucidate these relationships in human populations.

Sexual Behavioral Toxicity

Female sexual function demonstrates an intricate dependence on ovulatory cycling, with toxicological disruption of ovulation manifesting in altered sexual behavior patterns. Chemical-induced ovarian atrophy represents a significant mechanism through which xenobiotics can suppress female libido, highlighting the critical relationship between ovarian function and sexual desire. Pharmacological agents, particularly certain formulations of oral contraceptives, demonstrate the capacity to modulate female sexual response through various neuroendocrine mechanisms. Substances of abuse similarly exhibit complex effects on female sexual function, potentially disrupting multiple aspects of sexual response through both direct and indirect pathways. The antiandrogen cyproterone acetate, commonly prescribed for hirsutism management, exemplifies the profound impact of hormonal modulation on female sexuality, with its administration associated with significant reduction in sexual desire and overall sexual function through antagonism of androgenic pathways. This interconnection between endocrine disruption and sexual behavior underscores the broader implications of reproductive toxicants beyond their direct effects on fertility, emphasizing the need to consider behavioral endpoints in reproductive toxicity assessment.

Reproductive Toxicity Testing and Evaluation

Classification Criteria of Reproductive Toxicants

The classification of reproductive toxicants employs a comprehensive weight-of-evidence approach that integrates multiple lines of scientific evidence to systematically assess potential reproductive hazards. This rigorous evaluation framework synthesizes data from diverse sources, including human epidemiological studies, case reports, targeted reproductive toxicity investigations, and findings from sub-chronic and chronic animal studies. The assessment methodology carefully considers factors such as data consistency, biological plausibility, dose-response relationships, and the relevance of experimental models to human physiology. Through this integrative approach, substances are categorized based on their potential to induce adverse effects on various aspects of reproductive function, including gametogenesis, hormonal regulation, sexual function, fertility, and developmental processes. This systematic evaluation provides a scientifically robust foundation for regulatory decision-making and risk management strategies, ensuring that the identification and characterization of reproductive hazards reflect the totality of available scientific evidence rather than relying on isolated findings.

Reproductive toxicants are classified into categories based on the strength and source of evidence for their effects. The main categories are as follows:

Category 1: Known or Presumed Human Reproductive Toxicant

This category encompasses substances that are known to have adverse effects on human sexual function and fertility or development, or substances that animal studies (potential supplemented by other information) strongly indicate a likelihood of interfering with human reproduction. Category 1 is further subdivided based on the primary source of evidence:

Category 1A: Known Human Reproductive Toxicant

—Classification is primarily based on robust human evidence.

—Examples may include substances with clear epidemiological links to reproductive or developmental disorders in humans.

Category 1B: Presumed Human Reproductive Toxicant

—Classification is primarily based on data from experimental animal studies.

—The animal study data should provide clear evidence of adverse effects on sexual function, fertility, or development.

—These effects should occur in the absence of other toxic effects, or if they co-occur with other toxic effects, the reproductive effects should not be considered as a non-specific secondary consequence. However, the effects observed in animals should be deemed relevant to humans.

If mechanistic information raises significant doubts about the human relevance of the effects observed in animals, classification in Category 2 may be more appropriate.

Category 2: Suspected Human Reproductive Toxicant

Substances are classified in this category when there is evidence from human or animal studies (potentially supplemented by other information) suggesting adverse effects on sexual function, fertility, or development, but the evidence is not sufficiently convincing to place the substance in Category 1.

Key characteristics of Category 2 classification:

—The observed reproductive effects occur either in the absence of other toxic effects or in the presence of other toxic effects. However, the reproductive effects are not considered to be non-specific secondary consequences of these other effects.

—The evidence is not strong enough to warrant Category 1 classification. This may be due to three aspects. ①Limitations in study design or execution; ②Inconsistencies in results across studies; ③Uncertainties in the interpretation of data.

—When there are mechanistic considerations that raise doubt about the relevance of the effect for humans, Category 2 classification may be more appropriate than Category 1B.

Examples of substances that might fall into Category 2 include those where animal studies show reproductive effects, but there are questions about the relevance to humans or the robustness of the data.

Male Reproductive Toxicity Tests

The assessment of male reproductive toxicity requires a comprehensive, multiparametric approach that integrates diverse analytical methodologies to evaluate the potential reproductive effects of xenobiotic compounds. This systematic evaluation framework encompasses detailed semen analysis, reproductive endocrine profiling, assessment of testicular morphology and function, and in vitro testicular cell culture systems. These methodological approaches, particularly in vitro systems, prove invaluable in elucidating specific mechanistic pathways through which toxicants interact with reproductive tissues at the cellular and molecular levels.

The evaluation protocol incorporates detailed assessment of body and reproductive organ weights, with specific focus on the testes, epididymides, seminal vesicles, prostate, and pituitary gland. Gross anatomical examination is complemented by comprehensive histopathological analysis of reproductive tissues, enabling detection of structural alterations at both macroscopic and microscopic levels. These morphological assessments provide crucial information about target organ toxicity and potential mechanisms of reproductive impairment. Furthermore, sperm parameters serve as essential indicators of male reproductive function, encompassing quantitative measurements of sperm production and qualitative assessments of sperm morphology, motility, and viability.

The evaluation framework extends beyond structural analysis to include assessment of reproductive behavior, particularly mating behavior, which can be significantly altered by reproductive toxicants. Endocrine function is evaluated through measurement of key reproductive hormones, including GnRH, LH, FSH, testosterone, estradiol, and prolactin. These hormonal measurements provide crucial information about the functional status of the hypothalamic-pituitary-gonadal axis and its potential disruption by toxicant exposure.

Critical developmental endpoints are incorporated into the assessment protocol, including evaluation of testicular descent, preputial separation, onset of spermatogenesis, and anogenital distance. These parameters serve as sensitive indicators of developmental toxicity and can reveal perturbations in reproductive development resulting from exposure during critical developmental windows. External genital structure is carefully examined, as morphological abnormalities may indicate exposure to reproductive toxicants during crucial developmental periods. This comprehensive evaluation framework enables detailed characterization of male reproductive toxicity, facilitating both hazard identification and mechanistic understanding of reproductive toxicants, ultimately contributing to more effective risk assessment and regulatory decision-making processes.

Female Reproductive Toxicity Tests

The assessment of female reproductive toxicity presents unique challenges due to the inherent complexity of the female reproductive system, characterized by cyclical hormonal changes and distinct physiological states encompassing pregnancy and lactation. This complexity necessitates a comprehensive evaluation framework that integrates multiple detection methods, including detailed ovarian morphological assessment, functional evaluation of reproductive organs, and extensive reproductive endocrine profiling.

The evaluation protocol incorporates systematic assessment of body and reproductive organ weights, with particular emphasis on the ovaries, uterus, vagina, and pituitary gland. Comprehensive histopathological analysis of these reproductive tissues provides critical insights into structural and functional alterations that may result from toxicant exposure. These morphological assessments serve as fundamental indicators of reproductive system integrity and potential pathological changes induced by xenobiotic compounds.

Reproductive cycle parameters constitute essential indicators of female reproductive health and endocrine function. The evaluation encompasses detailed analysis of estrous cyclicity, follicular development dynamics, and ovulation patterns. These parameters provide crucial information about the functional status of the hypothalamic-pituitary-ovarian axis and its potential disruption by reproductive toxicants. Reproductive behavior assessment, particularly mating behavior, offers additional insights into the neurological and endocrine aspects of reproduction that may be affected by toxicant exposure.

Fertility indicators represent critical endpoints in female reproductive toxicity assessment. These include quantification of corpora lutea formation, evaluation of pre-and post-implantation loss, and detailed analysis of implantation and early embryonic development. The assessment protocol carefully monitors pregnancy-related parameters, including gestational duration and parturition outcomes, providing comprehensive data on reproductive success and potential developmental toxicity.

Post-natal evaluation extends to assessment of lactation efficiency, maternal behavior, and uterine function, including normal cyclical endometrial changes. The protocol also considers reproductive senescence, recognizing that certain toxicants may accelerate age-related decline in reproductive function. This longitudinal approach enables detection of both immediate and delayed effects of reproductive toxicants throughout the female reproductive lifespan.

Comprehensive Evaluation of Reproductive Toxicity

A thorough assessment of reproductive toxicity demands a holistic, multigenerational approach that extends beyond immediate reproductive capacity to encompass offspring viability, developmental outcomes, and potential transgenerational effects. This comprehensive framework integrates multiple assessment strategies to evaluate both direct reproductive impacts and subtle, long-term consequences that may manifest across generations.

The implementation of diverse study designs forms the cornerstone of comprehensive reproductive toxicity evaluation. One-, two-, and multiple-generation studies enable detailed examination of reproductive effects across successive generations, revealing both immediate impacts and inherited consequences of toxicant exposure. Continuous breeding studies provide crucial insights into cumulative effects of prolonged exposure on reproductive function, while three-segment reproductive toxicity studies offer targeted assessment of specific developmental windows and their unique susceptibilities to toxicant exposure.

Animal exposure models that encompass the complete reproductive cycle represent the gold standard in reproductive toxicity evaluation. These models facilitate simultaneous assessment of multiple endpoints across various life stages during continuous toxicant exposure, enabling detection of stage-specific effects that might remain unidentified in more limited study designs. This approach proves particularly valuable in identifying developmental stage-specific vulnerabilities and delayed manifestations of reproductive toxicity that may only become apparent after extended exposure periods.

The integration of these complementary study designs enables comprehensive characterization of reproductive toxicity profiles, incorporating both immediate and delayed effects across multiple generations. This thorough approach proves essential for several reasons: it facilitates identification of subtle reproductive impairments that might be missed in more limited assessments; it reveals potential transgenerational effects that could impact population health over extended periods; and it provides crucial data for evidence-based regulatory decision-making regarding chemical safety and pharmaceutical development.

One-Generation and Multi-Generation Reproductive Toxicity Study

Traditional three-segment reproductive toxicity studies prove insufficient for comprehensive evaluation of reproductive effects from chronic exposure to exogenous chemicals, including pharmaceuticals, food additives, pesticides, and endocrine-disrupting compounds. Multi-generation reproductive toxicity studies have emerged as essential tools for assessing long-term and transgenerational effects on reproductive function. These studies are classified based on the number of breeding generations directly exposed to test substances, enabling evaluation of cumulative and transgenerational impacts that may remain undetected in single-generation assessments.

One-Generation Reproductive Toxicity Study (OECD 415)

The one-generation reproductive study (OECD 415) involves direct exposure of parental (F_0) animals and indirect exposure of first filial (F_1) generation through in utero and lactational transfer. This protocol evaluates dose-related abnormalities, fertility effects, clinical manifestations, growth parameters, and mortality rates through F_1 weaning. While providing valuable insights into parental reproductive function and establishing no-observed-effect levels (NOEL), this study's offspring assessment remains limited to basic parameters of growth and survival. Integration with subchronic, teratogenic, and other toxicological data enhances the interpretation of results for human risk assessment.

Extended One-Generation Reproductive Toxicity Study (OECD 443)

The extended one-generation reproductive toxicity study (OECD 443) represents a significant advancement in reproductive toxicity assessment. This protocol incorporates toxicokinetic evaluation during pregnancy and lactation, alongside comprehensive assessment of developmental neurotoxicity and immunotoxicity. The study examines dose-response relationships for various endpoints, including organ-specific effects, fertility parameters, reproductive performance, and gender-specific alterations. Evaluation integrates physicochemical properties, toxicokinetic and toxicodynamic data, structural analog information, and previous toxicity findings. This enhanced protocol provides detailed insights into reproductive toxicity throughout the reproductive cycle while optimizing animal usage compared to traditional multi-generation studies.

▶ Two-Generation Reproductive Toxicity Study (OECD 416)

The two-generation reproductive toxicity study (OECD 416) represents the most comprehensive assessment framework, enabling evaluation of reproductive effects across multiple generations through continuous exposure of F_0 and F_1 parental generations. This protocol typically employs rodent models exposed from post-weaning through reproductive maturation, examining effects on fertility, offspring viability, reproductive organ development, and various toxicological endpoints across generations. The study design facilitates detection of subtle reproductive alterations and transgenerational effects through detailed assessment of reproductive parameters, developmental markers, and pathological changes in both generations (Table 16-1).

Table 16-1 One-, Extended One -, or Two-Generation Reproductive Studies

Factors	One-Generation Reproductive Toxicity Study (OECD 415)	Extended One-generation Reproductive Toxicity Study (OECD 443)	Two-Generation Reproductive Toxicity Study (OECD 416)
Animal species	Rat or mouse	Rat(preferred)	Rat(preferred)
Age of animals	Parental (P) male: 5-9 weeks old; Parental (P) female: after at least five days of acclimatization	approximately 90 days after mating	Parental (P) males and females: 5-9 weeks old; F_1 males and females: begin at weaning
Number and sex	About 20 pregnant	At least 20 pregnant	At least 20 pregnant
Dose levels	Minimum three dose levels	Minimum three dose levels	Minimum three dose levels
Route of administration	—	most relevant for human exposure	Oral(preferred) diet, drinking water, gavage
Experimental schedules	at least 2 weeks before mating; throughout mating and pregnancy	10 weeks before mating; throughout mating, gestation and lactation	at least 10 weeks before mating; throughout mating and pregnancy
Mating procedure	1 : 1 (one male to one female) or 1 : 2 (one male to two females)	1 : 1 paring	1 : 1 paring

(continue)

Factors	One-Generation Reproductive Toxicity Study (OECD 415)	Extended One-generation Reproductive Toxicity Study (OECD 443)	Two-Generation Reproductive Toxicity Study (OECD 416)
Observations	Gross necropsy; histopathology	Clinical observations; Body weight and food/water consumption; Oestrous cycles; Mating and pregnancy; Offspring parameters; Assessment of potential developmental neurotoxicity; Assessment of potential developmental immunotoxicity; Follow-up assessment of potential reproductive toxicity; Clinical biochemistry / Haematology; Sperm parameters; Gross necropsy; Organ weight and tissue preservation(P、F_1 adult animals and F1 weanlings); Histopathology(P and F_1)	Clinical observations; Body weight and food/water consumption of parent animals; Oestrus cycle; Sperm parameters; Offspring; Gross necropsy; Organ weights; Histopathology; Weanlings

This chapter provides an overview of reproductive toxicology, elucidating the adverse effects, mechanisms, and toxicity assessment of reproductive toxicants. The intricate regulation of sexual behavior and function is principally regulated by the hypothalamic-pituitary-gonadal axis. It is crucial to note that alterations in the endocrine function, often resulting from impacts on the nervous system, can significantly affect sexual behavior and reproductive outcomes. Human reproductive system disorders encompass a wide range of conditions, including but not limited to infertility, sexual dysfunction, menstrual cycle irregularities, and adverse pregnancy outcomes. These disorders can have profound impacts on individual health, quality of life, and population dynamics.

In the assessment of reproductive toxicity, multi-generation reproduction studies represent the gold standard approach. These studies are particularly valuable as they provide comprehensive information not only about reproductive parameters in the parental generation but also about the development, growth, and survival of offspring across multiple generations. This longitudinal approach allows for the detection of subtle, cumulative, or transgenerational effects that might be missed in shorter-term studies.

While the results of such studies can, to some extent, be extrapolated to humans, it is important to acknowledge the limitations of animal models and the need for careful interpretation when applying these findings to human risk assessment. Factors such as interspecies differences in physiology, metabolism, and exposure scenarios must be taken into account.

In conclusion, the field of reproductive toxicology is critical for understanding and mitigating the risks posed by environmental chemicals and pharmaceuticals to human and wildlife reproduction. Ongoing research in this area is essential for developing better testing strategies, improving risk assessment methodologies, and ultimately protecting reproductive health across species.

(Chen Tao)

CHAPTER 17

Nanotoxicology

Introduction

Nanotechnology and Nanomaterials

Nanotechnology, as defined by the United States National Nanotechnology Initiative (NNI), involves the understanding and control of matter at the nanoscale. Unique phenomena emerge at this scale that enable novel applications across various fields, which has positioned nanotechnology as one of the most dynamic and rapidly expanding areas of research, with significant implications for everyday life. The evolution of nanotechnology has led to the development of nanomaterials (NMs), an extraordinary class of materials characterized by at least one dimension in the range of 1 to 100 nm. The European Commission stipulates that for a material to be classified as a nanomaterial, at least 50% of its particles must measure 100 nm or less in size distribution. NMs can be categorized from different perspectives. Based on their mode of production, NMs can be classified into natural, incidental, and engineered nanomaterials (ENMs). From a dimensional viewpoint, NMs include zero-dimensional (0D) nanostructures such as nanodots; one-dimensional (1D) nanostructures like nanorods, nanofibers, and nanowires; two-dimensional (2D) nanostructures such as nanosheets; and three-dimensional (3D) structures like nanocomposites and complex hierarchical architectures. Additionally, based on their composition, NMs are typically divided into organic, inorganic, and hybrid materials (Figure 17-1).

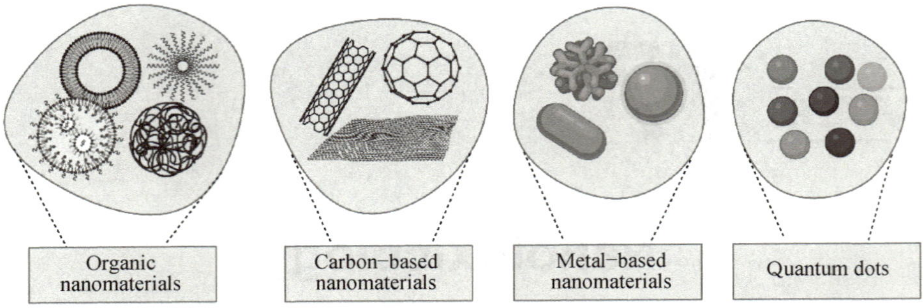

Figure 17-1 **The common types of NMs**

ENMs, in particular, exhibit four distinctive phenomena: the small size effect, surface effect, quantum size effect, and quantum tunneling effect. These properties impart exceptional optical, acoustic, thermal, electrical, magnetic, mechanical, and catalytic characteristics that differ significantly from their bulk counterparts.

Nanotoxicology

The rapid growth of nanotechnology has revolutionized multiple sectors, including energy, environment, aerospace, defense, and biomedicine. In the medical field, NMs have shown particular promise as drug delivery system (DDS), leveraging their exceptionally high specific surface area to enhance therapeutic efficacy and mitigate side effects of drug payload. However, the widespread application of NMs has also raised public concerns regarding their potential toxicity and unintended consequences of exposure. Given the diverse range of NMs currently in use or under development, understanding their toxic action is crucial for ensuring safe application and sustainable development. Unfortunately, research into the adverse environmental and health effects of NMs lags behind their rapid development. This disparity is particularly pronounced in developing countries, where occupational health practices may be suboptimal, and potentially put workers at increased risk. Consequently, strengthening nanosafety research strategies and improving the biosafety profiles of NMs are essential for the sustainable advancement of nanotechnology.

The discipline of nanotoxicology, formally established by the National Academy of Sciences (NAS) in 1983, represents a specialized branch of toxicology dedicated to investigating the adverse effects of NMs on biological systems and the environment. Since 2003, investigations into nanotoxicity and nanosafety have remained at the forefront of scientific inquiry. For NMs intended for human applications, particularly those with potential for systemic exposure, comprehensive toxicological characterization is essential to evaluate potential adverse effects and ensure safety in biomedical applications. Despite significant advances, substantial gaps persist in risk assessment methodologies and the development of standardized safety evaluation protocols. The urgency for expanded nanotoxicological research intensifies as the applications of nanotechnology continue to diversify and expand. As preventive medicine assumes an increasingly crucial role in public health, the biosafety evaluation of NMs presents both unprecedented opportunities and significant technical challenges. Addressing these challenges is fundamental to realizing the full potential of nanotechnology while minimizing risks to human and the environment.

Physicochemical Factors Relevant for Toxicity

Unlike traditional environmental chemicals, NMs possess attributes of both larger particles and molecules, making their toxicological evaluation more complex. Their toxicity is influenced by multiple physicochemical properties, including size, morphology and dimensions, hydrophilicity/hydrophobicity, agglomeration and hetero-agglomeration, surface charge, impurities, and their propensity for chemical transformation and biopersistence. These characteristics significantly affect how NMs interact with biological and environmental systems.

Size

At nanoscale dimensions, NMs exhibit dramatically increased surface-to-volume ratios, leading to enhanced surface defects, vacancies, and dangling chemical bonds that significantly augment their chemical and redox reactivity. Consequently, NMs demonstrate substantially higher surface area, surface energy, and reactivity compared to their microscale counterparts. For instance, a 1 nm spherical particle presents 1000-fold greater surface area than its 1 μm counterpart. Generally, specific surface area positively correlates with toxicity potential. The size distribution of NMs critically influences their exposure patterns, transport mechanisms, and cellular uptake pathways. Depending on their size, NMs can enter cells through various mechanisms, including passive diffusion, direct physical penetration, or active receptor-mediated processes such as endocytosis or phagocytosis. Notably, NMs that are smaller than 50 nm can penetrate cells and subcellular organelles through passive diffusion.

Morphology and Dimensions

The morphological characteristics and dimensional parameters of NMs significantly influence their biodistribution, cellular internalization, toxicity potential, and elimination pathways. The aspect ratio is particularly crucial in determining toxicity outcomes. High-aspect-ratio NMs that are rigid and elongated can be recognized by macrophages; however, when their length exceeds macrophage dimensions, incomplete clearance may occur, potentially leading to lysosomal disruption and inflammasome activation, resulting in pro-inflammatory cytokine release. For example, single-walled carbon nanotubes (SWCNTs) demonstrate the ability to translocate from alveolar spaces to lung interstitium, promoting collagen deposition and fibrosis.

Hydrophilicity/Hydrophobicity

The surface hydrophilicity/hydrophobicity balance of NMs critically influences their environmental behavior and biological interactions. Enhanced hydrophilicity facilitates aqueous suspension, while hydrophobic characteristics promote lipid membrane interactions and cellular penetration. In biological environments, NMs readily acquire molecular coatings, such as serum albumin or pulmonary surfactants, which modify their stability and biological identity. In therapeutic applications, surface modification with biocompatible molecules like polyethylene glycol (PEG) is commonly employed to enhance colloidal stability through steric stabilization.

Agglomeration and Hetero-agglomeration

Although particle size serves as a defining characteristic for NMs at critical stages (e. g. during synthesis or delivery), this parameter exhibits substantial variability in environmental settings due to various physicochemical processes including dissolution, precipitation, agglomeration, and hetero-agglomeration. This dynamic behavior presents significant challenges in monitoring and predicting particle size distributions under realistic exposure conditions.

Agglomeration refers to the phenomenon whereby two or more particles of similar composition form loose associations through physical interactions, whereas hetero-agglomeration describes the formation of weak associations between particles of dissimilar compositions. NMs demonstrate a marked propensity for agglomerate formation in both dry and aqueous environments—an inherent consequence of their nanoscale dimensions, which result in intermolecular attractive forces that significantly exceed gravitational or other dispersive forces. The magnitude of interparticle attractive forces is governed by multiple parameters, including particle size, morphology, density, chemical composition, electronic structure, and surface charge characteristics. In aqueous media, van der Waals interactions and hydrophobic forces predominantly mediate the agglomeration of numerous types of NMs. To achieve stable dispersions of non-agglomerated NMs, researchers typically employ one of two strategies: ① Surface modification with macromolecular coatings such as polyethylene glycol (PEG) to provide steric stabilization; ② Introduction of surface charges to generate electrostatic repulsion between particles.

Surface Charge

The surface charge of NMs strongly influences the mode and type of interactions with biotic systems. A common indicator of surface charge is the "zeta potential (ζ)", which is the electrical potential at the outer surface of the liquid shell that travels with the particle during its motion. Cationic NMs are especially cytotoxic because they induce membrane damage, especially in lysosomes where the "proton sponge effect" leads to accumulation of water and chloride ions (Cl^-) and osmotic rupture.

Impurities

Industrial NMs are synthesized through various chemical processes and are purified to differing degrees. It is common for NMs to contain residual surfactants, ions, acids, bases, and other potential reaction contaminants. For instance, carbon nanotubes (CNTs) are synthesized in the presence of metal catalysts, usually iron, nickel, or cobalt, and may contain redox-active metal residues that can undergo redox cycling and iron-catalyzed generation of highly reactive ·OH via Fenton chemistry. It has been reported that release of yttrium ions (Y^{3+}) in trace levels from CNTs can displace Ca^{2+} from voltage-gated calcium channels, with implications for neuronal activity.

Chemical Transformation and Biopersistence

NMs undergo various transformations throughout their lifecycle, from manufacturing to environmental release and biological interactions. These transformations encompass dissolution, degradation, and formation of new chemical species through reactions with environmental constituents. The case of nanosilver exemplifies such transformations, involving oxidative dissolution, ion release, secondary particle formation, and conversion to sulfides or selenides. The extent and location of these transformations significantly influence toxicological outcomes.

Biopersistence, determined by mechanical clearance efficiency and dissolution kinetics, represents a crucial factor in environmental and biological toxicity assessment. While some metal oxide NMs demonstrate limited biopersistence due to enhanced dissolution in the presence of natural organic matter, others, particularly carbon-based NMs, exhibit high biopersistence. This characteristic raises concerns regarding potential bioaccumulation and long-term biological effects. For instance, certain commercial CNTs have demonstrated toxicological profiles reminiscent of asbestos fibers, emphasizing the importance of biopersistence in risk assessment.

"Nano-Bio" Interface

The extensive surface area of NMs provides a significant interface for interactions with diverse biological molecules, including proteins, lipids, nucleic acids, ions, and so on. This complex interplay between NMs and biological entities constitutes the "nano-bio" interface, a fundamental concept critical to elucidating the behavior and biological effects of NMs in living systems.

Protein Corona Formation

A key aspect of the nano-bio interface is the formation of "protein corona", a term proposed in 2007 to describe the spontaneous self-assembly and layering of proteins onto NMs surfaces when they enter biological fluids. Due to the unique surface characteristics of NMs, many serum proteins, also known as opsonins, can be deposited on their surfaces or enter the NMs to form dynamic protein coronas. These protein-functionalized NMs become recognizable to the immune system, facilitating their uptake by phagocytic cells.

The composition and structure of the protein corona can significantly influence the biological identity and fate of NMs in vivo. It's important to note that the protein corona is not a static entity but rather a dynamic structure that evolves over time, with proteins constantly associating and dissociating based on their affinity for the surface of NMs and their relative abundance in the biological medium.

Effects of Protein Adsorption on the Properties of NMs

Protein adsorption can markedly alter the physicochemical properties of NMs, including ① Surface charge: the adsorption of protein can neutralize or reverse the original surface charge of NMs; ② Hydrodynamic size: the protein layer increases the effective size of the NMs; ③ Surface hydrophobicity: proteins can mask or alter the hydrophobic/hydrophilic character of the surface of NMs; ④ Radius of curvature: the protein layer can change the effective curvature of the surface of NMs. These alterations in properties of NMs can significantly affect their distribution, cellular uptake, and biological fate in vivo.

Consequences of Interactions Between Proteins and NMs

The consequences of protein adsorption to NMs are complex, including: ① Protein denaturation: the interaction with surface of NMs may cause proteins to lose their native structure; ② Fibrillation or aggregation: some proteins may form fibrils or aggregates upon interaction with NMs; ③ Altered enzyme activity: the function of enzymes may be enhanced or inhibited when adsorbed to NMs; ④ Changes in biodistribution of NMs: the protein corona can influence how NMs are distributed in the body and their cellular uptake. Specific examples of proteins-NMs interactions have been extensively studied, particularly with plasma proteins. For instance, the adsorption of fibrinogen to NMs is of particular concern due to the potential to induce blood clot formation, a significant pathological consequence.

Implications for Drug Delivery and Biodistribution

The interaction of NMs with plasma proteins has profound implications for their use in DDS and their overall biological fate. The effects of the protein corona lie in three aspects. ① Circulation time: protein-coated NMs may have altered blood circulation time compared to bare NMs; ② Organ distribution: the protein corona can influence which organs the NMs accumulate in; ③ Clearance: protein-coated NMs may be more readily recognized by the mononuclear phagocyte system (MPS), leading to their removal from the circulatory system.

Understanding and manipulating these interactions opens up possibilities for tailoring the properties of NMs to achieve desired outcomes in drug delivery applications. For example, ① Extending blood circulation: by modifying the surface properties of NMs, it's possible to reduce protein adsorption and thereby extend their circulation time; ② Enhancing targeting: the protein corona can be engineered to promote accumulation of NMs in specific tissues or organs; ③ Controlling immune recognition: by manipulating the protein corona, it's possible to modulate how the immune system recognizes and responds to NMs.

"ADME" of NMs

Absorption of NMs

Absorption refers to the process by which NMs and their loaded drugs enter the bloodstream from various exposure routes. The primary portals of entry include the gastrointestinal (GI) tract, respiratory tract, and skin upon direct exposure to NMs. Intravenous injection allows NMs to directly enter the blood without an absorption process. In the bloodstream, the circulatory ability of NMs, their persistence, and their capacity to target pathological tissues such as tumors are determined by their size, colloid stability, ionic strength, and targeting moiety modification. However, absorption through non-intravenous administration routes (oral, inhalation and transdermal) requires NMs to pass through biological barriers. These routes also allow NMs to be transported to local lymph nodes before entering the bloodstream.

Oral administration is one of the most important and widely used delivery methods for

NMs, second only to intravenous injection. NMs can be absorbed into the blood through chemical and enzymatic barriers in the GI tract, as well as through absorption barriers in the intestinal epithelium. This occurs via several mechanisms, including passive cross-cell diffusion, paracellular pathway transport, carrier-mediated transcytosis, and M cell absorption. M cell-mediated absorption appears to be more conducive to NMs uptake, as it allows NMs to enter the intestinal lymphatic system, bypassing the first-pass effect. Subsequently, they can enter systemic circulation via the portal vein or the intestinal lymphatic pathway. For inhalation exposure, NMs in the lungs are primarily absorbed by macrophages and lymphatic uptake across the lung barrier. They may be cleared by alveolar macrophages or accumulate in lymph nodes within the pulmonary microenvironment. The skin itself presents the most significant obstacle for transdermal administration of NMs. To penetrate the skin, NMs must pass through the epidermis and dermis, with the stratum corneum (SC) being the main barrier. Two potential pathways exist for skin penetration: transepidermal pathway (across the SC) and transappendageal pathways (via the eccrine ducts and hair follicles). The transepidermal pathway is widely recognized as the primary route for cutaneous penetration. However, accumulating evidence demonstrates that the transappendageal pathway serves as an alternative and effective route for the skin permeation of macromolecules, nanoparticles, and microparticles. For instance, imidazole-based ionic liquid microemulsions have been shown to enhance nanomaterial absorption in vivo through dual mechanisms: disrupting the tightly packed keratinocyte arrangement and modulating the surface properties of the SC. Intramuscular and subcutaneous injections allow NMs to diffuse through connective tissue and capillary and lymphatic endothelial cell spaces. They are then rapidly transported through the membrane pores into systemic circulation, where they are mainly absorbed by macrophages and lymphocytes. Some of these NMs are phagocytized, while others enter the circulatory system through capillary lymph vessels.

Notably, while these absorption mechanisms have been summarized based on various administration routes, most studies are in vitro and lack systemic and holistic data. Therefore, these absorption pathways and mechanisms should be further verified through real-time in vivo experiments, which would require advanced in vivo tracer technology. Additionally, tracking both intact and disintegrated NMs could demonstrate differences between in vitro and in vivo methods.

Distribution of NMs

Distribution is defined as the process of transporting NMs and their payload from the blood to tissues, intercellular fluid, and cells. Several factors may affect the distribution profiles of NMs, including blood flow, vascular permeability, plasma protein content, the

MPS, complement system, and biological barriers.

At the tissue level, NMs are distributed throughout the body via blood circulation. The long-circulating nature of NMs in the blood prevents rapid clearance and provides sufficient time for drug accumulation at the target area. For example, compared to free ^{131}I that rapidly distributes throughout the body, ^{131}I carried by reduced graphene oxide (RGO) can be effectively delivered to the target site, enhancing internal radiotherapy of breast cancer while minimizing radiation damage to healthy tissues. Studies have shown that neutral and hydrophilic materials can escape macrophage uptake, prolonging the circulation time of NMs in vivo and promoting their accumulation in target tissues. Additionally, specific proteins can be utilized to modulate the surface chemistry of NMs, altering the composition of protein coronas, extending circulation time, enhancing biocompatibility, and reducing toxicity. Biokinetic studies have demonstrated that NMs rapidly distributed to organs with major reticuloendothelial system (RES) functions, particularly the liver, spleen and bone marrow. For instance, it is estimated that 30% - 90% of conventional NMs without functional modifications accumulate in the liver. Opsonization, a process introduced in 1903, tags particles with opsonins such as antibodies, complement system, making them more readily ingested by the MPS. However, opsonization can also mask target ligands on the surface of NMs, potentially decreasing their specificity to target tissues. This non-specific accumulation of NMs in the body not only reduces pharmacological effects but also increases safety risks. Despite generally low translocation rates of NMs from the portal of entry to secondary organs and efficient clearance mechanisms, continuous exposure may result in redistribution, leading to significant accumulation in some secondary organs.

At the cellular level, target cells may recognize untargeted NMs through surface scavenger receptors, lectin receptors, and Toll-like receptors that recognize hydrophobic domains. Conversely, NMs can also be designed to target specific cell surface receptors, triggering internalization via clathrin, caveolae, or lipid rafts. Following endocytosis or phagocytosis, NMs typically follow a well-defined intracellular pathway, often leading to fusion with lysosomes. The kinetics and mechanisms of cell uptake vary depending on the target cell, size, shape, and surface modifications of NMs. Most NMs are stored in membrane-bound vesicles, endosomes, or phagosomes.

Metabolism of NMs

Metabolism of NMs includes any process where the nanomaterial loses its original form, including degradation, transformation, and biotransformation. The metabolic fate of NMs is highly dependent on their inherent stability and biological reactivity. Biodegradable organic NMs are generally broken down into more hydrophilic, low molecular weight metabolites, which are subsequently excreted via renal or biliary routes. For inorganic NMs, metabolic fate is more variable: some inert metal-based NMs may remain relatively stable in vivo, whereas other inorganic NMs can undergo reactions with various biomolecules via oxidation, reduction, hydrolysis, or binding processes.

It is crucial to note that not all biodegradable NMs are inherently safe. Nanosilver, for example, can undergo two main metabolic pathways: the dissolution and release of Ag^{+} ions, and the transformation into silver sulfide. From a biological perspective, both enzymatic and non-enzymatic processes can lead to the metabolism of inorganic NMs. The resulting metabolites may have significant biological activity, including effects on drug transporters and metabolic enzymes, potentially leading to toxicity.

Elimination of NMs

The primary routes of elimination for NMs are renal and hepatic pathways, directly impacting their efficacy, circulation time, and potential side effects. Renal filtration is governed by strict size limitations: ① NMs with a hydrodynamic diameter (HD) of less than 5.5 nm can be efficiently removed through urine; ② Positively charged NMs with an HD larger than 8 nm can also be partially excreted in urine; ③ Larger, degradable NMs may be broken down into low molecular weight metabolites in the body and subsequently cleared by the kidneys. However, it should be noted that renal accumulation of these metabolites may contribute to renal dysfunction or kidney damage.

The hepatobiliary system is the primary route for removing NMs that have not undergone renal clearance. Fecal excretory clearance pathways consist of several inputs: one is mucociliary clearance of deposited particles from the airways into the GI tract; another is via hepatobiliary clearance of blood-borne NMs via liver and bile into the small intestine. In the liver, both Kupffer cells and hepatocytes are involved in NMs metabolism, albeit with different roles: ① Kupffer cells phagocytose and degrade intracellular NMs to achieve elimination; ② NMs that avoid phagocytosis by Kupffer cells can enter into hepatocytes and undergo bile excretion. Like renal clearance, bile excretion also heavily depends on the hydrodynamic diameter and surface charges of NMs, with hepatocytes more prone to take up positively charged NMs. Generally, hepatobiliary excretion is slower than renal clearance, occurring over a period ranging from hours to months.

Toxicity Mechanisms and Research Methods

The toxicity of NMs is a complex and multifaceted issue that requires comprehensive study at various levels of biological organization. While measurements of impacts at the community and ecosystem level are less common for NMs compared to traditional chemical toxicants, significant progress has been made in understanding their effects on human beings and animals. Oxidative stress has emerged as a primary mechanism by which NMs exert toxicity. NMs have been observed to generate excess reactive oxygen species (ROS), leading to a cascade of cellular events, involing in lipid peroxidation, inactivating structural proteins, enzymes, ion pumps, and DNA damage. The specific cellular response to NMs depends on several factors, including type of NMs, dose, duration of exposure, and the target cells. These factors can activate cell-type-specific signaling pathways, potentially leading to cell proliferation, apoptosis, stress-related signaling, and calcium-mediated signal transduction events. Dysregulation of calcium ion homeostasis is particularly important and can arise from several mechanisms: ① Influx across a damaged plasma membrane; ② Release of Ca^{2+} ions from Ca-based NMs; ③ Disruption of intracellular calcium stores in organelles like the mitochondria and endoplasmic reticulum. Sustained elevation in intracellular calcium concentrations can ultimately induce cell death through necrosis.

Worthy to notice, the toxicity of NMs is closely linked to their physicochemical properties, which are determined by their structure, size, composition, and morphology. These properties can significantly influence the biological interactions and potential adverse effects of NMs. To accurately identify and characterize the hazard associated with NMs, both in vitro and in vivo studies are essential. Results should be derived from well-designed dose-response relationships. Key considerations for designing such studies include: ① Careful characterizations of the structure and physicochemical properties of NMs; ② Determination of the most relevant exposure route; ③ Justification of the dosing regimen; ④ Selection of appropriate target cells, tissues, or animal species; ⑤ Choice of suitable endpoints. Additionally, the inclusion of reference NMs can be valuable for ranking unknown NMs against known positive and/or negative controls.

In vivo toxicological studies are particularly important as they allow for a full evaluation of exposure-dose-response relationships. This information is crucial for predicting human equivalent exposure concentrations or occupational exposure limits (OELs) in risk assessment. However, it is important to acknowledge the limitations of these studies: Anatomical and physiological differences between experimental animals and humans; and Challenges in extrapolating from high-dose, short-term exposures to chronic, low-dose scenarios typically encountered in human environmental exposures. Most current studies employ a variety of cellular toxicity assays using relatively high concentrations for toxicological evaluation. This approach may not accurately reflect real-world exposure scenarios, where humans are typically exposed to low doses of NMs over extended periods. To address these challenges and improve our understanding towards toxicities of NMs, there is an ongoing need to develop additional tools for toxicology testing. ① In silico models: computational approaches to predict toxicities of NMs based on physicochemical properties and structural characteristics; ② Advanced in vitro systems: development of 3D cell cultures, organoids, and microfluidic devices to better mimic in vivo conditions; ③ Improved *in vivo* models: refinement of animal models and development of humanized animal models to better predict human responses; ④ High-throughput screening methods: to rapidly assess the potential toxicity of a wide range of NMs; ⑤ Long-term, low-dose exposure studies: to better understand the effects of chronic exposure to NMs at environmentally relevant concentrations. These advancements will help to bridge the gap between *in vitro* and *in vivo* studies, improve the accuracy of risk assessments, and ultimately enhance our ability to predict and assess the risks of human exposure to NMs.

Limitations and Future Directions

As nanotechnology continues to advance at a rapid pace, it is imperative that research efforts ensure its sustainable integration into human society, with due considerations given to ethical and safety concerns. Nanotoxicology plays a pivotal role in this process, being indispensable in addressing emerging challenges and safeguarding human health and the environment from potential hazards associated with NMs.

Despite significant progress, the field of nanotoxicology still faces several key limitations. ① Limited scope of study: to date, most nanotoxicology research has focused on a relatively narrow range of simple NMs with existing or potential high manufacturing volume. As nanotechnology evolves, there is an urgent need to expand this focus to include more complex and newly developed NMs, particularly as these materials approach commercialization; ② Challenge in risk assessment: acquiring comprehensive toxicological profiles for the multitude of newly-developed NMs anticipated in the coming decades presents a significant challenge. Ongoing efforts in the risk assessment of NMs are valuable and must be continued and expanded to keep pace with the rapid development of diverse NMs; ③ Methodology gaps: there is a lack of well-established methodologies for identification of critical effects, extrapolation of toxicokinetics and toxicity data from in vitro to in vivo system, and translating findings across species. These gaps highlight the need for additional studies to fully evaluate the potential risk of NMs across different sectors of applications; ④ Limited expertise: the field of nanotoxicology requires further expansion of its research community to address the growing complexity and diversity of NMs.

Recognizing the concept of "Leading science and technology, safe products" as a national strategic goal in many countries, product safety is increasingly recognized as a critical factor in both national development and economic success. Globally, there is a growing focus on the biosafety of NMs, as evidenced by the fact that many nations, including China, are actively engaging in research on this topic, underscoring the global recognition of the importance of understanding and mitigating the potential risks associated with nanotechnology. The environmental health effects of NMs and occupational health protection have emerged as strategic priorities in the nanotechnology development strategies of numerous countries, indicating a concerted effort to promote safe applications and sustainable development. Future research initiatives should focus on several key areas: ① Embracing interdisciplinary approaches that integrate nanotoxicology with materials science, environmental science, and public health to develop a comprehensive understanding of NMs interactions with biological systems; ② Developing advanced testing methods such as high-throughput screening, improved in vitro models (e. g. 3D cell cultures, organoids), and more robust in silico prediction tools to facilitate more efficient and accurate assessment of toxicities of NMs; ③ Establishing standardized protocols and reference materials to ensure consistency and comparability of nanotoxicology studies across different laboratories and countries; ④ Conducting comprehensive life cycle assessments for NMs to fully understand their potential environmental and health impacts from production through disposal.

(Zhong Xiaoyan)

CHAPTER 18

Toxic Effects of Radiation and Radioactive Materials

Introduction

The advancement of nuclear science and technology has brought significant progress to human society, with applications spanning agriculture, industry, military affairs, and medicine. However, the expanding utilization of nuclear and radiation technologies has concomitantly increased human exposure to ionizing radiation, raising concerns about potential health consequences. The occurrence of nuclear and radiation accidents has drawn unprecedented global attention to the safety of nuclear and radiation practices. Incidents resulting in acute radiation syndrome and associated fatalities underscore the critical need for a comprehensive understanding of the biological effects of ionizing radiation and the development of effective mitigation strategies.

Radiation toxicology investigates the detrimental effects of ionizing radiation and radioactive substances on living organisms. This discipline seeks to elucidate the mechanisms by which radiation induces adverse effects across various levels of biological organization, from the molecular and cellular to the tissue and systemic levels. This knowledge is paramount for assessing and mitigating the health risks posed by ionizing radiation exposure, and informs the development of effective countermeasures, including medical interventions and public health policies.

This chapter provides a comprehensive and contemporary overview of the biological effects of radiation and radioactive materials, aiming to enhance understanding of radiation-induced biological responses and improve risk management strategies associated with ionizing radiation exposure.

Source and Characteristics of Ionizing Radiation

The Nature of Ionizing Radiation

Radiation is defined as the emission or transmission of energy through space or a material medium in the form of waves or particles. Radiation can be categorized into two main types based on its ability to ionize matter: ionizing radiation and non-ionizing radiation.

Ionizing radiation is characterized by its ability to remove electrons from atoms or molecules, thereby creating ions. This process occurs when the radiation possesses sufficient energy, typically greater than 10 electron volts (eV). Ionizing radiation comprises two main categories: electromagnetic ionizing radiation and particulate ionizing radiation. Electromagnetic ionizing radiation includes X-rays and gamma rays (γ-rays), which are high-energy photons capable of penetrating matter. Particulate ionizing radiation consists of subatomic particles with varying masses and charges. This category includes alpha particles (α), which are essentially helium nuclei; beta particles (β), which can be either electrons (negative beta particles) or positrons (positive beta particles); neutrons (n), which are uncharged particles; protons (p), which are positively charged particles; and heavy charged particles, such as accelerated ions of elements heavier than hydrogen. Each of these types of ionizing radiation interacts with matter in unique ways, leading to different patterns of energy deposition and biological effects.

Non-ionizing radiation refers to types of electromagnetic radiation that do not have sufficient energy to ionize atoms or molecules. This includes radio waves, microwaves, infrared, visible light, and some ultraviolet radiation. While non-ionizing radiation can cause thermal effects and excite electrons to higher energy states, it does not produce charged ions when passing through matter. Common sources of non-ionizing radiation include cell phones, Wi-Fi routers, microwave ovens, and the sun. Although non-ionizing radiation can have biological effects, particularly at high intensities, it generally poses lower health risks compared to ionizing radiation. However, the discussion of non-ionizing radiation is beyond the scope of this chapter, which focuses primarily on the toxicology of ionizing radiation.

Sources of Ionizing Radiation

Ionizing radiation originates from two primary sources: natural and artificial. While public concern often focuses on artificial radiation sources, it is important to note that natural background radiation contributes significantly to the overall radiation exposure of the general population.

Natural Radiation: Natural radiation sources can be categorized into three main types, cosmic rays, cosmogenic radionuclides, and primordial radionuclides.

Cosmic rays originate from outer space and consist of primary and secondary components. Primary cosmic rays, mainly composed of protons, alpha particles, and heavy nuclei, interact with atmospheric elements to produce secondary cosmic rays. These secondary particles, including neutrons, protons, muons, and photons, are the principal cosmic radiation reaching the Earth's surface.

Cosmogenic radionuclides are produced by nuclear reactions between cosmic rays and atmospheric or terrestrial nuclei. The most significant cosmogenic radionuclides for human exposure are ^{3}H, ^{7}Be, ^{14}C, and ^{22}Na, primarily ingested through food and water.

Primordial radionuclides have existed since Earth's formation and include three natural radioactive series (uranium, thorium, and actinium) and single-decay nuclides like ^{40}K and ^{87}Rb. These are found in soil, building materials, and food.

Radon, particularly ^{222}Rn, and its decay products constitute the primary source of natural radiation exposure for humans. Human activities have altered the natural distribution of uranium, leading to diverse radon sources. These include terrestrial and marine releases, as well as emissions from the nuclear industry, coal combustion, and building materials.

Artificial radiation: In addition to natural radiation, humans are exposed to artificial radiation sources through various practical activities. These sources of artificial radiation arise from human-made or processed natural sources. The primary sources of artificial radiation today include nuclear weapons: The production, testing, and use of nuclear weapons generate significant amounts of artificial radiation; Nuclear energy: The production of nuclear energy involves processes that release controlled amounts of artificial radiation; Nuclear technology applications: This includes medical diagnostic and therapeutic procedures using radiation, such as X-rays radiography computed tomography (CT) scans, as well as the use of radioactive pharmaceuticals; Nuclear accidents: Incidents like the Chernobyl disaster result in considerable radiation exposure; Radiation from radioactive waste: Waste generated from nuclear reactors and accelerators is another source of artificial radiation.

Additionally, certain human activities can lead to increased exposure to natural radiation sources. These activities include the mining and utilization of coal, oil, and other naturally occurring radioactive materials, energy production from coal-fired power plants, and frequent air travel. Understanding these sources and their impact is crucial for managing radiation exposure and ensuring public safety.

Generation of Ionizing Radiation

Ionizing radiation arises from two fundamental processes: nuclear processes and non-nuclear processes.

Nuclear processes are intimately linked to the atomic nucleus and involve nuclear reactions or nuclear decay. The atomic nucleus, despite occupying only one ten-thousandth of the atom's size, accounts for over 99.9% of its mass and carries a positive charge equal in magnitude to the sum of the negatively charged electrons orbiting it. Composed of protons and neutrons, the nucleus of unstable atoms, known as radioactive nuclides, can spontaneously emit various types of radiation. Alpha particles (α), consisting of two protons and two neutrons, are emitted by heavy radioactive nuclides such as uranium and plutonium isotopes. These particles have a short range and weak penetration power but possess strong ionizing effects. Beta particles are high-speed electrons emitted by the nucleus of radioactive isotopes like ^{131}I and ^{90}Sr. They have greater penetration power than alpha particles but less than gamma rays. Gamma rays are high-energy electromagnetic waves emitted by excited nuclei. They exhibit the highest penetration power among these three types of radiation but have the weakest ionizing ability. Neutrons, uncharged particles with significant penetration ability, are also emitted in some nuclear processes and can induce radioactivity in other materials through collisions.

Non-nuclear processes generate ionizing radiation through interactions involving extra-nuclear electrons or the acceleration of particle beams. X-rays, a prime example, are produced when high-speed electrons interact with matter, either through bremsstrahlung (deceleration radiation) or by electron transitions between atomic energy levels. The resulting X-ray spectrum includes both continuous (bremsstrahlung) and discrete (characteristic) components. Particle accelerators can produce various forms of ionizing radiation, including electron beams, proton beams, and heavy ion beams. Heavy ions, defined as atomic nuclei with atomic numbers greater than 2 that have been partially or fully stripped of their electrons, are of particular interest in radiation research and therapy due to their unique interaction properties with matter.

The Modes of Ionizing Radiation Impact on the Human Body

Ionizing radiation sources encompass a wide range of substances and devices capable of emitting ionizing radiation. These sources can be broadly categorized into sealed sources, unsealed sources, and radiation-generating devices. Sealed sources contain radioactive materials securely encased or consolidated within a solid coating, minimizing the risk of environmental contamination. In contrast, unsealed sources lack permanent containment, potentially leading to workplace or environmental contamination during use. This distinction is crucial, as unsealed sources may allow radionuclides to enter the human body through various pathways. Radiation-generating devices, such as X-ray machines, accelerators, and neutron generators, produce ionizing radiation without the use of radioactive materials.

The impact of ionizing radiation on the human body can be classified into two primary modes: internal irradiation and external irradiation. Internal irradiation occurs when radionuclides enter the body through inhalation, ingestion, skin absorption, or wound contamination. This form of exposure is particularly concerning as it results in continuous irradiation of internal organs and tissues. The duration of internal exposure depends on both the physical half-life of the radionuclide and its biological retention time within the body. Irradiation persists until the radionuclide decays to a stable form or is completely eliminated from the body through natural processes or medical intervention.

External irradiation results from exposure to radiation sources outside the body. This can occur in various scenarios, including medical procedures like radiation therapy, occupational exposures, or environmental sources. A key characteristic of external irradiation is its immediate cessation upon removal from the radiation source. However, it's important to note that while the active irradiation stops, biological effects may continue to manifest over time.

Physicochemical Basis of Ionizing Radiation-Induced Damage

Ionizing radiation is characterized by its ability to remove electrons from atoms or molecules, a process known as ionization. When ionizing radiation interacts with biological systems, it initiates a complex series of events that can lead to significant effects at the molecular, cellular, and organismal levels. The fundamental mechanism underlying these effects involves the transfer of energy from radiation to matter, specifically to the atoms and molecules that constitute living tissues.

Direct Effects and Indirect Effects

The biological effects of ionizing radiation can be broadly categorized into two main types: direct effects and indirect effects.

Direct effects occur when radiation energy is absorbed directly by large biological molecules, such as DNA, proteins, or lipids. This absorption leads to ionization and excitation of these molecules, resulting in structural alterations that can compromise their biological function. This immediate interaction between radiation and critical cellular components is termed direct action.

Indirect effects involve a more complex pathway. Ionizing radiation primarily interacts with water molecules, which are abundant in biological systems. This interaction triggers the radiolysis of water, producing highly reactive free radicals and other reactive oxygen species (ROS). These unstable molecules then diffuse and interact with nearby biological molecules, inducing secondary physical and chemical changes. This process, known as indirect action, is responsible for a significant portion of radiation-induced damage in biological systems.

The relative contribution of direct effects and indirect effects depends on various factors, including the type and energy of radiation, the presence of oxygen, and the target molecule's characteristics. For instance, high-LET (Linear Energy Transfer) radiation, such as alpha particles, tends to cause more direct effects, while low-LET radiation, like X-rays or gamma rays, predominantly induces indirect effects through water radiolysis.

Time Course of Biological Effects Induced by Ionizing Radiation

Ionizing radiation interacts with biological systems through a complex series of physical, chemical, and biological processes, occurring across vastly different timescales. The initial interaction, known as the physical stage, takes place within an incredibly brief period of 10^{-18} to 10^{-13} seconds. During this phase, energy is transferred from the radiation to atoms and molecules in the biological system, resulting in excitation or ionization. The spatial distribution of these events is largely determined by the type and energy of the incident radiation. This physical stage is immediately followed by the physico-chemical stage, lasting from 10^{-13} to 10^{-10} seconds, during which rapid chemical reactions occur. Most notably, the radiolysis of water leads to the formation of free radicals such as hydroxyl radicals, hydrogen atoms, and hydrated electrons. These highly reactive species can diffuse over short distances and interact with critical biological molecules. The ensuing chemical stage, spanning from 10^{-10} to 10^{-6} seconds, involves interactions between these free radicals and cellular components, potentially leading to the formation of peroxides, breakage of chemical bonds, and other molecular alterations. DNA, proteins, and lipids are particularly susceptible to these chemical modifications. The final biological stage encompasses the cellular and tissue responses to radiation-induced damage, including the activation of repair mechanisms. If these repair processes are unsuccessful or incomplete, cellular dysfunction or death may occur. Moreover, long-term effects such as mutations or cancer induction may manifest over extended periods. This comprehensive understanding of the stages involved in radiation-induced damage provides crucial insights into the underlying mechanisms of biological effects and informs the development of radioprotective strategies and therapies for radiation-induced injuries.

Biological Effects of Ionizing Radiation

Molecular Biological Effects of Ionizing Radiation

The biological effects of ionizing radiation primarily stem from energy transfer to biomolecules, with DNA being the most critical target. Radiation-induced DNA damage manifests mainly as strand breaks and crosslinks, each with distinct characteristics and implications for cellular function.

DNA strand breaks occur as single-strand breaks (SSB) and double-strand breaks (DSB), with DSB typically occurring at a frequency of 1/20 to 1/10 that of SSB. The ratio of SSB to DSB is influenced by the LET of the radiation, with high-LET radiation like neutrons producing proportionally more DSB than low-LET radiation such as X-rays or gamma rays.

Oxygen concentration in the cellular environment also plays a crucial role, enhancing strand break formation by increasing the production of hydroxyl radicals.

The pattern of DNA base damage varies with radiation dose. At low doses (<10 Gy), guanine is most susceptible to damage, followed by adenine, thymine, and cytosine. However, at higher doses (40–80 Gy), this order changes, with thymine becoming most vulnerable. These patterns reflect the complex interplay between radiation energy, molecular structures, and cellular conditions.

DNA crosslinking, another significant form of radiation damage, typically occurs at doses between 20–100 Gy. This type of damage can severely impair DNA function by preventing strand separation necessary for replication and transcription.

In response to radiation-induced DNA damage, cells employ a variety of repair mechanisms. These include base excision repair, nucleotide excision repair, single-strand break repair, and double-strand break repair pathways such as homologous recombination and non-homologous end joining. The efficiency and fidelity of these repair processes significantly influence cell survival and the potential for mutation or carcinogenesis. While DNA repair mechanisms often successfully restore genomic integrity, some damage may persist, leading to cellular adaptations or, in severe cases, cell death.

Cellular Biological Effects of Ionizing Radiation

The radiosensitivity of cells refers to their varying response to ionizing radiation under identical exposure conditions. This sensitivity generally follows the *Bergonie & Tribondeau Law*, which states that radiosensitivity is directly proportional to a cell's division rate and inversely proportional to its differentiation level. However, exceptions exist, such as lymphocytes, which are highly radiosensitive despite being differentiated.

Cells can be broadly categorized based on their radiosensitivity. Highly sensitive cells include lymphocytes, hematopoietic cells, and intestinal epithelial cells. Moderately sensitive cells include ganglion and muscle cells, while cartilage and bone cells are relatively insensitive. Tumors also exhibit varying radiosensitivity, with malignant lymphomas being highly sensitive and melanomas being resistant.

Ionizing radiation significantly impacts cellular processes, particularly the cell cycle. Post-irradiation, cells experience DNA synthesis inhibition and cell cycle arrests, allowing time for DNA repair or clearance. This response is crucial for maintaining genetic stability.

Radiation can induce various forms of cell death, including necrosis, apoptosis, autophagic cell death, and mitotic catastrophe. Proliferative death occurs when cells lose their ability to divide after several post-irradiation mitotic cycles. Interphase death involves cells dying without division, while autophagic cell death is characterized by the degradation of cellular components through autophagy. Mitotic catastrophe results from aberrant cell division due to radiation-induced DNA damage or spindle disruption.

Carcinogenic Effects of Radiation

Radiation-induced carcinogenesis is a complex, multi-stage process initiated by the interaction of ionizing radiation with biological systems. This interaction triggers genomic instability and disrupts cellular signaling pathways. The primary mechanism begins with radiation-induced DNA damage, which can lead to gene mutations and initiate the transformation of normal cells into cancerous ones.

It's crucial to understand that carcinogenesis is not determined by a single gene or radiation-specific genes, but rather is a stochastic process involving multiple genes in the progeny of irradiated cells.

Various factors influence radiation carcinogenesis, including the type of radiation (e. g. X-rays, gamma rays, neutrons, alpha or beta particles), dose and dose rate. External exposure and internal contamination by radioactive nuclei can both contribute to carcinogenic effects. Non-radiation factors, such as genetic predisposition and age of organism at exposure, also play significant roles in determining the likelihood and severity of radiation-induced cancers.

A key characteristic of radiation carcinogenesis is the presence of a latency period between exposure and cancer manifestation. This period varies depending on the cancer type: leukemia typically has a latency of 3–5 years, thyroid cancer has a latency of 10–15 years, while lung and breast cancers may take 15–20 years or longer to develop. Recent studies have provided compelling evidence that even long-term exposure to low-dose radiation can increase the risk of leukemogenesis, highlighting the potential risks associated with chronic low-level radiation exposure.

Acute Radiation Syndrome (ARS)

Acute Radiation Syndrome, also known as radiation sickness, is a severe condition resulting from exposure to high doses of ionizing radiation (>1 Gy) over a short period. This exposure can be from external sources such as X-rays, gamma rays, and neutrons, or internal contamination, with external sources occurring more frequently.

ARS can occur in various scenarios, including nuclear accidents, warfare, or medical mishaps. Symptoms vary depending on the radiation dose and can include fatigue, dizziness, skin lesions, bleeding, hair loss, vomiting, and diarrhea. Long-term effects may include an increased risk of cancer and genetic mutations.

The severity of ARS correlates with the radiation dose received. Based on the affected organ systems and dose ranges, ARS is classified into three types:

(1) Bone Marrow Syndrome (1–10 Gy): This type primarily affects the hematopoietic system, leading to decreased blood cell counts, infections, and bleeding. It progresses through four stages: prodromal, latent, manifest illness, and recovery or death. The severity is categorized as mild, moderate, severe, or extremely severe.

(2) Gastrointestinal Syndrome (10 – 50 Gy): This more severe form of ARS is characterized by damage to the gastrointestinal tract. Symptoms include severe vomiting, diarrhea, and electrolyte imbalances. The syndrome progresses through initial, latent, and manifest illness phases.

(3) Cerebrovascular Syndrome (> 50 Gy): This most severe form of ARS involves damage to the central nervous system. Symptoms include impaired consciousness, ataxia, seizures, and tremors. It rapidly progresses through initial and manifest illness phases.

The Biological Effects of Internal Irradiation by Radioactive Nuclides

Radiation toxicology investigates the biological effects of radioactive nuclides within the body, encompassing their absorption, distribution, metabolism, and excretion. This field aims to establish safe exposure limits and develop protective measures to minimize the risks associated with radioactive contamination.

Disposition of Radioactive Nuclides within the Body

The metabolism of radioactive nuclides in the body is influenced by their inherent physical and chemical properties, route of entry, and tendency to accumulate in specific tissues. Nuclides can enter the body through ingestion, inhalation, skin absorption, or wounds, with inhalation being the most common. Once internalized, nuclides may distribute uniformly throughout the body or concentrate in specific organs like radioactive iodine in the thyroid.

Elimination occurs through multiple routes, including gastrointestinal, respiratory, and urinary systems. The rate of elimination is characterized by the effective half-life (T_e), which considers both radioactive decay (physical half-life, T_p) and biological clearance (biological half-life, T_b).

The effective half-life can be calculated using the following formula:

$$T_e = \frac{T_p \cdot T_b}{T_p + T_b}$$

Where: T_e is the effective half-life. T_p is the physical half-life of the radioactive nuclide, which is a constant for a given isotope and represents the time required for half of the radioactive atoms to decay. T_b is the biological half-life, defined as the time required for half of a radionuclide to be eliminated from the body through biological processes, varies with the specific nuclide, the type of tissue, and the biological processes involved in the elimination of the nuclide from the body.

Internal irradiation exerts its effects through both direct and indirect mechanisms. Direct effects involve energy deposition from emitted particles or rays, directly ionizing and damaging biomolecules. Indirect effects arise from the interaction of radiation with water molecules, generating ROS and free radicals that damage DNA, proteins, and lipids. The severity of these effects depends on factors like radiation type and energy, oxygen concentration, and the presence of antioxidants. The impact of radioactive nuclides is characterized by sustained duration, typically assessed over six effective half-lives, and can exert both radiological and chemical toxicity.

The biological impact of internal irradiation is influenced by a multitude of factors. The physicochemical properties of the nuclide, including its physical state, solubility, and chemical form, affect its absorption, distribution, and retention within the body. Intrinsic biological factors, such as species, age, sex, and overall health, can also significantly influence susceptibility to radiation damage. For instance, younger individuals are generally more radiosensitive, and certain elements may exhibit sex-specific patterns of accumulation and toxicity. Additionally, the route of exposure, dose and dose rate, and the presence of other stressors (e. g. chemical toxins) can modify the biological response to internal irradiation.

Effects of Internal Irradiation of Radioactive Nuclides

Radioactive nuclides are classified into four toxicity levels based on their annual limit of intake (ALI): extremely toxic, highly toxic, moderately toxic, and low toxicity. This classification aids in risk management and radiation protection strategies.

Effects of internal irradiation can be categorized as short-term effects (occurring within weeks) or long-term effects (manifesting months to years after exposure). They can also be classified as somatic effects (affecting the irradiated individual) or genetic effects (impacting offspring).

From a radiation protection perspective, internal irradiation effects are divided into deterministic effects and stochastic effects. Deterministic effects have a dose threshold and their severity increases with dose. They result from high-dose radiation damage to cell populations. Stochastic effects, such as genetic mutations and some cancers, have no dose threshold, and their probability of occurrence increases with dose.

Diagnosis and Medical Treatment of Internal Radiation Disease

Diagnostic Criteria for Internal Radiation Disease

Internal radiation disease arises from the systemic and localized damage caused by the intake of radioactive nuclides. Clinical manifestations can be diverse, ranging from non-specific symptoms like fatigue, nausea, and hematopoietic abnormalities to organ-specific damage depending on the nuclide's biodistribution.

Confirmation of the disease requires meeting one of the following criteria: ① A single or short-term entry into the body with a cumulative effective dose equivalent possibly exceeding 1.0 Sv with documented personal dose records and health records; ② Continuous, repeated intakes over an extended period, leading to a dose intake many times higher than the annual limit.

Medical Treatment of Internal Radiation Disease

Medical treatment for internal contamination focuses on mitigating further uptake, enhancing elimination, and managing clinical symptoms. Treatment strategies are tailored to the specific radioactive nuclide, considering its properties and route of entry. Immediate actions may involve decontamination procedures such as gastric lavage for ingested nuclides or nasal irrigation for inhaled particles. Additionally, enhancing natural elimination pathways through increased fluid intake, diuretics, or specific medications that bind to and sequester the radioactive material may be employed. Supportive care, including blood transfusions, antibiotics, and medications to manage symptoms, plays a critical role in patient management. Overall, treatment emphasizes a multi-faceted approach to minimize the long-term consequences of internal radiation exposure.

Radiation Protection

Radiation protection is a fundamental discipline in nuclear science and technology, dedicated to safeguarding the health of individuals, future generations, and the environment from the potential harms of ionizing radiation.

Principles of Radiation Protection

The foundation of radiation protection is built upon three fundamental principles: justification of radiation practices, optimization of protection measures, and adherence to personal dose limits.

Every activity involving radiation exposure must be justified, ensuring that the total benefit outweighs the total cost and risk. The principle of optimization, often referred to as ALARA (As Low As Reasonably Achievable), mandates that radiation exposure be minimized by all practical means, taking into account economic and social factors. Finally, dose limits are established to define acceptable boundaries for radiation exposure. For occupational exposure, the effective dose limit is an average of 20 mSv per year over a period of 5 consecutive years, with a maximum of 50 mSv in any single year. The public dose limit is 1 mSv per year, averaged over 5 years.

Protective Measures for external Radiation Exposure

Protecting against external radiation exposure primarily involves minimizing the time spent near a radiation source, maximizing distance from the source, and employing appropriate shielding. Radiation intensity decreases rapidly with increasing distance, so even small increases in distance can drastically reduce exposure. When working with radioactive materials, shielding provides a barrier to absorb or attenuate radiation before it reaches individuals. The choice of shielding material hinges on the type and energy of the radiation emitted. Alpha particles are easily stopped by a sheet of paper, beta particles require denser materials, such as plastic or aluminum for shielding. High-energy photons, such as X-rays and gamma rays, require much denser materials like lead or concrete for effective attenuation.

Neutron radiation is more challenging to shield against and often requires a combination of hydrogenous materials (e. g. water, polyethylene) to slow down neutrons, and neutron absorbers like boron to capture neutrons.

Protective Measures for Internal Radiation Exposure

Internal radiation protection focuses on preventing the uptake of radioactive substances into the body. This can be achieved through a combination of engineering controls, personal protective equipment, and stringent handling procedures. Isolating radioactive materials during handling, using fume hoods or glove boxes, prevents their release into the work environment. Dilution, by increasing ventilation or adding a non-radioactive carrier to a solution, can also effectively reduce the concentration of radioactive material in air or water, thereby minimizing potential uptake. Personal protective equipment, such as gloves, lab coats, and respirators, provides a barrier against skin contact or inhalation. The rigorous decontamination procedures to remove any radioactive contamination from personnel or equipment are equally important. Finally, responsible radioactive waste management is paramount for long-term protection. This includes minimizing waste generation, proper waste segregation and storage.

(Cao Yi)

CHAPTER 19

Chronotoxicology

Introduction

Survival of the fittest is the law of survival for all organisms on Earth. In order to adapt to various periodic changes in the environment, different organisms exhibit periodically recurring characteristics in physiology, behavior and other aspects, which are known as biological rhythms. Chronobiology refers to the science that studies the biochemical, physiological, and behavioral rhythms and their mechanisms produced by organisms as it adapts to periodic changes in the environment.

Rhythmic events can be represented by parameters such as period, phase and amplitude (Figure 19-1). ① Period: Biological clocks are free-running. Period is the amount of time it takes to complete a cycle. Period is typically measured from peak to peak, but it can be measured from any specific position on the curve. ② Phase: Phase is the relative position on the trace (e. g. the peak) in relation to a specific time (e. g. the time at the beginning of dark conditions). If one rhythmic event precedes another in terms of peak or trough occurrence, it is considered to have an advanced phase, whereas a delayed occurrence indicates a delayed phase. ③ Amplitude: Amplitude is the measurement of the recorded power from the midline of the curve to either the peak or the trough. The amplitude level may reflect the strength of the biological rhythm.

Different biological rhythms have different cycle lengths, which can be categorized into three types according to the duration of the rhythmic cycles: ① **Ultradian Rhythm**,

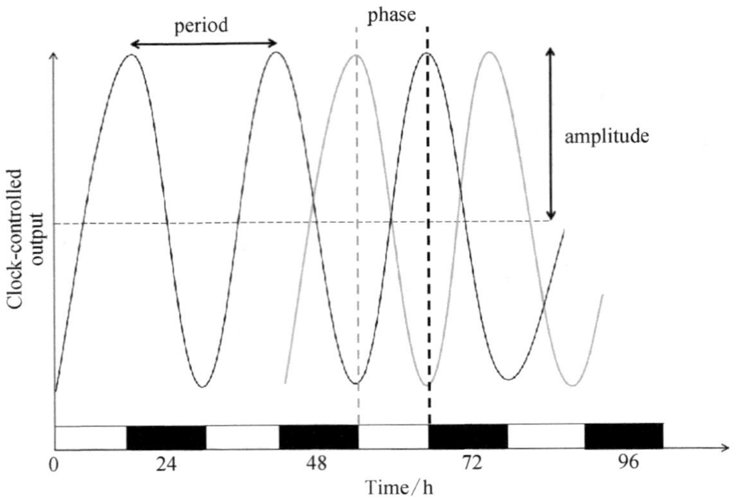

Figure 19-1 **Characteristics of a circadian rhythm**

characterized by a cycle shorter than 20 hours, ranging from a few hours to minutes or even seconds, such as heart rate, respiration, etc. ② **Infradian Rhythm**, characterized by a cycle significantly longer than 24 hours, typically exceeding 28 hours and possibly extending over days, months or even longer. Menstrual cycles, seasonal reproduction, hibernation and migration are examples of infradian rhythms, among others. ③ **Circadian Rhythm**, also called diurnal rhythm, with a cycle approximately 24 hours, including feeding behaviors, regulation of the sleep-wake cycle, and metabolic homeostasis. In this chapter, biological rhythm refers to circadian rhythm, while the biological clock refers specifically to the circadian clock.

Chronotoxicology, a branch of chronobiology, is the scientific study of the interaction and its mechanisms between exogenous harmful factors and endogenous biological rhythms. Chronotoxicology focuses on two main aspects. Firstly, it applies the theories and methods of chronobiology to study the influence of an organism's endogenous biological rhythms on the action and metabolism of toxicants in the body. Secondly, it examines the disruptive effects of toxicants on the body's biological rhythms, with particular emphasis on the temporal impacts of these substances and the intricate time-dose and time-effect relationships underlying their toxic effects. This approach provides a comprehensive understanding of the temporal dynamics of toxicity and its complex interaction with biological rhythms.

Given the profound influence of biological rhythms on the physiological functions and behavioral patterns of organisms, the study of chronotoxicology is of immense importance in elucidating the biological effects and toxicities of toxicants. Such studies provide valuable insights for more accurate risk assessment and prediction, ultimately leading to the formulation of more precisely targeted and effective preventive and therapeutic interventions.

Time is a fundamental physical quantity that measures the duration of events and the intervals between them. It is perceived as the continuous, progressive movement or flow of existence and events from the past through the present to the future. Time is often measured using clocks and calendars, which are devices and systems that represent, track, and display the passage of time.

In physics, time is considered as one of the seven fundamental physical quantities, and it is used to describe change in other physical quantities, such as position, velocity, and acceleration. The International System (SI) of Units defines the second as the base unit of time.

In philosophy, time has been a subject of much debate and speculation, with different views on its nature, origin, and relation to the universe. Some philosophers argue that time is an illusion or a construct of the human mind, while others view it as an objective, physical reality.

In daily life, time is an essential aspect of human activity and organization. We use time to plan events, schedule appointments, and coordinate actions. Time also plays a role in our perception of reality and the ordering of events.

In biology, time refers to the internal timing mechanism that regulates various biological processes and behaviors in organisms. It is a system of biological oscillations that enables organisms to anticipate and adapt to the cyclic changes in their environment, such as the day-night cycle.

Synopsis of Circadian Clock

The circadian clock (from the Latin "circa diem" or about a day), as a mechanism for regulating time in organisms, is an invisible "timekeeper" with an endogenous rhythm close to 24 hours that affects many physiological processes and aspects of daily life. A mismatch between the endogenous biological clock and the exogenous light-dark cycle can cause significant distress and dysfunction.

In mammals, the master circadian pacemaker, located in the suprachiasmatic nucleus (SCN) of the anterior hypothalamus generates circadian rhythmicity and orchestrates numerous subsidiary local clocks in other regions of the brain and peripheral tissues. Regardless of their location, these circadian clocks are cell-autonomous and self-sustaining, implicating rhythmic oscillations in a variety of biochemical and metabolic processes. A group of core clock genes provide interlocking molecular feedback loops that drive the circadian rhythm even at the single-cell level. In addition to the core transcription/translation feedback loops, post-translational modifications also contribute to the fine regulation of molecular circadian clocks.

Basic Properties of the Circadian Clock

Endogenous Rhythms

Since de Mairian's experiments in 1729, numerous studies in a wide variety of species have consistently demonstrated the existence of self-sustaining circadian rhythms that approximate a 24-hour cycle. Organisms such as plants, Neurospora crassa, cockroaches, fruit flies, and mice exhibit physiological or behavioral patterns aligned with this near-24-hour rhythm, even under constant environmental conditions. This highlights the endogenous nature of circadian rhythms, which persist independently of external cues. Free-running periodicity under constant conditions is often described by circadian time (CT), a standardized 24-hour phase in a circadian cycle that represents an estimate of the organism's subjective time.

Temperature Compensation

Temperature compensation is quantified by the Q_{10} coefficient, which represents the comparison of reaction rates at temperatures that differ by 10 ℃. For many species across large phylogenetic groups, the Q_{10} values of their circadian rhythm periods typically fall within the range of 0. 8 to 1. 2, indicating that the rate of the clock remains nearly constant across physiologically acceptable stable temperatures. The critical role of temperature compensation is particularly pronounced in poikilothermic animals, whose internal clocks must maintain 24-hour rhythmicity across a wide temperature range.

Entrainment

Circadian rhythms can be entrained or synchronized by environmental cues called zeitgebers (time-givers). Zeitgebers include light, mealtimes, work schedules, exercise, and social activities, etc. The primary zeitgeber for organisms on Earth is light, and specialized photoreceptive and phototransduction mechanisms have evolved in almost all biological clock systems. Consequently, changes in the zeitgeber time (e. g. traveling to another time zone) result in the resetting and phase shifting of internal rhythmicity. Chronobiologists define time based on these environmental cycles and call it zeitgeber time (ZT). In a 24-hour cycle with 12 hours of light and 12 hours of darkness, ZT0 corresponds to "lights on" and ZT12 to "lights off". Time points from 0 to 12 represent daytime, while those from 12 to 24 (equivalent to 0) represent nighttime.

Physiological Basis of the Circadian Clock

The mammalian circadian clock system consists of three basic components: input signals (environmental timing cues), a central oscillator (pacemaker), and output signals (apparent rhythm). The central oscillator generates the endogenous biological rhythm and can be synchronized with the environment via cues of input pathways such as light or temperature. Output pathways transmit the clock rhythms to downstream targets and drive overt rhythmic activities (Figure 19-2).

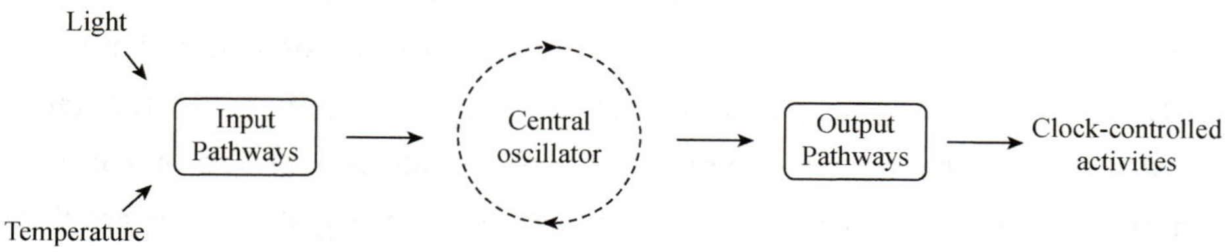

Figure 19-2 Components of the mammalian circadian system

Pacemaker of the Circadian Clock

In mammals, light is detected primarily by the eyes. Extensive behavioral studies in laboratory animals, including mice, rats and hamsters, have shown that these animals maintain a circadian rhythm of approximately 24 hours, even in the absence of external cues such as light-dark cycles or constant darkness. These observations provide compelling evidence for the existence of a "master circadian oscillator" that regulates the intrinsic circadian rhythmicity within the mammalian body.

To identify the central pacemaker responsible for this circadian rhythm, anatomical studies have shown that the suprachiasmatic nucleus (SCN) of the hypothalamus serves as a direct target for retinal fibres. In particular, selective disruption of the SCN results in a complete loss of circadian rhythmicity. Conversely, transplantation of a healthy SCN into a mutant animal restores circadian rhythmicity. Based on these findings, the SCN is currently recognized as the master circadian oscillator responsible for generating the circadian rhythm in mammals.

In addition, the circadian rhythm generated within the SCN is likely to be translated into neural or hormonal signals that have far-reaching effects on the behavior, physiology, and metabolic processes of the whole animal. These signals ensure that various bodily functions are synchronized with the external environment, allowing mammals to adapt and thrive in their respective habitats.

Peripheral Clocks

In addition to the central pacemaker, numerous subsidiary circadian clocks exist outside the SCN in peripheral tissues (including the liver, heart, lung and muscle) and even in immortalized cell lines maintained ex vivo for long periods of time. It is now considered that these peripheral clocks play tissue-or organ-specific roles in the regulation of circadian rhythms. Unlike the central pacemaker located in the SCN, these peripheral oscillators are not directly synchronized by light. Instead, they are controlled by output signals from the SCN or other external stimuli, such as food, which regulate the circadian rhythmicity of local peripheral clocks.

In brief, changes in light due to the day/night cycle are detected directly by the eyes. The light information is transported by the retinohypothalamic tract (RHT) to SCN in the anterior hypothalamus. The SCN acts as a master circadian oscillator where circadian rhythmicity is generated. The generated circadian rhythmicity is translated into output pathways that control the behavior, physiology and metabolism of the organisms. These environmental signals, the master circadian oscillator and the output rhythms are three basic components of the circadian clock system (Figure 19-3).

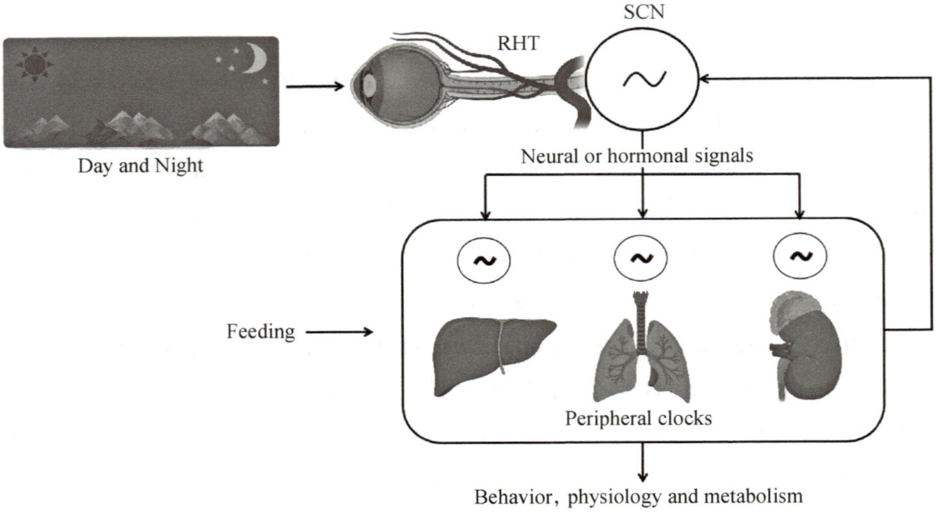

Figure 19-3 **Illustration of the circadian clock system**

Molecular Basis of the Circadian Clock

Transcriptional Feedback Loops

The molecular clock mechanism in mammals is currently understood as two interlocking regulatory feedback loops (Figure 19-4). In the first loop, the positive effectors are CLOCK and BMAL1 (brain and muscle ARNT-like protein 1). CLOCK and BMAL1 are bHLH-PAS (basic helix-loop-helix; *Per-Arnt-Single-minded*, named after the proteins in which the domains were first characterized) domain-containing transcription factors that form heterodimers in the cytoplasm, enter the nucleus, and bind to the E-box sequence in the promoters of the genes encoding negative elements. BMAL1 contains both nuclear localization and nuclear export signals that allow it to shuttle between the nucleus and cytoplasm to promote the nuclear translocation of CLOCK. In mammals, the negative arm of this feedback loop consists of a combination of the *Period* (in mice, *Per*1, *Per*2, and *Per*3) and *Cryptochrome* (*Cry*1 and *Cry*2) genes. CRYs form heterodimers with the PER proteins, enter the nucleus, and inhibit the activity of CLOCK/BMAL1 complexes. Without CLOCK/BMAL1 to activate the transcription of the *Per* and *Cry* genes, levels of *Per* and *Cry* transcripts, and their respective protein products decrease. The degradation of PER and CRY is induced by progressive phosphorylation by casein kinase 1δ (CK1δ) and CK1ε, which leads to the release of CLOCK/BMAL1 inhibition and the cycle starts again.

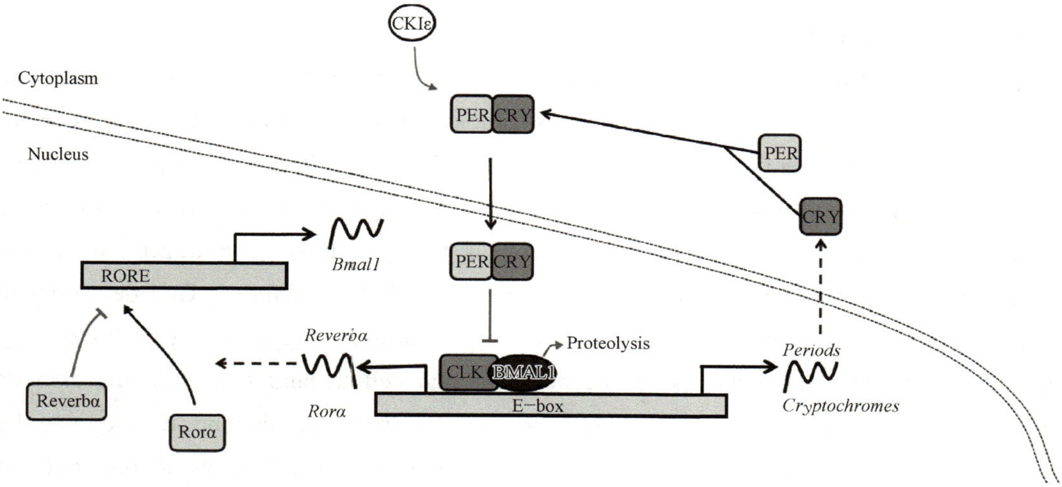

Figure 19-4 Transcription/translation regulatory feedback loops. Several core clock genes form interlocking molecular feedback loops

In this molecular clock, the bHLH-PAS-containing transcription factors BMAL1 and CLOCK act as positive regulators. Upon heterodimerization, they translocate into the nucleus, where they bind to the E-box enhancer element in the promoter region of downstream clock genes such as *Periods* (*Pers*) and *Cryptochromes* (*Crys*). Rhythmically expressed PER and CRY form a heterocomplex. In the nucleus, PER and CRY from a negative feedback loop by repressing their own transcriptional activation by the CLOCK/BMAL1 heterodimer. The CLOCK/BMAL1 heterodimer also induces the transcription of the nuclear receptors *Reverbα* and *Rorα*. *Reverbα* and *Rorα* form another feedback loop by repressing and activating Bmal1 transcription, respectively.

A second feedback loop regulates the expression of the Bmal1 gene. CLOCK/BMAL1 heterodimers enter the nucleus and bind to the E-box sequences in the promoter regions of genes encoding the retinoic acid-related orphan nuclear receptors REV-ERBα and RORα, which compete for the ROR element (RORE) in the Bmal1 promoter. The ROR family (α, β, and γ) of proteins activates Bmal1 expression, and REV-ERBα and REV-ERBβ repress Bmal1 expression. This regulation of Bmal1 maintains a robust rhythm of activity in vivo.

Influence of the Circadian Clock on Toxicant Effects

Chronotoxicology of Chemicals

Several studies have shown that the toxic effects of exogenous chemicals on the body display temporal variations depending on the time of exposure to the toxins. Even under identical conditions, the toxic responses of animals to the same dose of chemicals can vary significantly in terms of the degree of toxicity, simply because of the difference in the time of exposure. This variability can range from high sensitivity at one point in time to no response at another, exemplifying the "all or none" phenomenon.

Circadian systems have been implicated in regulating the absorption, distribution, metabolism, and excretion (ADME) of exogenous chemicals. Each of these processes contributes to determining the blood levels of these chemicals. Therefore, the time of day when an animal is exposed to exogenous chemicals, as well as the synchronization of peripheral molecular clocks in key organs such as the gut, liver, and target tissue, can significantly influence the chemical levels and their bioavailability. The development trajectory of chronotoxicology in China is similar to that of toxicology, starting with the study of drugs, especially chemotherapeutic agents. Through cell dynamics and pharmacokinetic experiments, circadian rhythmic parameters related to drug efficacy and toxicity can be obtained. It has been found that drugs such as the anthracycline antibiotics doxorubicin and pirarubicin have lower toxicity and higher efficacy when administered in the morning. Furthermore, platinum compounds such as cisplatin, carboplatin and oxaliplatin are less toxic and more effective when given in the afternoon and evening. Antimetabolites such as 5-Fu, FUDR, Ara-C, 6-MP, and MTX are best tolerated in the evening or during the night. In addition, mortality from Harringtonine poisoning is higher during the dark period. Pharmacokinetic studies have also shown that the toxicity of methotrexate and florfenicol to mice is greater during the light period, with a larger area under the blood concentration curve and a lower clearance rate, while the opposite is true during the dark period. These findings suggest that circadian differences in toxicity are closely linked to environmental timing cycles and diurnal changes in metabolism and transport within the body. Through these studies, it is possible to select appropriate diurnal dosing times and schedules to achieve the goals of reducing drug doses, decreasing toxicity, and improving therapeutic effects.

Since the late 1980s, Chinese toxicologists have been systematically studying the interaction between pesticides and the biological rhythms of animals. Their initial studies focused on acute temporal toxicity, administering fixed doses of pesticides at different times within a 24-hour period and monitoring animal mortality. For example, exposure to the 1605 pesticide revealed a peak in mortality at 8 pm and a trough at 8 am, indicating a clear relationship between toxicity and exposure time. Similar patterns were observed for DDVP exposure. These findings underscore the importance of applying diurnal timing and animals' internal sensitivity rhythms when conducting toxicity tests. The chronotoxicity of pesticides is based on observations of the diurnal sensitivity of insects to specific insecticides. By exploiting this diurnal variation, timed application strategies can be developed to maximize insecticidal efficacy while minimizing pesticide use, thereby optimizing both economic returns and pest control. However, it's also important to take the rhythmic differences and similarities between animals, humans, and insects into account. This ensures a balance between enhancing pesticidal efficacy and ensuring safety, a delicate balance that toxicologists must navigate carefully.

It is widely believed that LD_{50} (LC_{50}) provides a relatively stable measure of toxicity. However, numerous animal studies have shown that the LD_{50} (LC_{50}) values of many drugs and toxins vary diurnally. One study investigated the temporal changes in the toxicity of valproic acid and its effects on mice. Under identical conditions, mice injected with an LD_{50} of the substance showed a mortality rate of 40% at 9 HALO (hours after light onset). However, this rate increased significantly to 93. 33% when the injection was given at 17 HALO. Similarly, when mice were injected with an LD_{50} of florfenicol at different times of the day, the highest mortality rate was observed at 16 HALO, which was 2. 5 times higher than the lowest rate observed at 4 HALO. Cosine analysis confirmed that the mortality rates caused by the LD_{50} showed significant diurnal variation.

Volatile organic compounds (VOCs) are solvents commonly found in occupational and environmental settings. Previous research on chloroform, CCl_4, and 1, 1-dichloroethylene has shown circadian rhythms in the susceptibility of rats to liver damage. In a recent experiment, fed and fasted male Sprague-Dawley rats were given CCl_4 every 2–4 hours for 24 hours. Peaks in markers of liver injury were observed near the beginning of the dark/active cycle. Blood acetone, CYP2E1 activity and binding of CCl_4 metabolites to liver proteins also showed circadian patterns. Fasted rats showed more pronounced fluctuations. Hepatic glutathione was lowest at the peak of CCl_4 sensitivity. Acetone dose-response experiments showed strong correlations with CYP2E1 induction and CCl_4-induced liver injury. Pretreatment with diallylsulfide suppressed CYP2E1 and abolished the circadian rhythm of CCl_4 susceptibility. These findings suggest that food abstinence during sleep triggers lipolysis and acetone formation, which induces CYP2E1, leading to a diurnal increase in CCl_4 metabolic activation and acute liver injury.

The above phenomenon extends to various VOCs and lipophilic compounds that are metabolized by CYP2E1 to cytotoxic or mutagenic metabolites. Their toxicity and carcinogenic potential vary significantly depending on the time of exposure due to the animal circadian rhythms. It is therefore essential to assess these chemicals at the animals' peak periods of sensitivity to obtain accurate assessments. Experimental protocols must take into account light/dark cycles and treatment times to ensure reliable results. In addition, further research is needed to determine whether other P450 isoenzymes exhibit diurnal rhythms, as this could have significant implications for understanding and assessing the health risks associated with VOCs and other chemicals.

Chronotoxicology of Physical Factors

The response of both neoplastic and normal tissue to radiotherapy exhibits significant diurnal variation. Research has demonstrated that mucositis, a treatment-limiting side effect of radiotherapy for brain tumor and cervical cancer, is more severe when radiotherapy is administered in the morning or evening. This finding suggests that the timing of radiotherapy sessions may be crucial in minimizing adverse effects while maintaining therapeutic efficacy.

The crystalline lens of the eye shows particular sensitivity to ionizing radiation. Studies indicate that damage to the lens epithelium can be mitigated by scheduling radiotherapy in the afternoon rather than in the morning. This temporal approach to treatment may help reduce the risk of radiation-induced cataracts, a common long-term side effect of cranial irradiation.

Auditory structures also display circadian rhythms in their response to physical stressors. The cochlea and inferior colliculus (IC) of mice possess an autonomously regulated circadian system. In a notable experiment, mice were exposed to noise [100 dB sound pressure level (SPL), 6-12 kHz octave band noise] for one hour at different times of the day. Results showed that exposure during the night (active phase for nocturnal animals) led to a greater threshold shift in auditory brainstem responses when measured two weeks post-exposure, compared to exposure during the day (inactive phase).

These findings underscore the importance of considering circadian rhythms in the planning and administration of radiotherapy and in assessing the risks of noise exposure. The field of chronotoxicology offers promising avenues for optimizing treatment schedules and developing strategies to minimize the adverse effects of physical factors on human health.

Disruptive Effects of Toxicants on the Circadian Clock

Environmental Chemicals Impacts on Circadian Rhythms

Circadian rhythms are sensitive to numerous external stimuli. These include changes in light-dark cycles, temperature variations, and increasingly recognized, exposure to environmental chemicals. A growing body of research demonstrates that these environmental chemicals can disrupt circadian rhythms, leading to significant health implications in both animals and humans. A comprehensive study utilizing the zebrafish larval model for circadian behavior screening analyzed over 60 synthetic aquatic chemicals at 100 μg/L exposure. This research identified several circadian disruptors:

(1) Phthalates: Diisopentyl phthalate (DIPP) increased the circadian period by 10.1% and amplitude by 49.6%.

(2) Neuroactive substances: Mirtazapine increased the period by 10.6% and amplitude by 63.1%.

(3) Biocides: Thiamethoxam increased amplitude by 100.3%.

The effect of DIPP was particularly pronounced. Further screening of eleven other phthalates revealed increases in circadian period for: benzyl butyl phthalate (7.9%), diisobutyl phthalate (3.7%) and diisohexyl phthalate (8.5%). These findings underscore the effectiveness of the zebrafish larval model in detecting circadian disruptors and highlight the potential widespread impact of environmental chemicals on biological rhythms.

Disruption of circadian rhythms can trigger disturbances in innate and adaptive immune processes and increase susceptibility to cancer, sepsis and bowel inflammation. In humans, circadian rhythm disruption has been associated with an increased risk of neurological, cardiometabolic, and immunological disorders. For example, several studies have shown that steroids such as dexamethasone (DEX) and 17β-estradiol (E2) can reset circadian rhythms in rodents, with E2 specifically shortening locomotor activity cycles. In zebrafish, DEX and prednisone significantly affect locomotor behavior, gonadal histology, and the circadian network. Progesterone exposure downregulates key circadian genes such as per1a and nr1d2a in zebrafish larvae. Heavy metals, including lead and cadmium, disrupt the circadian rhythm by altering clock gene expression, such as upregulation of rPer1/rPer2 and repression of rBmal1b. Lithium exposure induces changes in per1a, per1b, bmal1b, clock1a mRNA levels and signalling in zebrafish. PCBs increase circadian swimming activity by modulating circadian genes via the AhR pathway.

Physical Factors Disrupt the Circadian Rhythms

Research has shown that exposure to electromagnetic fields suppresses the expression of clock genes, including Ror-α, Bmal1 and Clock, leading to changes in the secretion of the reproductive hormone testosterone. Organs and cells exposed to radiation bring about dose-dependent effects on circadian rhythm, suggesting that radiation affects circadian cycles. One study focused on the effects of a 24-hour exposure (3 Gy of X-rays) on the circadian rhythm of testicular tissue and epididymal markers of reproductive function in mice. The animals were examined for epididymal sperm motility and the expression of clock gene mRNA, such as Clock, Bmal1, Ror-α, Ror-β, and Ror-γ. The results showed that mice exposed to infrared radiation exhibited disrupted circadian rhythms in reproductive markers, manifested by decreased sperm motility, increased daily sperm production (DSP), and reduced activity of testicular enzymes such as G6PDH, SDH, LDH, and ACP. In addition, infrared exposure downregulated the mRNA expression of five clock genes in the testes, altering the circadian rhythms.

In 2007, the International Agency for Research on Cancer (IARC) of the World Health Organization classified shift work (i. e. night work) that disrupts circadian rhythms as a potential carcinogen for shift workers. Shift or night workers are particularly vulnerable to the artificial light at night (ALAN). Research suggests that ALAN disrupts endogenous circadian clocks by suppressing melatonin secretion and downregulating key circadian rhythm-related genes, including CLOCK, BMAL1, PER2, and REV-ERB. This downregulation weakens the rhythmic amplitude, which is strongly associated with negative outcomes such as altered sleep patterns, accumulation of obesity, cardiovascular disease, increased breast cell proliferation and migration, increased neuroinflammation, and oxidative damage.

Chronotoxicology and Future Prospects

Chronotoxicology: An Emerging Field in Toxicological Research

Chronotoxicology is an innovative branch of toxicology that investigates the temporal aspects of toxicant exposure and their effects on biological systems. This field examines how the timing of exposure pollutants and other toxic substances influences their metabolism, expression of toxicity, and subsequent biological responses in organisms. Central to this discipline is the understanding of how the circadian clock, which regulates various physiological and behavioral rhythms, interacts with toxicological processes.

Key Aspects of Chronotoxicology

(1) Toxicokinetics and Toxicodynamics: Chronotoxicology focuses on how circadian rhythms modulate the four primary phases of toxicant interaction with the body: absorption, distribution, metabolism, and excretion. Additionally, it examines how circadian timing affects the intensity and duration of toxic responses.

(2) Therapeutic Implications: Understanding the temporal patterns of toxicant effects can lead to optimized drug treatments, potentially enhancing efficacy while minimizing side

effects.

(3) Circadian Disruption: Perturbations in normal circadian rhythms, such as those experienced by shift workers or individuals with sleep disorders, can alter toxicant processing and potentially increase the risk of adverse effects.

(4) Risk Assessment: Chronotoxicological research contributes to more accurate and comprehensive toxicity risk assessments, informing the establishment of safer exposure standards and prevention strategies.

(5) Novel Therapeutics: This field facilitates the development of innovative therapeutic approaches that consider circadian timing to mitigate toxic effects.

(6) Environmental and Human Health Protection: By elucidating the temporal aspects of toxicant-organism interactions, chronotoxicology contributes to better strategies for protecting both human and environmental health.

Significance and Future Prospect

Chronotoxicology holds considerable promise in various fields, including environmental science, medicine, and public health. Its interdisciplinary nature, incorporating elements of chronobiology, pharmacology, and toxicology, positions it as a pivotal area of research for improving our understanding of toxic effects.

As the field advances, it is likely to yield further insights into the complex interplay between time, biological rhythms, and toxic responses. These findings may lead to more personalized approaches in toxicology and medicine, taking into account individual variations in circadian rhythms and their impact on toxicant susceptibility.

In conclusion, chronotoxicology represents a significant advancement in toxicological research, offering new perspectives on how temporal factors influence the impact of toxic substances on living organisms. Its continued development promises to enhance risk assessment methodologies, improve therapeutic strategies, and ultimately contribute to better health outcomes and environmental protection.

(Zhang Jie)